HERE'S AMERICA'S FAVORITE
DIET GUIDE

CALORIES AND CARBOHYDRATES

THE BOOK THAT MAKES IT FUN
TO LOSE THOSE EXTRA POUNDS

Whether you aim to lose five pounds or fifty, the only safe, healthy way is to eat an adequate, well-balanced diet, choosing your calories from many different kinds of foods in order to ensure that you're getting sufficient vitamins, minerals, and other nutrients. CALORIES AND CARBOHYDRATES contains the most accurate and dependable caloric and carbohydrate counts for practically everything you will eat and drink—thousands and thousands of brand names and basic foods, including alcoholic beverages and take-out foods such as your favorites from McDONALD'S.

So diet—and enjoy it!

SIGNET Books of Interest

BARBARA KRAUS

CALORIES AND CARBOHYDRATES

NEWLY REVISED AND UPDATED

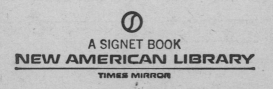

A SIGNET BOOK

NEW AMERICAN LIBRARY

TIMES MIRROR

For Rebecca K. Pecot

Library of Congress Catalog Card Number: 70-119037

Ⓞ

SIGNET TRADEMARK REG. U.S. PAT. OFF. AND FOREIGN COUNTRIES
REGISTERED TRADEMARK—MARCA REGISTRADA
HECHO EN CHICAGO, U.S.A.

SIGNET, SIGNET CLASSICS, MENTOR,
PLUME and MERIDIAN BOOKS
are published by The New American Library, Inc.,
1301 Avenue of the Americas, New York, New York 10019

First Printing, August, 1973
Second Revised Printing, July, 1975

8 9 10 11 12 13 14 15

PRINTED IN THE UNITED STATES OF AMERICA

CONTENTS

INTRODUCTION

This dictionary of foods lists several thousand brand-name products and basic foods with their caloric and carbohydrate content. The calorie yield of your diet versus the amount of energy you expend is the key to whether you maintain your ideal weight, gain too many pounds or lose weight.

Because of the relationship of weight to health, many individuals are "counting calories" at every meal. Interest has also been directed to the carbohydrate content of the diet in relation to weight control. Comprehensive information on these values in basic foods and brand-name products is not readily available in any one source. Nor is the information regularly reported in portions that are usually eaten or bought at the grocery store. To compound the problem, hundreds of new food items appear in our stores every year.

Arrangement of This Book

Foods are listed alphabetically by brand name or by the name of the food. The singular form is used for the entries, that is, blackberry instead of blackberries. Most items are listed individually though a few are grouped (see p. xiii), for example, all candies are listed together so that if you are looking for *Mars* bar, you look first under Candy, then under *M* in alphabetical order. But, if you are looking for a breakfast food such as Oatmeal, you will find it under *O* in the main alphabet. Many cross references are included to assist in finding items called by different names.

Under the main headings, it was often not possible nor even desirable to follow an alphabetical arrangement. For basic foods such as apricots, for example, the first entries are for the fresh product weighed with seeds as it is purchased in the store, then the fruit in small portions as they may be eaten or measured. These entries are followed by the processed products, canned (although it may actually be a bottle or jar), dehydrated, dried and frozen. This basic plan, with adaptations where necessary, was followed for fruits, vegetables and meats.

In almost all entries where data were available the U.S. Department of Agriculture figures are shown first. The Department values represent averages from several manufacturers and are shown for comparison with the values from individual companies or for use where particular brands are not available.

All brand-name products have been italicized and company names appear in parentheses.

Portions Used

The portion column is a most important one to read and note. Common household measures are used insofar as possible. For some items, the amounts given are those commonly purchased in the store, such as 1 pound of meat. These quantities can be divided into the number of servings used in the home and the nutritive values available to each person served can then be readily determined. Of course, any ingredients added in preparing such products must also be taken into account.

The smaller portions given are for foods as served or measured in moderate amounts, such as ½ cup of juice reconstituted, or 4 ounces of meat. Be sure to adjust the calories and carbohydrates to the actual portions you use. For example, if you serve 1 cup of juice instead of ½ cup, multiply the calories and carbohydrates shown for the smaller amount by 2.

Don't fool yourself about the size of portions you use. If you are serious about controlling the calories and carbohydrates in your diet, weigh your foods until you can accurately gauge the weight visually. Remember, the calories and carbohydrates go up with any increase in the weight of foods. Remember, too, that 4 ounces by weight may be very different from 4 fluid ounces or ½ cup. Ounces in the table are always ounces by weight unless specified as fluid ounces, or fractions of a cup or other volumetric measure. Foods that are fluffy in texture, such as flaked coconut and bean sprouts, vary greatly in weight per cup depending on how tightly they are packed into the cup. Such foods as canned green beans also vary when weighed with and without liquid, for example, canned green beans with liquid weigh 4.2 ounces for ½ cup, but drained beans weigh 2.5 ounces for the same ½ cup. Check the weights of your serving portions regularly. Bear in mind that you can cut calories and carbohydrates by cutting the serving size.

It was impossible to convert all the portions to a uniform basis. Some sources were only able to report data in terms of weights with no information on cup or other volumetric measures. I have shown small portions in quantities that might reasonably be expected to be served or measured in the home or institution. Package sizes are useful to show the composition of products as they are purchased and may be divided into the number of serving portions prepared from the entire product, taking into account any added ingredients.

You will find in the portion column the phrases "weighed with bone." or "weighed with skin and seeds" or other inedible parts. These descriptions apply to the products as you purchase them in the markets but the caloric values and the carbohydrate content as shown are for the amount of edible food after you discard the bone, skin, seed or other inedible part. The weight given in the "measure or quantity" column is to the nearest gram or fraction of an ounce.

Data on the composition of foods are constantly changing for many reasons. Better sampling and analytical methods, improvements in marketing procedures and changes in formulas of mixed products, all may alter values for carbohydrates and other nutrients as well as caloric values. Weights of packaged foods are frequently changed. It is essential to read label information to be informed about these matters and to make intelligent use of food tables.

I will be constantly revising and updating this book along with my individual calorie and carbohydrate annual guides (*The Barbara Kraus 1975 Calorie and Carbohydrate Guides to Brand Names and Basic Foods*) to help keep you as up-to-date as possible.

Calories

What is a calorie? It is not a nutrient nor is it a good guide to the nutritive value of a food. It is more like a yardstick to measure the energy that a food will yield in the body. You need energy for your body functions as well as for exercise. If your diet contains more calories than your body uses for these purposes, the extra "energy" will be stored as fat.

If your plan is to cut down on calories, the easiest way to do so is to consult the calorie column of this counter and keep an accurate count of your total intake of food and beverages for a period of seven days. If you have not gained or lost weight during that week divide that number by seven and you'll have your maintenance diet expressed in calories. To lose weight, you must reduce your daily or weekly intake of calories below this maintenance level. (To gain, increase the intake.)

One pound of fat is equal to 3500 calories. Add this number of calories to those you need to balance your energy requirements and you will gain one pound; subtract it, and you will lose a pound.

Carbohydrates

The carbohydrate column shows the amount of this nutrient in grams for the quantities of foods indicated in the portion column. Some dietitians are giving special attention to this nutrient at present in connection with weight control. Carbohydrates include sugars, starches, acids and other nutrients. The values in this book are total carbohydrates, by difference, the basis on which calories from carbohydrates are calculated in the U.S. diet.

Other Nutrients

Do not forget that other nutrients are extremely important in diet planning—protein, fat, minerals and vitamins. Calories yielded by alcohol must also be taken into consideration. From a nutrition viewpoint, perhaps the best advice that can be given to the dieter is to eat a varied diet with all classes of foods represented. Meat, fish, chicken, fats and oils, milk, vegetables, fruits and grain products are all important sources of essential nutrients and some foods from each of these classes of foods should be included in the diet every day. With the great abundance and variety of foods on the grocer's shelves, there is no reason why the dieter should not enjoy a tasty, nutritious and attractive diet. Just eat in moderation and there is no need to eliminate any one food altogether, except in special conditions under a doctor's directions. Choose wisely and eat well.

Sources of Data

Values in this dictionary are based on publications issued by the U.S. Department of Agriculture and on data submitted by manufacturers and processors. The U.S. Department of Agriculture issues basic tables on food composition for use in the United States. The commercial products from U.S.D.A. publications represent average values obtained on products of more than one company. The figures designated "home recipe" are based on recipes on file with the Department of Agriculture. Data on commercial products listed by brand name in this publication are based on values supplied by manufacturers and processors for their own individual products. Very few supermarket brand names, such as A & P's *Ann Page*, or private labels were included in this book inasmuch as they are not usually analyzed under these trade names. Every care has been taken to interpret the data and the descriptions supplied by the companies as fully and accurately as possible. Many values have been recalculated to different portions from those submitted in order to bring about greater uniformity among similar items.

Calories in these different sources are not always on a strictly uniform basis. In the Department of Agriculture, calories are calculated using specific factors, which make allowances for losses in digestion and metabolism. The technical explanation of these factors is given in Handbook 74 of the United States Department of Agriculture. Most manufacturers use average factors of 4, 9 and 4 for calories yielded by each gram of protein, fat and carbohydrate respectively; a factor of 7 is used as an average value to calculate the calories from one gram of alcohol. These differences in procedure will give somewhat different results for products of similar composition. Some manufacturers have adopted the values from U.S. Department of Agriculture publications as representative of their own products. In these cases, it will be apparent in the table that the data from the companies match exactly those from U.S.D.A. publications.

Analyses of foods to provide information on nutritive values are extremely expensive to conduct. Many small companies have not been able to afford to have their products analyzed and thus were unable to provide data for this book or were able to provide only the calories or only the carbohydrates. Other companies have simply never gotten around to having the analysis done. New requirements for labeling nutritive values of products may provide information on additional items in the future. Therefore, wherever data for carbohydrates were unavailable, blank spaces were left which may be filled in by the reader at a later time.

Bear in mind that small differences in calorie values on similar products of the same weight are not important in diet planning. They may be due to different methods of calculating the calories or to small differences in the nutritive values of the samples analyzed because no two foods ever have exactly the same composition. Some differences may also be due to the way the food was measured as noted in the case of green beans earlier.

Carbohydrates in this book are usually total carbohydrates by difference. A few manufacturers reported only "available carbohydrates." These values were omitted.

Foods Listed by Groups

Foods in the following classes are reported together rather than as individual items in the main alphabet: Baby Food; Bread; Cake Icing; Cake Icing Mix; Candy; Cheese; Cookie; Cookie Mix; Cracker; Gravy; Salad Dressing; and Sauce.

Barbara Kraus

ABBREVIATIONS AND SYMBOLS

(USDA) = United States Department of Agriculture
(HEW/FAO) = Health, Education and Welfare/Food and Agriculture Organization
* = prepared as package directs[1]
< = less than
& = and
" = inch
canned = bottles or jars as well as cans
dia. = diameter
fl. = fluid

liq. = liquid
lb. = pound
med. = medium
oz. = ounce
pkg. = package
pt. = pint
qt. = quart
sq. = square
T. = tablespoon
Tr. = trace
tsp. = teaspoon
wt. = weight

italics or name in parentheses = registered trademark, ®
Blank spaces indicate that no data are available.

EQUIVALENTS

By Weight
1 pound = 16 ounces
1 ounce = 28.35 grams
3.52 ounces = 100 grams

By Volume
1 quart = 4 cups
1 cup = 8 fluid ounces
1 cup = ½ pint
1 cup = 16 tablespoons
2 tablespoons = 1 fluid ounce
1 tablespoon = 3 teaspoons

---

[1]If the package directions call for whole or skim milk, the data given here are for whole milk, unless otherwise stated.

Food and Description	Measure or Quantity	Calories	Carbo- hydrates (grams)

A

ABALONE (USDA):
Raw, meat only	4 oz.	111	3.9
Canned	4 oz.	91	2.6

ABISANTE LIQUEUR
(Leroux) 100 proof	1 fl. oz.	87	1.0

AC'CENT
	¼ tsp. (1 gram)	3	0.

ACEROLA, fresh (USDA)
	½ lb. (weighed with seeds)	52	12.6

ALBACORE, raw, meat only (USDA)
	4 oz.	201	0.

ALCOHOLIC BEVERAGES (See individual listings)

ALEWIFE (USDA):
Raw, meat only	4 oz.	144	0.
Canned, solids & liq.	4 oz.	160	0.

ALEXANDER COCKTAIL MIX (Holland House)
	.6-oz. pkg.	69	16.0

ALMOND:
In shell:			
(USDA)	4 oz. (weighed in shell)	347	11.3
(USDA)	1 cup (2.8 oz.)	239	7.8
Shelled:			
Plain:			
Whole (USDA)	½ cup (2.5 oz.)	425	13.8
Whole (USDA)	1 oz.	170	5.5
Whole (USDA)	13-15 almonds (.6 oz.)	105	3.4
Chopped (USDA)	1 cup (4.5 oz.)	759	24.8
(Blue Diamond)	½ cup	504	19.4

(USDA): United States Department of Agriculture
(HEW/FAO): Health, Education and Welfare/Food and Agriculture Organization
* Prepared as Package Directs

Food and Description	Measure or Quantity	Calories	Carbo-hydrates (grams)
Blanched, salted (Blue Diamond)	½ cup	492	15.3
Chocolate-covered (See CANDY)			
Flavored (Blue Diamond) barbecue, cheese, French-fried, onion-garlic or smokehouse-style	1 oz.	180	9.5
Roasted:			
Diced (Blue Diamond)	1 oz.	176	5.5
Dry (Flavor House)	1 oz.	178	5.5
Dry (Planters)	1 oz.	191	5.5
Salted (USDA)	½ cup (2.8 oz.)	492	15.3
ALMOND EXTRACT:			
(Durkee)	1 tsp.	13	
(Ehlers)	1 tsp.	5	
(French's)	1 tsp.	12	
(Virginia Dare)	1 tsp. (4 grams)	10	0.
ALMOND MEAL, partially defatted (USDA)	1 oz.	116	8.2
ALPHABET SOUP MIX:			
*(Golden Grain)	1 cup	54	9.0
*(Goodman's)	8 oz.	43	
ALPHA-BITS, oat cereal (Post)	1 cup (1 oz.)	113	23.0
A.M., fruit juice drink (Mott's)	½ cup	62	15.2
AMARANTH, raw (USDA):			
Untrimmed	1 lb. (weighed untrimmed)	103	18.6
Trimmed	4 oz.	41	7.4
AMBROSIA, chilled, bottled (Kraft)	4 oz.	85	14.7
ANCHOVY PASTE, canned (Crosse & Blackwell)	1 T.	20	1.0
ANCHOVY, PICKLED, canned, with & without added oil (USDA)	7 anchovies (.5 oz.)	26	Tr.

Food and Description	Measure or Quantity	Calories	Carbo-hydrates (grams)
ANESONE LIQUEUR			
(Leroux) 90 proof	1 fl. oz.	86	2.8
ANGEL FOOD CAKE:			
Home recipe (USDA)	1/12 of 8" cake (1.4 oz.)	108	24.1
Loaf (Van de Kamp's)	10-oz. loaf	1006	
Ring, chocolate iced (Van de Kamp's)	7½" cake	2528	
ANGEL FOOD CAKE MIX:			
(USDA)	4 oz.	437	100.4
*(USDA)	1/12 of 10" cake (1.9 oz.)	137	31.5
(Betty Crocker):			
*1 step	1/16 of cake	111	26.2
*2 step	1/16 of cake	100	22.8
*Confetti	1/16 of cake	114	26.8
*Lemon custard	1/16 of cake	111	26.0
*Strawberry	1/16 of cake	115	27.1
*(Duncan Hines)	1/12 of cake (2 oz.)	131	29.6
*(Pillsbury) raspberry or white swirl	1/12 of cake	140	33.0
*(Swans Down)	1/12 of cake (1.8 oz.)	132	29.7
ANISE EXTRACT:			
(Durkee)	1 tsp.	16	
(Ehlers)	1 tsp.	12	
(French's)	1 tsp.	26	
(Virginia Dare)	1 tsp. (4 grams)	22	0.
ANISE SEED, dried			
(HEW/FAO)	½ oz.	58	6.3
ANISETTE LIQUEUR, red or white:			
(Bols) 50 proof	1 fl. oz.	111	13.9
(DeKuyper) 60 proof	1 fl. oz. (1.2 oz.)	95	11.4
(Garnier) 54 proof	1 fl. oz.	82	9.3
(Hiram Walker) 60 proof	1 fl. oz.	92	10.8

(USDA): United States Department of Agriculture
(HEW/FAO): Health, Education and Welfare/Food and Agriculture Organization

* Prepared as Package Directs

Food and Description	Measure or Quantity	Calories	Carbo-hydrates (grams)
(Leroux) 60 proof	1 fl. oz.	89	9.9
(Old Mr. Boston) 60 proof	1 fl. oz.	90	7.5
APPLE, any variety:			
Fresh (USDA):			
Eaten with skin	1 lb. (weighed with skin & core)	242	60.5
Eaten with skin	1 med., 2½″ dia. (about 3 per lb.)	80	20.0
Eaten without skin	1 lb. (weighed without skin & core)	211	55.0
Eaten without skin	1 med., 2½″ dia. (about 3 per lb.)	70	18.2
Pared, diced	1 cup (3.8 oz.)	59	15.4
Pared, quartered	1 cup (4.3 oz.)	66	17.2
Dehydrated:			
Uncooked (USDA)	1 oz.	100	26.1
Cooked, sweetened (USDA)	½ cup (4.2 oz.)	91	23.5
Dried (USDA):			
Uncooked	1 cup (3 oz.)	212	54.6
Uncooked (Del Monte)	1 cup (3 oz.)	238	56.7
Cooked, unsweetened	½ cup (4.3 oz.)	94	24.6
Cooked, sweetened	½ cup (4.9 oz.)	157	40.9
Frozen, sweetened, slices, not thawed (USDA)	10-oz. pkg	264	68.9
APPLE BROWN BETTY, home recipe (USDA)	1 cup (8.1 oz.)	347	68.3
APPLE BUTTER:			
(USDA)	1 T. (.6 oz.)	33	8.4
(Smucker's) cider	1 T. (.6 oz.)	37	9.2
(White House)	1 T.	28	7.6
*APPLE CAKE MIX, cinnamon:			
(Betty Crocker) pudding cake	⅛ of cake	223	44.5
(Betty Crocker) upside down	⅑ of cake	269	44.2
(Duncan Hines)	¹⁄₁₂ of cake (2.7 oz.)	202	35.0
APPLE CIDER:			
(USDA)	½ cup (4.4 oz.)	58	14.8
Cherry or sweet (Mott's)	½ cup	59	14.6

Food and Description	Measure or Quantity	Calories	Carbo-hydrates (grams)
APPLE DRINK, canned:			
(Del Monte)	6 fl. oz. (6.5 oz.)	84	23.6
(Hi-C)	6 fl. oz. (6.3 oz.)	90	22.7
(Wagner)	6 fl. oz.	90	22.5
APPLE DUMPLING, frozen (Pepperidge Farm)	1 dumpling (3.3 oz.)	276	30.7
APPLE FRITTERS, frozen (Mrs. Paul's)	8-oz. pkg.	474	64.0
APPLE FRUIT ROLL, frozen (Chun King)	1 oz.	64	10.1
APPLE JACKS, cereal (Kellogg's)	1 cup (1 oz.)	110	25.9
APPLE JELLY:			
Sweetened (Smucker's)	1 T. (.7 oz.)	49	12.5
Sweetened (White House)	1 T. (.7 oz.)	46	13.0
Dietetic or low calorie:			
(Dia-Mel)	1 T. (.5 oz.)	6	1.4
(Diet Delight)	1 T. (.6 oz.)	22	5.4
(Kraft)	1 oz.	34	8.5
(Louis Sherry)	1 T. (.4 oz.)	6	1.5
(Slenderella)	1 T. (.7 oz.)	25	6.4
(Tillie Lewis)	1 T. (.8 oz.)	11	3.5
APPLE JUICE:			
Canned:			
(USDA)	½ cup (4.4 oz.)	58	14.8
(Heinz)	5½-fl.-oz. can	88	21.7
(Mott's)	½ cup (4.4 oz.)	59	14.6
(Seneca)	½ cup (4.4 oz.)	61	14.8
(White House)	½ cup	58	15.0
*Frozen (Seneca)	½ cup (4.4 oz.)	61	14.8
APPLE NECTAR (Mott's)	½ cup (5 oz.)	63	15.9
APPLE PIE:			
Home recipe, 2 crusts (USDA)	⅛ of 9″ pie (5.6 oz.)	404	60.2
(Drake's)	2-oz. pie	204	25.5

(USDA): United States Department of Agriculture
(HEW/FAO): Health, Education and Welfare/Food and Agriculture Organization
* Prepared as Package Directs

Food and Description	*Measure or Quantity*	*Calories*	*Carbohydrates (grams)*
(Hostess)	4½-oz. pie	421	52.3
French (Hostess)	4½-oz. pie	447	56.1
(McDonald's)	1 serving (3 oz.)	269	30.7
(Tastykake)	4-oz. pie	380	58.6
French apple (Tastykake)	4½-oz. pie	451	64.3
Frozen:			
Baked (USDA)	5 oz.	361	56.8
(Banquet)	5 oz.	351	49.5
(Morton)	⅙ of 24-oz. pie	270	40.1
(Mrs. Smith's)	⅙ of 8″ pie (4.2 oz.)	302	40.0
(Mrs. Smith's) Dutch apple	⅙ of 8″ pie (4.2 oz.)	309	45.0
(Mrs. Smith's) natural juice	⅙ of 8″ pie (4.2 oz.)	340	46.7
(Mrs. Smith's) tart	⅙ of 8″ pie (4.2 oz.)	250	41.7
Tart (Pepperidge Farm)	1 tart (3 oz.)	276	32.8
APPLE PIE FILLING:			
(Comstock)	⅙ of 8″ pie	115	28.5
(Lucky Leaf)	8 oz.	248	60.8
(Wilderness)	21-oz. can	709	163.7
APPLESAUCE, canned:			
Sweetened:			
(USDA)	½ cup (4.5 oz.)	116	30.5
(Del Monte)	½ cup (4.6 oz.)	119	32.6
(Seneca) cinnamon	½ cup (4.5 oz.)	134	30.2
(Seneca) 100% McIntosh	½ cup (4.5 oz.)	116	30.2
(Stokely-Van Camp)	½ cup (4.2 oz.)	109	28.5
(White House)	½ cup (4.5 oz.)	110	28.2
Unsweetened, dietetic or low calorie:			
(USDA)	½ cup (4.3 oz.)	50	13.2
(Blue Boy)	4 oz.	43	10.4
(Diet Delight)	½ cup (4.4 oz.)	58	14.2
(Lucky Leaf)	4 oz.	49	11.6
(S and W) *Nutradiet*, low calorie	4 oz.	56	13.7
(Tillie Lewis)	½ cup (4.2 oz.)	51	12.2
(White House)	½ cup (4.3 oz.)	48	12.2
APPLESAUCE CAKE MIX:			
*Raisin (Duncan Hines)	⅑ of cake (2.7 oz.)	200	37.2
*Spice (Pillsbury)	1/12 of cake	200	36.0

Food and Description	Measure or Quantity	Calories	Carbohydrates (grams)
APPLE TURNOVER, frozen:			
(Pepperidge Farm)	1 turnover (3.3 oz.)	315	30.2
(Pillsbury)	1 turnover	150	23.0
APRICOT:			
Fresh (USDA):			
Whole	1 lb. (weighed with pits)	217	54.6
Whole	3 apricots (about 12 per lb.)	55	13.7
Halves	1 cup (5.5 oz.)	80	20.0
Canned, solids & liq.:			
Juice pack (USDA)	4 oz.	61	15.4
Light syrup (USDA)	4 oz.	75	19.1
Heavy syrup:			
Halves & syrup (USDA)	½ cup (4.4 oz.)	108	27.7
Halves & syrup (USDA)	4 med. halves with 2 T. syrup (4.3 oz.)	105	26.8
(Hunt's)	½ cup (4.5 oz.)	103	26.9
Extra heavy syrup (USDA)	4 oz.	114	29.5
Unsweetened or low calorie:			
Water pack, halves & liq. (USDA)	½ cup (4.3 oz.)	46	11.7
(Diet Delight) solids & liq.	½ cup (4.4 oz.)	60	14.9
(Libby's)	4 oz.	40	10.9
(S and W) *Nutradiet,* low calorie	2 whole (3.5 oz.)	32	7.2
(Tillie Lewis) solids & liq., unpeeled	½ of 8-oz. can	54	13.1
Dehydrated:			
Uncooked (USDA)	4 oz.	376	95.9
Cooked, solids & liq., sugar added (USDA)	4 oz.	135	34.6
Dried:			
Uncooked:			
(USDA)	14 large halves (½ cup or 2.8 oz.)	211	53.9

(USDA): United States Department of Agriculture
(HEW/FAO): Health, Education and Welfare/Food and Agriculture Organization
* Prepared as Package Directs

Food and Description	Measure or Quantity	Calories	Carbo-hydrates (grams)
(USDA)	10 small halves (¼ cup or 1.3 oz.)	99	25.3
(Del Monte)	½ cup (2.3 oz.)	154	39.2
Cooked (USDA):			
Sweetened	½ cup with liq. (12-13 halves, 5.7 oz.)	198	50.9
Unsweetened	½ cup with liq. (4.3 oz.)	104	26.4
Frozen, sweetened, not thawed (USDA)	10-oz. pkg.	278	71.2
APRICOT-APPLE JUICE & PRUNE (Sunsweet)	½ cup	63	16.0
APRICOT BRANDY (DeKuyper) 70 proof	1 fl. oz. (1.1 oz.)	85	6.9
APRICOT, CANDIED (USDA)	1 oz.	96	24.5
APRICOT JELLY, low calorie (Tillie Lewis)	1 T. (.5 oz.)	10	2.4
APRICOT LIQUEUR:			
(Bols) 60 proof	1 fl. oz.	96	8.9
(Hiram Walker) 60 proof	1 fl. oz.	82	8.2
(Leroux) 60 proof	1 fl. oz.	85	8.9
APRICOT NECTAR, canned			
Sweetened:			
(USDA)	½ cup (4.2 oz.)	68	17.5
(Del Monte)	½ cup (4.3 oz.)	68	18.0
(Dewco)	½ cup	68	
(Heinz)	5½-fl.-oz. can	90	21.0
(Sunsweet)	½ cup	75	18.0
Low calorie (S and W) *Nutradiet*	4 oz. (by wt.)	35	8.2
APRICOT PIE FILLING:			
(Comstock)	1 cup (10¾ oz.)	314	78.5
(Lucky Leaf)	8 oz.	316	77.6
(Wilderness)	21-oz. can	756	176.7
APRICOT & PINEAPPLE NECTAR, unsweetened (S and W) *Nutradiet*	4 oz. (by wt.)	35	8.5
APRICOT & PINEAPPLE PRESERVE:			
Sweetened (Bama)	1 T. (.7 oz.)	54	13.5

Food and Description	Measure or Quantity	Calories	Carbo-hydrates (grams)
Sweetened (Smucker's)	1 T	50	12.5
Low calorie (Tillie Lewis)	1 T. (.8 oz.)	12	3.2
APRICOT PRESERVE:			
Sweetened (Bama)	1 T. (.7 oz.)	51	12.7
Sweetened (Smucker's)	1 T. (.7 oz.)	41	12.5
Low calorie (Slenderella)	1 T. (.7 oz.)	28	7.1
APRICOT SOUR COCKTAIL:			
(National Distillers)			
Duet, 12½% alcohol	2 fl. oz.	48	1.6
(Party Tyme)	2 fl. oz.	66	5.7
12½% alcohol			
Dry mix (Party Tyme)	½-oz. pkg.	50	11.6
Liquid mix (Holland House)	2 fl. oz.	86	24.0
Liquid mix (Party Tyme)	2 fl. oz.	58	14.0
APRICOT SYRUP (Smucker's)	1 T. (.6 oz.)	45	11.6
AQUAVIT (Leroux) 90 proof	1 fl. oz.	75	Tr.
ARTICHOKE, Globe or French (See also **JERUSALEM ARTICHOKE**):			
Raw, whole (USDA)	1 lb. (weighed untrimmed)	85	19.2
Boiled, drained (USDA)	4 oz.	50	11.2
Frozen, hearts (Birds Eye)	5-6 hearts (3 oz.)	22	4.8
Marinated, drained (Sara Mia)	5 hearts (1.6 oz.)	65	2.5
ASPARAGUS:			
Raw, whole spears (USDA)	1 lb. (weighed untrimmed)	66	12.7
Boiled, drained (USDA):			
Whole spears	4 spears (½" at base, 2.1 oz.)	12	2.2
Cut spears, 1½"-2" pieces	1 cup (5.1 oz.)	29	5.2
Canned, regular pack:			
Green:			
Spears & liq. (USDA)	1 cup (8.6 oz.)	44	7.1
Spears only USDA)	1 cup (7.6 oz.)	45	7.3

(USDA): United States Department of Agriculture
(HEW/FAO): Health, Education and Welfare/Food and Agriculture Organization
* Prepared as Package Directs

Food and Description	Measure or Quantity	Calories	Carbo-hydrates (grams)
Spears only (USDA)	6 med. spears (3.4 oz.)	20	3.3
Liq. only (USDA)	2 T.	3	.7
Spears & liq. (Green Giant)	⅛ of 15-oz. can	24	3.3
Spears & liq. (Le Sueur)	¼ of 1-lb.-3-oz. can	23	3.1
Spears & liq. (Stokely-Van Camp)	1 cup (7.8 oz.)	40	6.6
Drained solids (Del Monte)	1 cup (7.6 oz.)	34	6.0
White:			
Spears & liq. (USDA)	1 cup (8.4 oz.)	43	7.9
Spears only (USDA)	6 med. spears (3.4 oz.)	21	3.5
Liq. only (USDA)	2 T.	3	.8
Spears & liq. (Del Monte)	1 cup (8 oz.)	34	6.8
Canned, dietetic pack:			
Green:			
Spears & liq. (USDA)	4 oz.	18	3.1
Drained solids (USDA)	4 oz.	23	3.5
Liq. only (USDA)	4 oz.	10	2.3
Spears & liq. (Blue Boy)	4 oz.	20	3.2
Spears & liq. (Diet Delight)	4 oz.	19	2.9
(S and W) *Nutradiet*	5 whole spears (3.5 oz.)	16	2.4
White, spears & liq. (USDA)	4 oz.	18	3.4
Frozen:			
Cuts & tips, not thawed (USDA)	4 oz.	26	4.1
Cuts & tips, boiled, drained (USDA)	½ cup (3.2 oz.)	20	3.2
Cuts (Birds Eye)	½ cup (3.3 oz.)	20	3.3
Cut spears in butter sauce (Green Giant)	⅓ of 9-oz. pkg.	45	3.7
Spears, not thawed (USDA)	4 oz.	27	4.4
Spears, boiled, drained (USDA)	4 oz.	26	4.3

Food and Description	Measure or Quantity	Calories	Carbohydrates (grams)
Spears (Birds Eye)	⅓ of a 10-oz. pkg.	22	3.6
Spears with Hollandaise sauce (Birds Eye)	⅓ of a 10-oz. pkg.	97	3.2
ASPARAGUS SOUP, Cream of, canned:			
Condensed (USDA)	8 oz. (by wt.)	123	19.1
*Prepared with equal volume water (USDA)	1 cup (8.5 oz.)	65	10.1
*Prepared with equal volume milk (USDA)	1 cup (8.5 oz.)	144	16.3
*(Campbell)	1 cup	80	10.7
ASTI WINE (Gancia) 9% alcohol	3 fl. oz.	126	18.0
AUNT JEMIMA SYRUP	¼ cup	212	54.0
AVOCADO, peeled, pitted (USDA):			
All commercial varieties:			
Whole	1 lb. (weighed with seed & skin)	568	21.4
Diced	½ cup (2.6 oz.)	124	4.7
Mashed	½ cup (4.1 oz.)	194	7.3
California varieties, mainly Fuerte:			
Whole	½ avocado (3⅛" dia.)	185	6.5
½-inch cubes	½ cup (2.7 oz.)	130	4.6
Florida varieties:			
Whole	½ avocado (3⅝" dia.)	195	13.4
½-inch cubes	½ cup (2.7 oz.)	97	6.7
*AWAKE (Birds Eye)	½ cup (4 oz.)	55	12.5
AYDS, vanilla or chocolate	1 piece (7 grams)	26	4.9

(USDA): United States Department of Agriculture
(HEW/FAO): Health, Education and Welfare/Food and Agriculture Organization
* Prepared as Package Directs

Food and Description	Measure or Quantity	Calories	Carbo-hydrates (grams)

B

BABY FOOD:
  Apple:

Food and Description	Measure or Quantity	Calories	Carbo-hydrates (grams)
& apricot, junior (Beech-Nut)	7¾ oz.	212	51.2
& apricot, strained (Beech-Nut)	4¾ oz.	123	29.7
& cranberry, junior (Heinz)	7¾ oz.	191	46.6
& cranberry, strained (Heinz)	4¾ oz.	124	30.7
& honey, junior (Heinz)	7½ oz.	155	36.9
& honey with tapioca, strained (Heinz)	4½ oz.	89	21.8
& pear, junior (Heinz)	7¾ oz.	180	43.7
& pear, strained (Heinz)	4½ oz.	108	26.4
Dutch, dessert, junior (Gerber)	7⁸⁄₁₀ oz.	207	47.8
Dutch, dessert, strained (Gerber)	4⁷⁄₁₀ oz.	126	28.5
Apple-apricot juice, strained (Heinz)	4½ fl. oz.	92	22.4
Apple Betty (Beech-Nut):			
Junior	7¾ oz.	234	55.2
Strained	4¾ oz.	147	34.8
Apple-cherry juice:			
Strained (Beech-Nut)	4⅕ fl. oz. (4.4 oz.)	74	18.4
Strained (Gerber)	4⅕ fl. oz. (4.6 oz.)	59	14.2
Strained (Heinz)	4½ fl. oz.	86	21.1
Apple-grape juice:			
Strained (Beech-Nut)	4⅕ fl. oz. (4.4 oz.)	81	20.1
Strained (Heinz)	4½ fl. oz.	89	22.3
Apple juice:			
Strained (Beech-Nut)	4⅕ fl. oz. (4.4 oz.)	57	14.4
Strained (Gerber)	4⅕ fl. oz. (4.6 oz.)	65	16.0
Strained (Heinz)	4½ fl. oz.	88	21.7
Apple pie, junior (Heinz)	7¾ oz.	219	49.5

Food and Description	Measure or Quantity	Calories	Carbo-hydrates (grams)
Apple pie, strained (Heinz)	4¾ oz.	133	30.0
Apple-pineapple juice, strained (Heinz)	4½ fl. oz.	92	22.5
Apple-prune & honey, junior (Heinz)	7½ oz.	181	43.8
Apple-prune & honey with tapioca, strained (Heinz)	4½ oz.	107	25.4
Apple-prune juice, strained (Heinz)	4½ fl. oz.	89	22.0
Applesauce:			
Junior (Beech-Nut)	7¾ oz.	197	47.7
Junior (Gerber)	7⁸⁄₁₀ oz.	185	44.6
Junior (Heinz)	7¾ oz.	182	44.7
Strained (Beech-Nut)	4¾ oz.	121	29.5
Strained (Gerber)	4⁷⁄₁₀ oz.	113	27.4
Strained (Heinz)	4½ oz.	98	24.0
& apricots, junior (Gerber)	7⁸⁄₁₀ oz.	197	47.0
& apricots, junior (Heinz)	7¾ oz.	174	41.6
& apricots, strained (Gerber)	4⁷⁄₁₀ oz.	120	29.2
& apricots, strained (Heinz)	4¾ oz.	98	23.8
& cherries, junior (Beech-Nut)	7¾ oz.	206	48.8
& cherries, strained (Beech-Nut)	4¾ oz.	127	29.3
& pineapple, junior (Gerber)	7⁸⁄₁₀ oz.	171	41.7
& pineapple, strained (Gerber)	4⁷⁄₁₀ oz.	109	26.4
& raspberries, junior (Beech-Nut)	7¾ oz.	243	57.8
& raspberries, strained (Beech-Nut)	4¾ oz.	143	34.6
Apricot with tapioca:			
Junior (Beech-Nut)	7¾ oz.	188	45.3
Junior (Gerber)	7⁸⁄₁₀ oz.	181	44.1

(USDA): United States Department of Agriculture
(HEW/FAO): Health, Education and Welfare/Food and Agriculture Organization
* Prepared as Package Directs

Food and Description	*Measure or Quantity*	*Calories*	*Carbohydrates (grams)*
Junior (Heinz)	7¾ oz.	224	55.0
Strained (Beech-Nut)	4¾ oz.	103	25.1
Strained (Gerber)	4⁷⁄₁₀ oz.	109	26.4
Strained (Heinz)	4¾ oz.	141	33.3
Banana:			
Strained (Heinz)	4½ oz.	105	25.0
& pineapple, junior (Heinz)	7¾ oz.	167	40.6
& pineapple, strained (Heinz)	4¾ oz.	102	25.0
& pineapple with tapioca, junior (Beech-Nut)	7¾ oz.	204	49.9
& pineapple with tapioca, junior (Gerber)	7⁸⁄₁₀ oz.	183	44.6
& pineapple with tapioca, strained (Beech-Nut)	4¾ oz.	129	30.2
& pineapple with tapioca, strained (Gerber)	4⁷⁄₁₀ oz.	114	27.4
Dessert, junior (Beech-Nut)	7¾ oz.	204	49.7
Pie, junior (Heinz)	7¾ oz.	207	45.0
Pie, strained (Heinz)	4¾ oz.	116	25.0
Pudding, junior (Gerber)	7⁸⁄₁₀ oz.	215	48.2
With tapioca, strained (Beech-Nut)	4¾ oz.	119	28.9
With tapioca, strained (Gerber)	4⁷⁄₁₀ oz.	118	28.8
Bean, green:			
Junior (Beech-Nut)	7½ oz.	62	12.5
Strained (Beech-Nut)	4½ oz.	40	7.8
Strained (Gerber)	4½ oz.	42	8.5
Strained (Heinz)	4½ oz.	37	6.4
Creamed with bacon, junior (Gerber)	7½ oz.	145	19.0
In butter sauce (Beech-Nut):			
Junior	7¼ oz.	94	16.8
Strained	4½ oz.	58	10.2
With potatoes & ham, casserole, toddler (Gerber)	6⅙ oz.	142	17.8
Beef:			
Junior (Beech-Nut)	3½ oz.	87	.3
Junior (Gerber)	3½ oz.	95	0.
Strained (Beech-Nut)	3½ oz.	101	.2

Food and Description	*Measure or Quantity*	*Calories*	*Carbohydrates (grams)*
Strained (Gerber)	3½ oz.	90	0.
Beef & beef broth:			
Junior (Heinz)	3½ oz.	99	0.
Strained (Heinz)	3½ oz.	92	0.
Beef & beef heart, strained (Gerber)	3½ oz.	85	.7
Beef dinner:			
Junior (Beech-Nut)	4½ oz.	120	7.3
Strained (Beech-Nut)	4½ oz.	134	7.7
& noodles:			
Junior (Beech-Nut)	7½ oz.	138	15.7
Junior (Gerber)	7½ oz.	109	16.7
Strained (Beech-Nut)	4½ oz.	79	9.4
Strained (Gerber)	4½ oz.	63	9.6
Strained (Heinz)	4½ oz.	59	9.3
With vegetables, junior (Gerber)	4½ oz.	106	7.9
With vegetables, strained (Gerber)	3½ oz.	106	8.0
With vegetables, strained (Heinz)	4¾ oz.	109	7.1
With vegetables & cereal, junior (Heinz)	4¾ oz.	110	5.8
Beef lasagna, toddler (Gerber)	6⅕ oz.	137	16.8
Beef liver, strained (Gerber)	3½ oz.	92	2.0
Beef liver soup, strained (Heinz)	4½ oz.	57	8.1
Beef stew, toddler (Gerber)	6⅕ oz.	122	15.2
Beet:			
Strained (Gerber)	4½ oz.	52	11.0
Strained (Heinz)	4½ oz.	60	12.7
Blueberry Buckle:			
Junior (Gerber)	7⁸⁄₁₀ oz.	187	45.7
Strained (Gerber)	4½ oz.	106	26.2
Butterscotch pudding:			
Junior (Gerber)	7½ oz.	198	39.7
Strained (Gerber)	4½ oz.	130	23.3
Caramel pudding			

(USDA): United States Department of Agriculture
(HEW/FAO): Health, Education and Welfare/Food and Agriculture Organization
* Prepared as Package Directs

Food and Description	Measure or Quantity	Calories	Carbo-hydrates (grams)
(Beech-Nut):			
Junior	7¾ oz.	215	48.8
Strained	4¾ oz.	131	29.7
Carrot:			
Junior (Beech-Nut)	7½ oz.	81	17.6
Junior (Gerber)	7½ oz.	69	14.9
Junior (Heinz)	7¾ oz.	86	19.0
Strained (Beech-Nut)	4½ oz.	47	10.4
Strained (Gerber)	4½ oz.	41	9.0
Strained (Heinz)	4½ oz.	52	11.6
In butter sauce (Beech-Nut):			
Junior	7½ oz.	119	24.2
Strained	4½ oz.	72	15.0
Carrot & pea, junior (Gerber)	7½ oz.	90	16.1
Cereal, dry:			
Barley (Gerber)	3 T. (7 grams)	27	5.3
Barley, instant (Heinz)	1 oz.	101	21.1
High protein (Gerber)	3 T. (7 grams)	27	3.3
High protein, instant (Heinz)	1 oz.	99	13.1
Hi-protein (Beech-Nut)	1 oz.	104	13.0
Mixed (Beech-Nut)	1 oz.	106	19.6
Mixed, honey (Beech-Nut)	1 oz.	106	19.9
Mixed (Gerber)	3 T. (7 grams)	27	5.3
Mixed (Heinz)	1 oz.	100	19.7
Mixed, honey (Beech-Nut)	1 oz.	106	20.0
Mixed, with banana (Gerber)	3 T. (7 grams)	28	5.5
Oatmeal (Beech-Nut)	1 oz.	109	19.1
Oatmeal (Gerber)	3 T. (7 grams)	28	4.7
Oatmeal, honey (Beech-Nut)	1 oz.	109	19.8
Oatmeal, instant (Heinz)	1 oz.	112	18.8
Oatmeal, with banana (Gerber)	3 T. (7 grams)	28	5.2
Rice (Beech-Nut)	1 oz.	107	21.7
Rice (Gerber)	3 T. (7 grams)	26	5.5
Rice, honey (Beech-Nut)	1 oz.	106	22.5
Rice, instant (Heinz)	1 oz.	101	21.5
Rice, with strawberry (Gerber)	3 T. (7 grams)	28	5.7
Cereal, or mixed cereal:			
With apple & banana,			

Food and Description	Measure or Quantity	Calories	Carbo-hydrates (grams)
strained (Heinz)	4¾ oz.	108	26.9
With applesauce & banana:			
Junior (Gerber)	7⁸⁄₁₀ oz.	180	40.6
Strained (Gerber)	4⁷⁄₁₀ oz.	113	24.4
With egg yolks & bacon:			
Junior (Beech-Nut)	7½ oz.	201	17.4
Junior (Gerber)	7½ oz.	159	15.1
Junior (Heinz)	7½ oz.	164	15.5
Strained (Beech-Nut)	4½ oz.	120	10.4
Strained (Gerber)	4½ oz.	92	9.0
Strained (Heinz)	4½ oz.	112	10.0
With fruit, strained (Beech-Nut)	4¾ oz.	113	26.0
High protein, with apple & banana, strained (Heinz)	4¾ oz.	132	25.8
Oatmeal with applesauce & banana:			
Junior (Gerber)	7⁸⁄₁₀ oz.	169	35.4
Strained (Gerber)	4⁷⁄₁₀ oz.	101	20.7
Oatmeal with fruit, strained (Beech-Nut)	4¾ oz.	99	20.6
Rice, with applesauce & banana, strained (Gerber)	4⁷⁄₁₀ oz.	94	21.3
Cheese:			
Cottage, creamed, with pineapple, junior (Beech-Nut)	7¾ oz.	186	35.7
Cottage, creamed, with pineapple, strained (Gerber)	4⁷⁄₁₀ oz.	179	23.3
Cottage, creamed, with pineapple juice, strained (Beech-Nut)	4¾ oz.	119	23.3
Cottage, with banana, junior (Heinz)	7¾ oz.	169	36.3
Cottage, with banana, strained (Heinz)	4½ oz.	97	20.9

(USDA): United States Department of Agriculture
(HEW/FAO): Health, Education and Welfare/Food and Agriculture Organization
* Prepared as Package Directs

Food and Description	Measure or Quantity	Calories	Carbohydrates (grams)
Cottage, dessert, with pineapple:			
Junior (Gerber)	7⁸⁄₁₀ oz.	200	37.4
Strained (Gerber)	4½ oz.	116	21.7
Cherry vanilla pudding (Gerber):			
Junior	7⁸⁄₁₀ oz.	191	43.3
Strained	4⁷⁄₁₀ oz.	117	29.8
Chicken:			
Junior (Beech-Nut)	3½ oz.	97	0.
Junior (Gerber)	3½ oz.	133	.5
Strained (Beech-Nut)	3½ oz.	97	.4
Strained (Gerber)	3½ oz.	131	.1
Chicken & chicken broth:			
Junior (Heinz)	3½ oz.	103	0.
Strained (Heinz)	3½ oz.	114	0.
Chicken dinner:			
Junior (Beech-Nut)	4½ oz.	105	9.0
Strained (Beech-Nut)	4½ oz.	110	9.3
Noodle, junior (Beech-Nut)	7½ oz.	95	15.5
Noodle, junior (Gerber)	7½ oz.	95	17.0
Noodle, junior (Heinz)	7½ oz.	123	15.7
Noodle, strained (Beech-Nut)	4½ oz.	58	9.7
Noodle, strained (Gerber)	4½ oz.	62	10.4
Noodle, strained (Heinz)	4½ oz.	70	9.2
With vegetables:			
Junior (Beech-Nut)	7½ oz.	98	17.6
Junior (Gerber)	4½ oz.	114	7.9
Junior (Heinz)	4¾ oz.	128	5.3
Strained (Beech-Nut)	4½ oz.	61	10.5
Strained (Gerber)	4½ oz.	111	7.7
Strained (Heinz)	4¾ oz.	124	5.8
Chicken soup:			
Junior (Heinz)	7½ oz.	113	17.6
Strained (Heinz)	4½ oz.	65	8.9
Cream of, junior (Gerber)	7½ oz.	118	19.6
Cream of, strained (Gerber)	4½ oz.	74	12.4
Chicken stew, toddler (Gerber)	6 oz.	130	15.0
Chicken sticks:			
Junior (Beech-Nut)	2½ oz.	146	1.6
Junior (Gerber)	2½ oz.	134	.8
Junior (Heinz)	1 jar	79	2.4

Food and Description	Measure or Quantity	Calories	Carbohydrates (grams)
Cookie, animal-shaped (Gerber)	1 cookie (6 grams)	29	4.3
Cookie, assorted (Beech-Nut)	½ oz.	61	9.5
Corn, creamed:			
Junior (Gerber)	7½ oz.	135	29.4
Junior (Heinz)	7½ oz.	153	34.0
Strained (Beech-Nut)	4½ oz.	123	26.5
Strained (Gerber)	4½ oz.	83	18.1
Strained (Heinz)	4½ oz.	92	20.4
Custard:			
Junior (Beech-Nut)	7¾ oz.	210	40.5
Junior (Heinz)	7¾ oz.	213	36.4
Strained (Beech-Nut)	4½ oz.	125	24.7
Strained (Heinz)	4½ oz.	122	21.6
Chocolate, junior (Gerber)	7⁸⁄₁₀ oz.	212	41.1
Chocolate, strained (Beech-Nut)	4½ oz.	138	27.8
Chocolate, strained (Gerber)	4½ oz.	126	24.4
Vanilla, junior (Gerber)	7½ oz.	207	39.7
Vanilla, strained (Gerber)	4½ oz.	116	23.4
Dutch apple dessert (See Apple, Dutch, dessert)			
Egg yolk:			
Strained (Beech-Nut)	3⅓ oz.	181	1.3
Strained (Gerber)	3⅓ oz.	187	0.
Strained (Heinz)	3¼ oz.	189	2.0
& bacon, strained (Beech-Nut)	3⅓ oz.	174	3.3
& ham, strained (Gerber)	3⅓ oz.	182	0.
Fruit (Heinz):			
Mixed, & honey, junior	7½ oz.	215	52.0
Mixed, & honey, strained	4½ oz.	105	24.7
Fruit dessert:			
Junior (Heinz)	7¾ oz.	207	50.9
Strained (Heinz)	4½ oz.	124	30.4

(USDA): United States Department of Agriculture
(HEW/FAO): Health, Education and Welfare/Food and Agriculture Organization
* Prepared as Package Directs

Food and Description	*Measure or Quantity*	*Calories*	*Carbohydrates (grams)*
Tropical, junior (Beech-Nut)	7¾ oz.	208	51.0
With tapioca:			
Junior (Beech-Nut)	7¾ oz.	221	53.2
Junior (Gerber)	7⁸⁄₁₀ oz.	204	49.7
Strained (Beech-Nut)	4¾ oz.	139	34.4
Strained (Gerber)	4⁷⁄₁₀ oz.	121	29.0
Fruit juice:			
Mixed, strained (Beech-Nut)	4⅕ fl. oz. (4.2 oz.)	79	19.0
Mixed, strained (Gerber)	4⅕ fl. oz. (4.6 oz.)	77	18.3
Ham:			
Junior (Gerber)	3½ oz.	116	.6
Strained (Beech-Nut)	3½ oz.	115	2.3
Strained (Gerber)	3½ oz.	113	.7
Ham dinner:			
Junior (Beech-Nut)	4½ oz.	122	6.4
Strained (Beech-Nut)	4½ oz.	137	7.8
With vegetables:			
Junior (Gerber)	4½ oz.	101	8.3
Junior (Heinz)	4¾ oz.	148	12.5
Strained (Gerber)	4½ oz.	102	8.5
Strained (Heinz)	4¾ oz.	124	6.7
Lamb:			
Junior (Beech-Nut)	3½ oz.	98	0.
Junior (Gerber)	3½ oz.	96	0.
Strained (Beech-Nut)	3½ oz.	92	0.
Strained (Gerber)	3½ oz.	96	0.
& noodles, junior (Beech-Nut)	7½ oz.	151	18.2
Lamb & lamb broth:			
Junior (Heinz)	3½ oz.	97	0.
Strained (Heinz)	3½ oz.	86	0.
Liver, with liver broth (Heinz)	3½ oz.	79	0.
Macaroni:			
Alphabets & beef casserole, toddler (Gerber)	6⅕ oz.	148	18.6
& bacon with vegetables, junior (Beech-Nut)	7½ oz.	197	20.0
& beef with vegetables, junior (Beech-Nut)	7½ oz.	136	15.5

Food and Description	Measure or Quantity	Calories	Carbo-hydrates (grams)
With tomato, beef & bacon:			
Junior (Gerber)	7½ oz.	134	21.9
Junior (Heinz)	7½ oz.	140	20.6
Strained (Gerber)	4½ oz.	80	11.9
Strained (Heinz)	4½ oz.	89	11.6
With tomato sauce, beef & bacon dinner, strained (Beech-Nut)	4½ oz.	108	11.0
MBF, concentrate (Gerber)	2 T. (1.2 oz.)	43	3.2
Meat sticks:			
Junior (Beech-Nut)	2½ oz.	135	.9
Junior (Gerber)	2½ oz.	116	1.0
Junior (Heinz)	1 jar	106	.3
Modilac, concentrate (Gerber)	2 T. (1.1 oz.)	40	4.8
Noodles & beef, junior (Heinz)	7½ oz.	111	16.4
Orange-apple juice, strained:			
(Beech-Nut)	4⅕ fl. oz. (4.4 oz.)	98	23.2
(Gerber)	4⅕ fl. oz. (4.6 oz.)	71	16.3
Orange-apple-banana juice, strained:			
(Gerber)	4⅕ fl. oz. (4.6 oz.)	86	20.2
(Heinz)	4½ fl. oz.	89	21.8
Orange-apricot juice, strained:			
(Beech-Nut)	4⅕ fl. oz. (4.4 oz.)	117	27.4
(Gerber)	4⅕ fl. oz. (4.6 oz.)	80	18.8
Orange-apricot juice drink, strained (Heinz)	4½ fl. oz.	73	17.5
Orange-banana juice, strained (Beech-Nut)	4⅕ fl. oz. (4.4 oz.)	122	28.4

(USDA): United States Department of Agriculture
(HEW/FAO): Health, Education and Welfare/Food and Agriculture Organization
* Prepared as Package Directs

Food and Description	Measure or Quantity	Calories	Carbohydrates (grams)
Orange juice, strained:			
(Beech-Nut)	4⅕ fl. oz.		
	(4.4 oz.)	64	14.5
(Gerber)	4⅕ fl. oz.		
	(4.6 oz.)	65	14.5
(Heinz)	4½ fl. oz.	69	16.2
Orange-pineapple dessert, strained (Beech-Nut)	4¾ oz.	161	38.5
Orange-pineapple juice, strained:			
(Beech-Nut)	4⅕ fl. oz.		
	(4.4 oz.)	104	24.7
(Gerber)	4⅕ fl. oz.		
	(4.6 oz.)	79	18.6
(Heinz)	4½ fl. oz.	72	17.5
Orange pudding, strained:			
(Gerber)	4⁷⁄₁₀ oz.	135	29.4
(Heinz)	4½ oz.	119	28.0
Pea:			
Strained (Beech-Nut)	4½ oz.	86	15.2
Strained (Gerber)	4½ oz.	62	10.1
Pea, creamed:			
Junior (Heinz)	7¾ oz.	158	24.9
Strained (Heinz)	4½ oz.	82	12.8
Pea, split (See Split pea)			
Peach:			
Junior (Beech-Nut)	7¾ oz.	197	46.9
Junior (Gerber)	7⁸⁄₁₀ oz.	189	44.4
Junior (Heinz)	7½ oz.	247	60.1
Strained (Beech-Nut)	4¾ oz.	119	28.3
Strained (Gerber)	4⁷⁄₁₀ oz.	111	26.9
Strained (Heinz)	4½ oz.	160	37.9
Peach cobbler:			
Junior (Gerber)	7⁸⁄₁₀ oz.	195	47.1
Strained (Gerber)	4⁷⁄₁₀ oz.	119	28.5
Peach & honey (Heinz):			
Junior	7½ oz.	155	37.0
With tapioca, strained	4½ oz.	94	22.1
Peach Melba (Beech-Nut):			
Junior	7¾ oz.	247	59.3
Strained	4¾ oz.	153	36.7
Peach pie:			
Junior (Heinz)	7¾ oz.	212	46.9
Strained (Heinz)	4¾ oz.	128	28.1
Pear:			
Junior (Beech-Nut)	7½ oz.	157	38.4

Food and Description	*Measure or Quantity*	*Calories*	*Carbo-hydrates (grams)*
Junior (Gerber)	7⁸⁄₁₀ oz.	164	39.4
Junior (Heinz)	7¾ oz.	167	40.0
Strained (Beech-Nut)	4½ oz.	96	23.0
Strained (Gerber)	4⁷⁄₁₀ oz.	100	24.3
Strained (Heinz)	4½ oz.	98	23.2
Pear & pineapple:			
Junior (Beech-Nut)	7½ oz.	167	40.7
Junior (Gerber)	7⁸⁄₁₀ oz.	167	39.5
Junior (Heinz)	7¾ oz.	158	38.0
Strained (Beech-Nut)	4½ oz.	100	24.3
Strained (Gerber)	4⁷⁄₁₀ oz.	102	24.6
Strained (Heinz)	4¾ oz.	104	24.9
Pineapple dessert, strained (Beech-Nut)	4¾ oz.	142	34.7
Pineapple-grapefruit juice drink, strained (Gerber)	4⅕ fl. oz. (4.6 oz.)	76	18.6
Pineapple juice, strained (Heinz)	4½ fl. oz.	72	16.6
Pineapple-orange dessert:			
Junior (Heinz)	7¾ oz.	204	49.3
Strained (Heinz)	4½ oz.	115	27.7
Pineapple pie:			
Junior (Heinz)	7¾ oz.	237	49.5
Strained (Heinz)	4¾ oz.	145	30.8
Plum with tapioca:			
Junior (Beech-Nut)	7¾ oz.	217	53.0
Junior (Gerber)	7⁸⁄₁₀ oz.	221	53.8
Strained (Beech-Nut)	4¾ oz.	141	34.4
Strained (Gerber)	4⁷⁄₁₀ oz.	134	32.7
Strained (Heinz)	4½ oz.	129	31.7
Pork:			
Junior (Beech-Nut)	3½ oz.	110	1.1
Junior (Gerber)	3½ oz.	113	0.
Strained (Beech-Nut)	3½ oz.	111	.4
Strained (Gerber)	3½ oz.	109	0.
Pork, with pork broth, strained (Heinz)	3½ oz.	93	0.
Potatoes, creamed, with ham, toddler (Gerber)	6 oz.	183	18.4
Pretzel (Gerber)	1 pretzel (5 grams)	19	3.9

(USDA): United States Department of Agriculture
(HEW/FAO): Health, Education and Welfare/Food and Agriculture Organization
* Prepared as Package Directs

Food and Description	*Measure or Quantity*	*Calories*	*Carbohydrates (grams)*
Prune-orange juice, strained:			
(Beech-Nut)	4⅕ fl. oz. (4.4 oz.)	95	22.8
(Gerber)	4⅕ fl. oz. (4.6 oz.)	101	23.6
(Heinz)	4½ fl. oz.	82	19.9
Prune with tapioca:			
Junior (Beech-Nut)	7¾ oz.	204	49.3
Junior (Gerber)	7⁸⁄₁₀ oz.	207	49.4
Strained (Beech-Nut)	4¾ oz.	129	31.1
Strained (Gerber)	4⁷⁄₁₀ oz.	122	29.3
Strained (Heinz)	4¾ oz.	140	33.7
Raspberry Cobbler:			
Junior (Gerber)	7⁸⁄₁₀ oz.	182	44.4
Strained (Gerber)	4½ oz.	103	25.2
Similac, ready-to-feed	1 fl. oz.	20	1.9
Spaghetti & meat balls, toddler (Gerber)	6⅕ oz.	137	21.5
Spaghetti, tomato sauce & beef:			
Junior (Beech-Nut)	7½ oz.	159	20.1
Junior (Gerber)	7½ oz.	148	27.2
Junior (Heinz)	7½ oz.	168	26.8
Strained (Heinz)	4½ oz.	96	14.6
Spinach, creamed:			
Junior (Gerber)	7½ oz.	99	14.1
Strained (Gerber)	4½ oz.	56	8.3
Strained (Heinz)	4½ oz.	56	8.3
Split pea with bacon, junior (Gerber)	7½ oz.	181	26.6
Split pea, vegetables & bacon:			
Junior (Heinz)	7½ oz.	213	23.6
Strained (Heinz)	4½ oz.	120	13.4
Split pea, vegetables & ham, junior (Beech-Nut)	7½ oz.	144	23.1
Squash:			
Junior (Beech-Nut)	7½ oz.	76	16.3
Junior (Gerber)	7½ oz.	65	13.4
Strained (Beech-Nut)	4½ oz.	46	9.7
Strained (Gerber)	4½ oz.	39	8.5
Strained (Heinz)	4½ oz.	50	10.5
In butter sauce (Beech-Nut):			

Food and Description	Measure or Quantity	Calories	Carbo-hydrates (grams)
Junior	7½ oz.	108	21.4
Strained	4½ oz.	64	12.7
Sweet potato:			
Junior (Beech-Nut)	7¾ oz.	136	31.3
Junior (Gerber)	7⁸⁄₁₀ oz.	158	35.9
Strained (Beech-Nut)	4¾ oz.	73	16.9
Strained (Gerber)	4⁷⁄₁₀ oz.	95	21.7
Strained (Heinz)	4½ oz.	84	18.8
In butter sauce (Beech-Nut):			
Junior	7¾ oz.	155	33.3
Strained	4½ oz.	91	19.5
Teething biscuit (Gerber)	1 piece (.4 oz.)	43	8.2
Teething ring, honey (Beech-Nut)	½ oz.	56	10.7
Tuna with noodles, strained (Heinz)	4½ oz.	55	9.3
Turkey:			
Junior (Beech-Nut)	3½ oz.	100	.7
Junior (Gerber)	3½ oz.	105	.1
Strained (Beech-Nut)	3½ oz.	104	1.0
Strained (Gerber)	3½ oz.	129	.3
Turkey dinner:			
Junior (Beech-Nut)	4½ oz.	88	8.4
Strained (Beech-Nut)	4½ oz.	106	10.8
With rice:			
Junior (Gerber)	7½ oz.	94	15.9
Strained (Beech-Nut)	4½ oz.	64	12.7
Strained (Gerber)	4½ oz.	60	9.7
With rice & vegetables, junior (Beech-Nut)	7½ oz.	87	17.0
With vegetables:			
Junior (Gerber)	4½ oz.	102	8.3
Strained (Gerber)	4½ oz.	97	7.8
Strained (Heinz)	4¾ oz.	94	7.9
Tutti frutti dessert (Heinz):			
Junior	7¾ oz.	187	44.6
Strained	4½ oz.	108	25.1
Veal:			
Junior (Beech-Nut)	3½ oz.	88	0.

(USDA): United States Department of Agriculture
(HEW/FAO): Health, Education and Welfare/Food and Agriculture Organization
* Prepared as Package Directs

Food and Description	Measure or Quantity	Calories	Carbo- hydrates (grams)
Junior (Gerber)	3½ oz.	99	0.
Strained (Beech-Nut)	3½ oz.	109	.1
Strained (Gerber)	3½ oz.	89	0.
Veal dinner:			
Junior (Beech-Nut)	4½ oz.	131	6.9
Strained (Beech-Nut)	4½ oz.	120	7.7
With vegetables:			
Junior (Gerber)	4½ oz.	85	9.4
Junior (Heinz)	4¾ oz.	109	7.1
Strained (Gerber)	4½ oz.	83	8.6
Strained (Heinz)	4¾ oz.	84	6.3
Veal & veal broth:			
Junior (Heinz)	3½ oz.	93	0.
Strained (Heinz)	3½ oz.	90	0.
Vegetables:			
Garden, strained (Beech-Nut)	4½ oz.	59	11.3
Garden, strained (Gerber)	4½ oz.	46	7.9
Mixed, junior (Gerber)	7½ oz.	89	18.4
Mixed, junior (Heinz)	7½ oz.	100	20.8
Mixed, strained (Gerber)	4½ oz.	49	10.9
Vegetables & bacon:			
Junior (Beech-Nut)	7½ oz.	157	18.0
Junior (Gerber)	7½ oz.	139	18.7
Junior (Heinz)	7½ oz.	153	16.3
Strained (Beech-Nut)	4½ oz.	92	9.7
Strained (Gerber)	4½ oz.	96	13.0
Strained (Heinz)	4½ oz.	65	9.0
Vegetables & beef:			
Junior (Beech-Nut)	7½ oz.	136	15.5
Junior (Gerber)	7½ oz.	110	14.7
Junior (Heinz)	7½ oz.	106	17.1
Strained (Beech-Nut)	4½ oz.	88	10.2
Strained (Gerber)	4½ oz.	68	8.6
Strained (Heinz)	4½ oz.	70	8.5
Vegetables & chicken (Gerber):			
Junior	7½ oz.	107	21.2
Strained	4½ oz.	54	9.0
Vegetables, dumplings, beef & bacon:			
Junior (Heinz)	7½ oz.	145	16.9
Strained (Heinz)	4½ oz.	79	10.3
Vegetables, egg noodles & chicken:			
Junior (Heinz)	7½ oz.	134	17.6

Food and Description	Measure or Quantity	Calories	Carbo- hydrates (grams)
Strained (Heinz)	4½ oz.	80	11.2
Vegetables, egg noodles & turkey, junior (Heinz)	7½ oz.	113	16.6
Vegetables & ham:			
Junior (Heinz)	7½ oz.	132	15.4
Strained (Beech-Nut)	4½ oz.	82	10.5
With bacon:			
Junior (Gerber)	7½ oz.	124	18.5
Strained (Gerber)	4½ oz.	71	9.8
Strained (Heinz)	4½ oz.	79	7.3
Vegetables & lamb:			
Junior (Beech-Nut)	7½ oz.	125	15.5
Junior (Gerber)	7½ oz.	108	16.2
Junior (Heinz)	7½ oz.	117	17.4
Strained (Beech-Nut)	4½ oz.	66	9.9
Strained (Gerber)	4½ oz.	64	9.9
Strained (Heinz)	4½ oz.	56	8.1
Vegetables & liver:			
Junior (Beech-Nut)	7½ oz.	98	16.7
Strained (Beech-Nut)	4½ oz.	56	10.0
With bacon:			
Junior (Gerber)	7½ oz.	107	17.9
Strained (Gerber)	4½ oz.	78	8.4
Vegetables & turkey (Gerber):			
Junior	7½ oz.	91	17.7
Strained	4½ oz.	58	11.0
Toddler	6⅛ oz.	161	18.0
Vegetable soup:			
Junior (Beech-Nut)	7½ oz.	85	18.2
Junior (Heinz)	7½ oz.	106	20.4
Strained (Beech-Nut)	4½ oz.	51	11.3
BAC ONION (Lawry's)	1 tsp. (4 grams)	14	2.1
BACO NOIR BURGUNDY WINE (Great Western) 12% alcohol	3 fl. oz.	69	2.1
BAC*Os (General Mills)	1 T.	29	1.0

(USDA): United States Department of Agriculture
(HEW/FAO): Health, Education and Welfare/Food and Agriculture
Organization
* Prepared as Package Directs

Food and Description	Measure or Quantity	Calories	Carbohydrates (grams)
BACON, cured:			
Raw:			
(USDA) slab	1 oz. (weighed with rind)	177	.3
(USDA) sliced	1 oz.	189	.3
(Hormel) Black Label	1 piece (.8 oz.)	125	.2
(Hormel) *Range Brand*	1 piece (1.6 oz.)	275	.5
(Wilson)	1 oz.	169	.3
Broiled or fried crisp (Oscar Mayer):			
Thin slice, drained	1 slice (4 grams)	24	.1
Medium slice, drained	1 slice (6 grams)	36	.1
Thick slice, drained	1 slice (.4 oz.)	67	.1
Canned (USDA)	1 oz.	194	.3
BACON BITS:			
(Wilson)	1 oz.	139	1.0
Imitation (Durkee)	1tsp. (2 grams)	8	.5
Imitation (French's) crumbles	1 tsp. (2 grams)	7	.4
Imitation (McCormick)	1 tsp. (2 grams)	8	.5
BACON, CANADIAN:			
Unheated:			
(Oscar Mayer)	1-oz. slice	45	0.
(Wilson)	1 oz.	42	.1
Broiled or fried (USDA)	1 oz.	79	Tr.
BAGEL:			
Egg (USDA)	3" dia. (1.9 oz.)	165	28.0
Garlic, onion or poppyseed (Lender's)	2-oz. bagel	161	31.5
Water (USDA)	3" dia. (1.9 oz.)	165	30.0
BAKING POWDER:			
Phosphate (USDA)	1 tsp. (5 grams)	6	1.4
SAS (USDA)	1 tsp. (4 grams)	5	1.2
Tartrate (USDA)	1 tsp. (4 grams)	3	.7
(Royal)	1 tsp. (4 grams)	5	1.3
BAKON DELITES (Wise):			
Regular	½ oz. bag	72	0.
Barbecue flavored	½ oz. bag	70	.3
BAMBOO SHOOT:			
Raw, trimmed (USDA)	4 oz.	31	5.9
Canned, drained (Chun King)	1 cup	64	2.4

Food and Description	Measure or Quantity	Calories	Carbohydrates (grams)
BANANA (USDA):			
Common:			
Fresh:			
Whole	1 lb. (weighed with skin)	262	68.5
Small size	4.9-oz. banana (7¾"x1¹¹⁄₃₂")	81	21.1
Medium size	6.2 oz. banana (8¾"x1¹³⁄₃₂")	101	26.4
Large size	7-oz. banana (9¾"x1⁷⁄₁₆")	116	30.2
Mashed	1 cup (about 2 med.)	189	49.3
Sliced	1 cup (1¼ med.)	124	32.4
Dehydrated, flakes (USDA)	½ cup (1.8 oz.)	170	44.3
Red, fresh, whole (USDA)	1 lb. (weighed with skin)	278	72.2
BANANA, BAKING (See PLANTAIN)			
BANANA CAKE MIX:			
*(Betty Crocker) layer	¹⁄₁₂ of cake	205	36.6
*(Duncan Hines)	¹⁄₁₂ of cake (2.7 oz.)	203	35.0
(Pillsbury)	¹⁄₁₂ of cake	180	34.0
BANANA CREAM PIE:			
(Tastykake)	4-oz. pie	485	82.4
Frozen (Banquet)	2½-oz. serving	185	25.0
Frozen (Morton)	¹⁄₁₆ of 16-oz. pie	190	25.9
Frozen (Mrs. Smith's)	¹⁄₁₆ of 8" pie (2.8 oz.)	214	28.3
BANANA CREAM PUDDING or PIE FILLING MIX:			
*Instant (Jell-O)	½ cup (5.3 oz.)	178	30.5
*Instant (Royal)	½ cup (5.1 oz.)	177	30.5
*Regular (Jell-O)	½ cup (5.2 oz.)	173	29.3
*Regular (My-T-Fine)	½ cup (5 oz.)	175	32.6
*Regular (Royal)	½ cup (5.1 oz.)	163	26.4

(USDA): United States Department of Agriculture
(HEW/FAO): Health, Education and Welfare/Food and Agriculture
　　　　　　　　Organization

* Prepared as Package Directs

Food and Description	Measure or Quantity	Calories	Carbohydrates (grams)
BANANA CUSTARD PIE, home recipe (USDA)	⅛ of 9″ pie (5.4 oz.)	336	46.7
BANANA LIQUEUR (Leroux) 56 proof	1 fl. oz.	92	11.4
BANANA PUDDING, canned (Del Monte)	5-oz. container	187	31.7
BANANA SOFT DRINK, high-protein (Yoo-Hoo)	6 fl. oz. (6.4 oz.)	100	18.9
B AND B LIQUEUR (Julius Wile) 86 proof	1 fl. oz.	94	5.7
BARBADOS CHERRY (See ACEROLA)			
BARBECUE DINNER MIX (Hunt's) *Skillet*	2-lb. 1-oz. pkg.	1404	247.1
BARBECUE SAUCE (See SAUCE, Barbecue)			
BARBECUE SEASONING (French's)	1 tsp. (2 grams)	7	.7
BARBERA WINE (Louis M. Martini) 12½% alcohol	3 fl. oz.	90	.2
BARDOLINO WINE, Italian red (Antinori) 12% alcohol	3 fl. oz.	84	6.3
BARLEY, pearled, dry: Light:			
(USDA)	¼ cup (1.8 oz.)	174	39.4
(Quaker-Scotch)	¼ cup (1.7 oz.)	173	37.4
Pot or Scotch (USDA)	2 oz.	197	43.8
BARRACUDA, raw, meat only (USDA)	4 oz.	128	0.
BARRELHEAD, soft drink (Canada Dry)	6 fl. oz.	79	19.8

Food and Description	Measure or Quantity	Calories	Carbo-hydrates (grams)
BASS (USDA):			
Black sea:			
Raw, whole	1 lb. (weighed whole)	165	0.
Baked, stuffed, home recipe	4 oz.	294	12.9
Smallmouth & largemouth, raw:			
Whole	1 lb. (weighed whole)	146	0.
Meat only	4 oz.	118	0.
Striped:			
Raw, whole	1 lb. (weighed whole)	205	0.
Raw, meat only	4 oz.	119	0.
Oven-fried	4 oz.	222	7.6
White, raw, meat only	4 oz.	111	0.
BAVARIAN PIE FILLING (Lucky Leaf)	8 oz.	306	51.8
BAVARIAN PIE or PUDDING MIX:			
*Cream (My-T-Fine)	½ cup (5 oz.)	175	32.5
*Custard, Rice-A-Roni	4 oz.	143	24.6
BAVARIAN-STYLE VEGE-TABLES (Birds Eye) frozen	⅓ of 10-oz. pkg.	135	11.8
BEAN, BAKED:			
Canned with brown sugar sauce:			
(B & M) red kidney	1 cup (8 oz.)	360	49.7
(Homemaker's) red kidney	1 cup (8 oz.)	337	50.2
Canned with pork:			
(Campbell) home style	1 cup	302	52.0
(Hunt's)	5-oz. can	169	35.3
(Van Camp)	1 cup (7.7 oz.)	286	41.8

(USDA): United States Department of Agriculture
(HEW/FAO): Health, Education and Welfare/Food and Agriculture Organization

* Prepared as Package Directs

Food and Description	Measure or Quantity	Calories	Carbo-hydrates (grams)
Canned with pork & molasses sauce:			
(USDA)	1 cup (9 oz.)	382	53.8
(B & M) Michigan pea	1 cup (7.9 oz.)	336	50.8
(Heinz) Boston-style	1 cup (8¾ oz.)	303	50.8
Canned with pork & tomato sauce:			
(Campbell)	1 cup	262	42.7
(Heinz)	1 cup (9¼ oz.)	293	48.5
(Libby's)	1 cup (9.3 oz.)	286	52.7
(Morton House)	½ of 8-oz. can	284	50.3
Canned with tomato sauce:			
(Heinz) *Campside,* smoky beans	1 cup (9½ oz.)	350	51.1
(Heinz) vegetarian	1 cup (9¼ oz.)	267	48.9
(Van Camp)	1 cup (8.1 oz.)	286	44.5
BEAN, BARBECUE (Campbell)	1 cup	287	51.1
BEAN, BAYO, BLACK or BROWN, dry (USDA)	4 oz.	384	69.4
BEAN, CALICO, dry (USDA)	4 oz.	396	72.2
BEAN, CHILI (See **CHILI**)			
BEAN & FRANKFURTER, canned:			
(Campbell) in tomato & molasses sauce	1 cup	364	35.7
(Heinz)	8¾-oz. can	399	38.0
BEANEE-WEENEE (Van Camp)	1 cup (7.8 oz.)	316	27.6
BEAN & FRANKFURTER DINNER, frozen:			
(Banquet)	10¾-oz. dinner	528	63.1
(Morton)	12-oz. dinner	547	78.2
(Swanson)	11½-oz. dinner	610	70.1
BEAN, GREEN or SNAP: Fresh (USDA):			
Whole	1 lb. (weighed untrimmed)	128	28.3
1½" to 2" pieces	½ cup (1.8 oz.)	17	3.7

Food and Description	Measure or Quantity	Calories	Carbo-hydrates (grams)
French-style	½ cup (1.4 oz.)	13	2.8
Boiled, drained, whole (USDA)	½ cup (2.2 oz.)	16	3.3
Boiled, drained, 1½" to 2" pieces (USDA)	½ cup (2.4 oz.)	17	3.7
Canned, regular pack:			
Solids & liq. (USDA)	½ cup (4.2 oz.)	22	5.0
Drained solids, whole (USDA)	4 oz.	27	5.9
Drained solids, cut (USDA)	½ cup (2.5 oz.)	17	3.6
Drained liq. (USDA)	4 oz.	11	2.7
Blue lake, solids & liq. (Libby's)	½ cup (5 oz.)	24	5.3
Cut, drained (Comstock)	½ cup (2.1 oz.)	13	2.4
Cut, French-style, or whole, solids & liq. (Green Giant)	¼ of 16-oz. can	19	3.5
French-style, drained (Comstock)	½ cup (2.1 oz.)	13	2.4
Seasoned, solids & liq. (Del Monte)	½ cup (4 oz.)	19	4.3
Solids & liq. (Stokely-Van Camp)	½ cup (3.9 oz.)	20	4.6
Canned, dietetic pack:			
Solids & liq. (USDA)	4 oz.	18	4.1
Drained solids (USDA)	4 oz.	25	5.4
Drained liq. (USDA)	4 oz.	9	2.0
Cut, solids & liq. (Blue Boy)	4 oz.	26	5.3
Solids & liq. (Diet Delight)	½ cup (4.2 oz.)	20	3.8
Cut (S and W) *Nutradiet*	4 oz.	18	3.6
Frozen:			
Cut or French-style, not thawed (USDA)	10-oz. pkg.	74	17.0
Cut or French-style, boiled, drained (USDA)	½ cup (2.8 oz.)	20	4.6
Cut (Birds Eye)	⅓ of 9-oz. pkg.	22	5.1
Whole (Birds Eye)	½ cup (3 oz.)	23	5.2

(USDA): United States Department of Agriculture
(HEW/FAO): Health, Education and Welfare/Food and Agriculture Organization

* Prepared as Package Directs

Food and Description	Measure or Quantity	Calories	Carbo- hydrates (grams)
(Blue Goose)	4 oz.	35	6.4
French-style (Birds Eye)	⅓ of 9-oz. pkg.	22	5.1
French-style, with sliced mushrooms (Birds Eye)	⅓ of 9-oz. pkg.	26	5.5
French-style, with toasted almonds (Birds Eye)	½ cup (3 oz.)	52	6.0
In butter sauce:			
(Birds Eye)	½ cup (3 oz.)	48	4.5
(Green Giant)	⅓ of 9-oz. pkg.	34	3.7
In mushroom sauce (Green Giant)	⅓ of 10-oz. pkg.	37	6.1
In mushroom sauce, casserole (Green Giant)	⅓ of 12-oz. pkg.	52	7.5
With onions & bacon (Green Giant)	⅓ of 9-oz. pkg.	37	4.4
BEAN, ITALIAN, frozen (Birds Eye)	⅓ of 10-oz. pkg.	23	4.1
BEAN, KIDNEY or RED:			
Dry:			
(USDA)	1 lb.	1556	280.8
(USDA)	½ cup (3.3 oz.)	319	57.6
(Sinsheimer)	1 oz.	99	17.6
Cooked (USDA)	½ cup (3.3 oz.)	109	19.8
Canned:			
Solids & liq. (USDA)	½ cup (4.5 oz.)	115	21.0
Drained solids (Butter Kernel)	½ cup	108	19.7
Red kidney & chili gravy (Nalley's)	4 oz.	120	18.5
BEAN LIMA, young:			
Raw, whole (USDA)	1 lb. (weighed in pod)	223	40.1
Raw, without shell (USDA)	1 lb. (weighed shelled)	558	100.2
Boiled, drained (USDA)	½ cup (3 oz.)	94	16.8
Canned, regular pack:			
Solids & liq. (USDA)	½ cup (4.4 oz.)	88	16.6
Drained solids (USDA)	½ cup (3 oz.)	84	15.9
Drained solids (Del Monte)	½ cup (3.1 oz.)	89	17.0
Solids & liq. (Stokely-Van Camp)	½ cup (4.1 oz.)	82	15.4
With ham (Nalley's)	4 oz.	132	14.3

Food and Description	Measure or Quantity	Calories	Carbo-hydrates (grams)
Canned, dietetic pack:			
Solids & liq., low sodium (USDA)	4 oz.	79	14.6
Drained solids, low sodium (USDA)	4 oz.	108	20.1
Solids & liq., unseasoned (Blue Boy)	4 oz.	79	12.6
Frozen:			
Baby butter beans (Birds Eye)	⅓ of 10-oz. pkg.	123	23.6
Baby limas, not thawed (USDA)	4 oz.	138	26.1
Boiled, drained solids (USDA)	½ cup (3 oz.)	101	19.2
(Birds Eye)	½ cup (3.3 oz.)	111	21.0
In butter sauce (Green Giant)	⅓ of 10-oz. pkg.	116	18.0
Tiny (Birds Eye)	½ cup (2.5 oz.)	83	16.2
Fordhooks:			
Not thawed (USDA)	4 oz.	116	22.1
Boiled, drained (USDA)	½ cup (3 oz.)	83	16.0
(Birds Eye)	⅓ of 10-oz. pkg.	94	17.9
BEAN, LIMA, MATURE:			
Dry:			
Baby (USDA)	½ cup (3.4 oz.)	331	61.4
Large (USDA)	½ cup (3.1 oz.)	304	56.3
(Sinsheimer)	1 oz.	92	17.5
Boiled, drained (USDA)	½ cup (3.4 oz.)	131	24.3
BEAN, MUNG, dry (USDA)	½ cup (3.7 oz.)	357	63.3
BEAN 'N BEEF (Campbell)	1 cup	259	34.8
BEAN, PINTO:			
Dry (USDA)	½ cup (3.4 oz.)	335	61.2
Dry (Sinsheimer)	1 oz.	99	17.6

(USDA): United States Department of Agriculture
(HEW/FAO): Health, Education and Welfare/Food and Agriculture
                        Organization

* Prepared as Package Directs

Food and Description	Measure or Quantity	Calories	Carbohydrates (grams)
BEAN, RED (See **BEAN, KIDNEY** or **BEAN, RED MEXICAN**)			
BEAN, RED MEXICAN, dry (USDA)	4 oz.	396	72.2
BEAN, REFRIED, canned (Gebhardt)	½ cup	120	
BEAN SALAD, MIXED:			
(Hunt's) Snack Pack	5-oz. can	111	23.7
(Le Sueur)	¼ of 1-lb. 1-oz. can	86	17.1
BEAN, SEMI-MATURE, in brine (B&M)	½ of 8¾-oz. can	155	25.9
BEAN SOUP, canned:			
*(Manischewitz)	1 cup	111	17.6
*With bacon (Campbell)	1 cup (8 oz.)	152	19.4
With pork, condensed (USDA)	8 oz. (by wt.)	304	39.3
*With pork, prepared with equal volume water (USDA)	1 cup (8.8 oz.)	168	21.8
With smoked ham (Heinz) *Great American*	1 cup (8¾ oz.)	201	24.5
*With smoked pork (Heinz)	1 cup (8½ oz.)	157	20.1
BEAN SOUP, BLACK, canned:			
*(Campbell)	1 cup	91	13.9
(Crosse & Blackwell)	6½ oz. (½ can)	96	15.5
*BEAN SOUP, LIMA, canned (Manischewitz)	8 oz. (by wt.)	93	15.3
BEAN SOUP MIX (Lipton) *Cup-a-Soup*	1.1-oz. pkg.	111	19.4
BEAN SOUP, NAVY, dehydrated (USDA)	1 oz.	93	17.8
BEAN SPROUT:			
Mung:			
Raw (USDA)	½ lb.	80	15.0
Raw (USDA)	½ cup (1.6 oz.)	16	3.0
Boiled, drained (USDA)	½ cup (2.2 oz.)	17	3.2

Food and Description	Measure or Quantity	Calories	Carbohydrates (grams)
Soy:			
Raw (USDA)	½ lb.	104	12.0
Raw (USDA)	½ cup (1.9 oz.)	25	2.9
Boiled, drained (USDA)	4 oz.	43	4.2
Canned (Chun King)	1 cup	39	2.5
BEAN, WAX (See BEAN, YELLOW)			
BEAN, WHITE, dry:			
Raw:			
Great Northern (USDA)	½ cup (3.1 oz.)	303	54.6
Navy or pea (USDA)	½ cup (3.7 oz.)	354	63.8
Navy or pea (Sinsheimer)	1 oz.	99	17.6
White (USDA)	1 oz.	96	17.4
Cooked:			
Great Northern (USDA)	½ cup (3 oz.)	100	18.0
Navy or pea (USDA)	½ cup (3.4 oz.)	113	20.4
All other white (USDA)	4 oz.	134	24.0
BEAN, YELLOW or WAX:			
Raw, whole (USDA)	1 lb. (weighed untrimmed)	108	24.0
Boiled, drained, 1″ pieces (USDA)	½ cup (2.9 oz.)	18	3.7
Canned, regular pack:			
Solids & liq. (USDA)	½ cup (4.2 oz.)	23	5.0
Drained solids (USDA)	½ cup (2.2 oz.)	15	3.2
Drained liq. (USDA)	4 oz.	12	2.8
Drained solids (Butter Kernel)	½ cup (3.9 oz.)	20	4.6
Drained (Comstock)	½ cup (2.2 oz.)	16	2.9
Solids & liq. (Del Monte)	½ cup (4 oz.)	18	3.5
Solids & liq. (Green Giant)	½ of 8.5-oz. can	19	3.5
Solids & liq. (Stokely-Van Camp)	½ cup (4.1 oz.)	32	4.6
Canned, dietetic pack:			
Solids & liq. (USDA)	4 oz.	17	3.9
Drained solids (USDA)	4 oz.	24	5.3

(USDA): United States Department of Agriculture
(HEW/FAO): Health, Education and Welfare/Food and Agriculture Organization

* Prepared as Package Directs

Food and Description	Measure or Quantity	Calories	Carbo-hydrates (grams)
Drained liq. (USDA)	4 oz.	8	1.6
Solids & liq. (Blue Boy)	4 oz.	24	5.0
Frozen:			
Cut, not thawed (USDA)	4 oz.	32	7.4
Boiled, drained (USDA)	4 oz.	31	7.0
Cut (Birds Eye)	⅓ of 9-oz. pkg.	24	5.4
BEAUJOLAIS WINE, French Burgundy:			
(Barton & Guestier) St. Louis, 11% alcohol	3 fl. oz.	60	.1
(Chanson) St. Vincent, 11% alcohol	3 fl. oz.	78	6.3
(Cruse) 12% alcohol	3 fl. oz.	72	
BEAUNE WINE:			
Clos de Feves, French Burgundy (Chanson) 12% alcohol	3 fl. oz.	84	6.3
St. Vincent, French Burgundy (Chanson) 12% alcohol	3 fl. oz.	84	6.3
BEAVER, roasted (USDA)	4 oz.	281	0.
BEECHNUT:			
Whole (USDA)	4 oz. (weighed in shell)	393	14.0
Shelled (USDA)	4 oz. (weighed shelled)	644	23.0

BEEF. Values for beef cuts are given below for "lean and fat" and for "lean only." Beef purchased by the consumer at the retail store usually is trimmed to about one-half-inch layer of fat. This is the meat described as "lean and fat." If all the fat that can be cut off with a knife is removed, the remainder is the "lean only." These cuts still contain flecks of fat

Food and Description	Measure or Quantity	Calories	Carbohydrates (grams)
known as "marbling" distributed through the meat. Cooked meats are medium done. Choice grade cuts (USDA):			
Brisket:			
Raw	1 lb. (weighed with bone)	1284	0.
Braised:			
Lean & fat	4 oz.	467	0.
Lean only	4 oz.	252	0.
Chuck:			
Raw	1 lb. (weighed with bone)	984	0.
Braised or pot-roasted:			
Lean & fat	4 oz.	371	0.
Lean only	4 oz.	243	0.
Dried (See **BEEF, CHIPPED**)			
Fat, separable, cooked	1 oz.	207	0.
Filet mignon. There are no data available on its composition. For dietary estimates, the data for sirloin steak, lean only, afford the closest approximation.			
Flank:			
Raw	1 lb.	653	0.
Braised	4 oz.	222	0.
Foreshank:			
Raw	1 lb. (weighed with bone)	531	.0.
Simmered:			
Lean & fat	4 oz.	310	0.
Lean only	4 oz.	209	0.
Ground:			
Lean:			
Raw	1 lb.	812	0.
Raw	1 cup (8 oz.)	405	0.

(USDA): United States Department of Agriculture
(HEW/FAO): Health, Education and Welfare/Food and Agriculture
    Organization
* Prepared as Package Directs

Food and Description	Measure or Quantity	Calories	Carbo-hydrates (grams)
Broiled	4 oz.	248	0.
Regular:			
Raw	1 lb.	1216	0.
Raw	1 cup (8 oz.)	606	0.
Broiled	4 oz.	324	0.
Heel of round:			
Raw	1 lb.	966	0.
Roasted:			
Lean & fat	4 oz.	296	0.
Lean only	4 oz.	204	0.
Hindshank:			
Raw	1 lb. (weighed with bone)	604	0.
Simmered:			
Lean & fat	4 oz.	409	0.
Lean only	4 oz.	209	0.
Neck:			
Raw	1 lb. (weighed with bone)	820	0.
Pot-roasted:			
Lean & fat	4 oz.	332	0.
Lean only	4 oz.	222	0.
Plate:			
Raw	1 lb. (weighed with bone)	1615	0.
Simmered:			
Lean & fat	4 oz.	538	0.
Lean only	4 oz.	252	0.
Rib roast:			
Raw	1 lb. (weighed with bone)	1673	0.
Roasted:			
Lean & fat	4 oz.	499	0.
Lean only	4 oz.	273	0.
Round:			
Raw	1 lb. (weighed with bone)	863	0.
Broiled:			
Lean & fat	4 oz.	296	0.
Lean only	4 oz.	214	0.
Rump:			
Raw	1 lb. (weighed with bone)	1167	0.
Roasted:			
Lean & fat	4 oz.	393	0.

Food and Description	Measure or Quantity	Calories	Carbo- hydrates (grams)
Lean only	4 oz.	236	0.
Steak, club:			
Raw	1 lb. (weighed without bone)	1724	0.
Broiled:			
Lean & fat	4 oz.	515	0.
Lean only	4 oz.	277	0.
One 8-oz. steak (weighed without bone before cooking) will give you:			
Lean & fat	5.9 oz.	754	0.
Lean only	3.4 oz.	234	0.
Steak, porterhouse:			
Raw	1 lb. (weighed with bone)	1603	0.
Broiled:			
Lean & fat	4 oz.	527	0.
Lean only	4 oz.	254	0.
One 16-oz. steak (weighed with bone before cooking) will give you:			
Lean & fat	10.2 oz.	1339	0.
Lean only	5.9 oz.	372	0.
Steak, ribeye, broiled:			
One 10-oz. steak (weighed before cooking without bone) will give you:			
Lean & fat	7.3 oz.	911	0.
Lean only	3.8 oz.	258	0.
Steak, sirloin, double-bone:			
Raw	1 lb. (weighed with bone)	1240	0.
Broiled:			
Lean & fat	4 oz.	463	0.
Lean only	4 oz.	245	0.
One 16-oz. steak (weighed before cooking with bone) will give you:			

(USDA): United States Department of Agriculture
(HEW/FAO): Health, Education and Welfare/Food and Agriculture Organization
* Prepared as Package Directs

Food and Description	Measure or Quantity	Calories	Carbo- hydrates (grams)
Lean & fat	8.9 oz.	1028	0.
Lean only	5.9 oz.	359	0.
One 12-oz. steak (weighed before cooking with bone) will give you:			
Lean & fat	6.6 oz.	767	0.
Lean only	4.4 oz.	268	0.
Steak, sirloin, hipbone:			
Raw	1 lb. (weighed with bone)	1585	0.
Broiled:			
Lean & fat	4 oz.	552	0.
Lean only	4 oz.	272	0.
Steak, sirloin, wedge & round-bone:			
Raw	1 lb. (weighed with bone)	1316	0.
Broiled:			
Lean & fat	4 oz.	439	0.
Lean only	4 oz.	235	0.
Steak, T-bone:			
Raw	1 lb. (weighed with bone)	1596	0.
Broiled:			
Lean & fat	4 oz.	536	0.
Lean only	4 oz.	253	0.
One-16 oz. steak (weighed before cooking with bone) will give you:			
Lean & fat	9.8 oz.	1315	0.
Lean only	5.5 oz.	348	0.
BEEFAMATO COCKTAIL (Mott's)	½ cup	49	10.7
BEEFARONI, canned (Chef Boy-Ar-Dee)	⅛ of 40-oz. can	206	27.9
BEEF & BEEF STOCK (Bunker Hill)	15-oz. can	920	0.
BEEF BOUILLON, cubes or powder:			
(Croyden House)	1 tsp. (5 grams)	12	2.2
(Herb-Ox)	1 cube (4 grams)	6	.5

Food and Description	Measure or Quantity	Calories	Carbo-hydrates (grams)
(Herb-Ox)	1 packet (4 grams)	8	.8
*(Knorr Swiss)	6 fl. oz.	13	
(Maggi)	1 cube or 1 tsp.	7	.5
(Steero)	1 cube	6	.5
(Wyler's)	1 cube (4 grams)	7	.4
(Wyler's)	1 envelope (5 grams)	11	1.4
(Wyler's) no salt	1 cube (4 grams)	10	1.6
BEEF & CABBAGE, frozen, (Mrs. Paul's)	12-oz. pkg.	432	27.5
BEEF, CHIPPED Uncooked:			
(USDA)	½ cup (2.9 oz.)	166	0.
(Armour Star)	1 oz.	48	0.
Cooked (Oscar Mayer)	1 slice (5 grams)	7	.1
Cooked, creamed, home recipe (USDA)	½ cup (4.3 oz.)	188	8.7
Canned, creamed (Swanson)	½ cup	96	5.8
Frozen, creamed (Banquet)	5 oz.	126	9.2
BEEF, CHOPPED, canned:			
(Armour Star)	12-oz. can	1042	4.4
(Hormel)	12-oz. can	867	2.0
*Freeze dry (Wilson)	4 oz.	198	0.
BEEF, CORNED (See CORNED BEEF)			
BEEF DINNER, frozen:			
(Banquet)	11-oz. dinner	312	20.9
(Swanson)	11½-oz. dinner	371	30.3
(Swanson) 3-course	15-oz. dinner	567	57.8
Chopped (Banquet)	11-oz. dinner	443	32.8
Chopped sirloin (Swanson)	10-oz. dinner	447	40.0
Chopped (Weight Watchers)	18-oz. dinner	665	6.2
Sliced (Morton)	11-oz. dinner	290	18.7
Sliced (Morton) 3-course	16-oz. dinner	636	68.1
Steak & carrot (Weight Watchers)	10-oz. luncheon	412	8.0

(USDA): United States Department of Agriculture
(HEW/FAO): Health, Education and Welfare/Food and Agriculture Organization

* Prepared as Package Directs

Food and Description	Measure or Quantity	Calories	Carbo-hydrates (grams)
Steak & cauliflower (Weight Watchers)	11-oz. luncheon	431	11.2
BEEF & EGGPLANT, frozen (Mrs. Paul's)	12-oz. pkg.	418	31.7
BEEF GOULASH:			
Canned (Heinz)	8½-oz. can	253	20.1
Seasoning mix (Lawry's)	1 pkg. (1.7 oz.)	127	24.1
BEEF & GREEN PEPPER, frozen (Mrs. Paul's)	12-oz. pkg.	384	31.7
BEEF, GROUND (see **BEEF, Ground**)			
BEEF, GROUND, SEASONING MIX:			
With onion (Durkee)	1⅛-oz. pkg.	92	19.9
With onion (French's)	1⅛-oz. pkg.	79	17.5
BEEF HASH, ROAST:			
Canned (Hormel)	7½ oz.	390	9.0
Frozen (Stouffer's)	11½-oz. pkg.	460	21.7
BEEF JERKY:			
Cow-Boy-Jo's	¼-oz. piece	24	.4
(General Mills)	¼-oz. piece	25	.3
(Lowrey's)	¼-oz. piece	21	1.0
BEEF PATTIES:			
Burgundy sauce (Morton House)	⅓ of 12½-oz. can	154	8.9
*Freeze dry (Wilson)	4 oz.	216	3.4
BEEF PIE:			
Baked, home recipe (USDA)	4¼″ pie (8 oz. before baking)	558	42.7
Frozen:			
(Banquet)	8-oz. pie	409	40.9
(Morton)	8-oz. pie	368	34.0
(Stouffer's)	10-oz. pie	572	42.9
(Swanson)	8-oz. pie	434	38.6
(Swanson) deep dish	1-lb. pie	703	56.8
BEEF, POTTED (USDA)	1 oz.	70	0.

Food and Description	Measure or Quantity	Calories	Carbo-hydrates (grams)
BEEF PUFFS, hors d'oeuvres, frozen (Durkee)	1 piece (½ oz.)	47	3.1
BEEF, ROAST, canned:			
(USDA)	4 oz.	254	0.
(Wilson) *Tender Made*			
BEEF, SLICED, with barbecue sauce (Banquet)	5-oz. bag	152	13.0
BEEF SOUP, canned:			
*(Campbell)	1 cup	99	10.5
*(Campbell) *Chunky*	1 cup	185	18.8
*Barley (Manischewitz)	1 cup	83	11.2
Bouillon, condensed (USDA)	8 oz. (by wt.)	59	5.0
*Bouillon, prepared with equal volume water (USDA)	1 cup (8.5 oz.)	31	2.6
Broth:			
Condensed (USDA)	8 oz. (by wt.)	59	5.0
*Prepared with equal volume water (USDA)	1 cup (8.5 oz.)	31	2.6
(College Inn)	1 cup	19	5.2
(Swanson)	1 cup	18	.2
*Cabbage (Manischewitz)	1 cup	62	9.0
Consomme:			
Condensed (USDA)	8 oz. (by wt.)	59	5.0
*Prepared with equal volume water (USDA)	1 cup (8.5 oz.)	31	2.6
*(Campbell)	1 cup	33	2.6
Noodle:			
Condensed (USDA)	8 oz. (by wt.)	129	13.2
*Prepared with equal volume water (USDA)	1 cup (8.5 oz.)	67	7.0
*(Campbell)	1 cup	67	8.2
*(Heinz)	1 cup (8½ oz.)	74	6.7
*(Manischewitz)	8 oz. (by wt.)	64	8.0
*Curly, with chicken (Campbell)	1 cup	77	9.3
With dumplings (Heinz) *Great American*	1 cup (8¾ oz.)	109	11.1

(USDA): United States Department of Agriculture
(HEW/FAO): Health, Education and Welfare/Food and Agriculture
               Organization
* Prepared as Package Directs

Food and Description	Measure or Quantity	Calories	Carbo-hydrates (grams)
Sirloin burger (Campbell)			
Chunky	1 cup	162	14.3
*Vegetable (Manischewitz)	8 oz. (by wt.)	59	8.9
BEEF SOUP MIX:			
*Barley (Wyler's)	6 fl. oz.	54	9.3
Broth (Lipton) *Cup-a-Soup*	1 pkg. (8 grams)	19	3.6
*Noodle, with vegetable			
(Lipton)	1 cup	66	11.2
*(Wyler's)	6 fl. oz.	37	7.0
*BEEF STEAK, freeze dry			
(Wilson)	4 oz.	199	0.
BEEF STEW:			
Home recipe (USDA)	1 cup (8.6) oz.)	218	15.2
Canned:			
(Armour Star)	24-oz. can	590	38.8
(Austex)	15½-oz. can	347	31.2
(B&M)	1 cup (7.9 oz.)	152	15.2
(Bunker Hill)	15-oz. can	422	18.0
(Heinz)	8½-oz. can	253	24.2
(Hormel) *Dinty Moore*	8 oz.	190	13.6
(Libby's)	8 oz.	154	15.2
(Morton House)	24-oz. can	725	53.8
(Nalley's)	8 oz.	218	18.8
(Swanson)	1 cup	181	15.9
(Van Camp)	1 cup (9.2 oz.)	204	18.4
(Wilson)	15½ oz.	343	30.8
Dietetic (Claybourne)	8-oz. can	365	18.4
*Freeze dry (Wilson)	8 oz.	268	17.9
Frozen, buffet (Banquet)	2-lb. pkg.	720	82.2
BEEF STEW SEASONING MIX:			
(Durkee)	1¾-oz. pkg.	99	22.1
(French's)	1⅞-oz. pkg.	133	28.5
(Kraft)	1 oz.	51	1.3
(Lawry's)	1⅜-oz. pkg.	131	24.2
BEEF STOCK BASE (French's)	1 tsp. (4 grams)	9	1.7
BEEF STROGANOFF (See STROGANOFF)			

Food and Description	Measure or Quantity	Calories	Carbo-hydrates (grams)
BEER, canned:			
Regular:			
Black Horse Ale, 5% alcohol	12 fl. oz. (12.7 oz.)	162	13.8
Black Label, 4.9% alcohol	12 fl. oz.	140	11.3
Buckeye, 4.6% alcohol	12 fl. oz.	144	11.0
Budweiser, 4.9% alcohol	12 fl. oz.	156	12.3
Budweiser, 3.9% alcohol	12 fl. oz.	137	11.9
Busch Bavarian:			
4.9% alcohol	12 fl. oz.	156	12.3
3.9% alcohol	12 fl. oz.	137	11.9
Eastside Lager	12 fl. oz.	145	
Hamm's	12 fl. oz.	151	13.3
Heidelberg, 4.6% alcohol	12 fl. oz.	133	10.7
Knickerbocker, 4.6% alcohol	12 fl. oz.	160	13.7
Meister Brau Premium, 4.6% alcohol	12 fl. oz.	144	11.0
Meister Brau Premium Draft, 4.6% alcohol	12 fl. oz.	144	11.0
Michelob, 4.9% alcohol	12 fl. oz.	160	12.8
Narraganset, 4.7% alcohol	12 fl. oz.	155	14.4
North Star, regular, 4.8% alcohol	12 fl. oz.	165	14.9
North Star, 3.2 low gravity	12 fl. oz.	142	13.6
Pabst Blue Ribbon	12 fl. oz.	150	
Pfeifer, regular, 4.8% alcohol	12 fl. oz.	165	14.9
Pfeifer, 3.2 low gravity	12 fl. oz.	142	13.6
Red Cap Ale, 5.6% alcohol	12 fl. oz.	153	10.8
Rheingold, 4.6% alcohol	12 fl. oz.	160	13.7
Schlitz	12 fl. oz.	155	14.7
Schmidt, regular or extra special, 4.8% alcohol	12 fl. oz. (12.7 oz.)	165	14.9

(USDA): United States Department of Agriculture
(HEW/FAO): Health, Education and Welfare/Food and Agriculture Organization

* Prepared as Package Directs

Food and Description	Measure or Quantity	Calories	Carbohydrates (grams)
Schmidt, 3.2 low gravity	12 fl. oz. (12.7 oz.)	142	13.6
Stag, 4.8% alcohol	12 fl. oz.	137	11.3
Tuborg USA, 4.8% alcohol	12 fl. oz.	140	12.1
Utica Club	12 fl. oz.	150	
Yuengling Premium	12 fl. oz.	144	15.1
Low carbohydrate:			
Dia-beer	12 fl. oz.	145	4.2
Dia-beer	7 fl. oz.	85	2.8
Gablinger's 4.5% alcohol	12 fl. oz.	99	.2
Meister Brau Lite, 4.6% alcohol	12 fl. oz.	96	1.4
BEER, NEAR:			
Kingsbury, 0.4% alcohol	12 fl. oz. (12 oz.)	62	15.0
Metbrew, 0.4% alcohol	12 fl. oz. (12.5 oz.)	73	13.7
BEET:			
Raw (USDA)	1 lb. (weighed with skins, without tops)	137	31.4
Raw, diced (USDA)	½ cup (2.4 oz.)	29	6.6
Boiled, drained (USDA):			
Whole	2 beets (2″ dia., 3.5 oz.)	32	7.2
Diced	½ cup (3 oz.)	27	6.1
Slices	½ cup (3.6 oz.)	33	7.3
Canned, regular pack:			
Solids & liq. (USDA)	½ cup (4.3 oz.)	42	9.7
Drained solids (USDA):			
Whole	½ cup (2.8 oz.)	30	7.0
Diced	½ cup (2.9 oz.)	30	7.2
Sliced	½ cup (3.1 oz.)	33	7.7
Drained liq. (USDA)	4 oz.	29	7.0
Drained solids (Butter Kernel)	½ cup (4.1 oz.)	38	9.1
Solids & liq.:			
(Del Monte)	½ cup (4 oz.)	30	7.0
Slices (Libby's)	½ cup (4 oz.)	34	8.1
(Stokely-Van Camp)	½ cup (4.1 oz.)	39	9.0
Harvard, solids & liq. (Greenwood's)	½ cup (3.8 oz.)	50	11.2
Pickled, drained solids (Greenwood's)	½ cup (2.9 oz.)	40	8.7

Food and Description	Measure or Quantity	Calories	Carbo-hydrates (grams)
Canned, dietetic pack:			
Solids & liq. (USDA)	4 oz.	36	8.8
Drained solids (USDA)	4 oz.	42	9.9
Drained liq. (USDA)	4 oz.	28	6.7
Whole (Blue Boy)	10 small (3.5 oz.)	43	9.3
Pickled, solids & liq. (Del Monte)	½ cup (4 oz.)	75	18.8
Diced, solids & liq. (Blue Boy)	4 oz.	25	5.1
Sliced (Blue Boy)	10 slices (3.5 oz.)	32	7.0
Sliced (S and W) *Nutradiet*	4 oz.	32	7.3
(Tillie Lewis)	½ cup (4.3 oz.)	46	9.0
Frozen, sliced, in orange-flavor glaze (Birds Eye)	½ cup (3.3 oz.)	54	14.9
BEET GREENS (USDA):			
Raw, whole	1 lb. (weighed untrimmed)	61	11.7
Boiled, leaves & stems, drained	½ cup (2.6 oz.)	13	2.4
BENEDICTINE LIQUEUR (Julius Wile) 86 proof	1 fl. oz.	112	10.3
BERNKASTELER, German Moselle wine (Deinhard) 11% alcohol	3 fl. oz.	60	1.0
BERRY FROST (Annie Green Springs) 9% alcohol	3 fl. oz.	69	7.3
BERRY PIE (Hostess)	4½-oz. pie	421	52.3
BEVERAGE (See individual listings)			
BIANCA DELLA COSTA TOSCANA, white wine (Antinori) 12½% alcohol	3 fl. oz.	87	6.3
BIF (Wilson) luncheon meat	3 oz.	272	1.5

(USDA): United States Department of Agriculture
(HEW/FAO): Health, Education and Welfare/Food and Agriculture
Organization
* Prepared as Package Directs

Food and Description	Measure or Quantity	Calories	Carbo- hydrates (grams)
BIG MAC (McDonald's)	1 hamburger (6.5 oz.)	561	42.2
BIG WHEEL (Hostess)	1.3-oz. cake	185	21.5
BIRCH BEER, soft drink:			
(Canada Dry)	6 fl. oz.	82	20.4
(Yukon Club)	6 fl. oz.	89	22.3
BISCUIT:			
Baking powder, home recipe (USDA)	1 oz. biscuit (2" dia.)	103	12.8
Egg (Stella D'oro):			
Dietetic	1 piece (.4 oz.)	42	6.6
Regular	1 piece (.4 oz.)	42	6.9
Roman	1 piece (1.1 oz.)	135	19.2
Sugared	1 piece (.5 oz.)	59	11.0
BISCUIT DOUGH, refrigerated:			
(Borden):			
Big 10's	1 biscuit (.9 oz.)	82	11.2
Buttered Up	1 biscuit (.9 oz.)	90	11.8
Buttermilk	1 biscuit (.8 oz.)	57	10.1
Gem	1 biscuit (.9 oz.)	82	11.2
Southern style	1 biscuit (.8 oz.)	57	10.1
(Pillsbury):			
Baking powder:			
1869 Brand	1 biscuit	80	9.0
Heat 'N Serve, *1869 Brand*	1 biscuit	100	12.0
Tenderflake	1 biscuit	60	8.0
Buttermelts	1 biscuit	60	9.0
Buttermilk	1 biscuit	60	11.0
Buttermilk, extra light	1 biscuit	55	10.5
Country style	1 biscuit	60	11.0
Flaky, *Hungry Jack*	1 biscuit	80	11.5
Oven-ready, *Ballard*	1 biscuit	60	11.0
BISCUIT MIX:			
Dry, with enriched flour (USDA)	1 oz.	120	19.5
*Baked from mix, with added milk (USDA)	1-oz. biscuit	92	14.8
Bisquick (Betty Crocker)	1 cup	503	79.4
BI-SICLE (Popsicle Industries)	3 fl. oz.	116	

Food and Description	Measure or Quantity	Calories	Carbo-hydrates (grams)
BITTER LEMON, soft drink:			
(Canada Dry)	6 fl. oz.	77	19.2
(Hoffman)	6 fl. oz.	85	21.3
(Schweppes)	6 fl. oz.	96	23.6
BITTER ORANGE, soft drink			
(Schweppes)	6 fl. oz.	92	22.6
BITTERS (Angostura)	½ tsp. (5 grams)	7	1.0
BLACKBERRY:			
Fresh (includes boysenberry, dewberry, youngberry):			
With hulls (USDA)	1 lb. (weighed untrimmed)	250	55.6
Hulled (USDA)	½ cup (2.6 oz.)	42	9.4
Canned, regular, solids & liq.:			
Juice pack (USDA)	4 oz.	61	13.7
Light syrup (USDA)	4 oz.	82	19.6
Heavy syrup (USDA)	½ cup (4.6 oz.)	118	28.9
Extra heavy syrup (USDA)	4 oz.	125	30.7
Canned, low calorie, solid & liq. (S and W) *Nutradiet*	4 oz.	50	11.2
Frozen (USDA):			
Sweetened, not thawed	4 oz.	109	27.7
Unsweetened, not thawed	4 oz.	55	12.9
BLACKBERRY BRANDY			
(DeKuyper) 70 proof	1 fl. oz. (1.1 oz.)	85	6.9
BLACKBERRY JAM:			
Sweetened (Smucker's)	1 T.	53	13.3
Low calorie (Dia-Mel)	1 T. (.5 oz.)	6	1.4
Low calorie (Diet Delight)	1 T. (.6 oz.)	22	5.5
BLACKBERRY JELLY, low calorie (Slenderella)	1 T. (.7 oz.)	25	6.4
BLACKBERRY LIQUEUR:			
(Bols) 60 proof	1 fl. oz.	96	8.9
(Hiram Walker) 60 proof	1 fl. oz.	100	12.8

(USDA): United States Department of Agriculture
(HEW/FAO): Health, Education and Welfare/Food and Agriculture
         Organization
* Prepared as Package Directs

Food and Description	Measure or Quantity	Calories	Carbo-hydrates (grams)
BLACKBERRY PIE:			
Home recipe (USDA)	⅛ of 9″ pie (5.6 oz.)	384	54.4
(Tastykake)	4-oz. pie	386	60.1
Frozen (Banquet)	5-oz. serving	376	55.5
BLACKBERRY PIE FILLING:			
(Comstock)	1 cup (10¾ oz.)	438	108.5
(Lucky Leaf)	8 oz.	258	62.4
BLACKBERRY SOUR COCKTAIL, liq. mix			
(Holland House)	1½ fl. oz.	75	18.0
BLACKBERRY SYRUP			
(Smucker's)	1 T. (.6 oz.)	45	11.6
BLACKBERRY WINE (Mogen David) 12% alcohol	3 fl. oz.	135	18.7
BLACK-EYED PEA, frozen (See also **COWPEA**):			
Cooked, drained (USDA)	½ cup (3 oz.)	111	20.1
(Birds Eye)	½ cup (2.5 oz.)	92	15.7
BLACK RUSSIAN COCKTAIL, liq. mix (Holland House)	1½ fl. oz.	138	34.5
BLANCMANGE (See **VANILLA PUDDING**)			
BLINTZE, frozen (Aunt Leah's):			
Apple, blueberry or cherry	1 blintze (2.5 oz.)	80	
Cheese	1 blintze (2.5 oz.)	70	
BLOOD PUDDING or **SAUSAGE** (USDA)	1 oz.	112	.1
BLOODY MARY MIX:			
Dry (Bar-Tender's)	1 serving (9 grams)	26	5.7
Dry (Holland House)	1 serving (.5 oz.)	56	14.0
Liq. (Sacramento)	5½-fl.-oz. can	39	9.1
BLUEBERRY:			
Fresh, whole (USDA)	1 lb. (weighed untrimmed)	259	63.8
Fresh, trimmed (USDA)	½ cup (2.6 oz.)	45	11.2

Food and Description	Measure or Quantity	Calories	Carbo-hydrates (grams)
Canned, solids & liq. (USDA):			
Syrup pack, extra heavy	½ cup (4.4 oz.)	126	32.5
Water pack	½ cup (4.3 oz.)	47	11.9
Frozen:			
Sweetened, solids & liq. (USDA)	½ cup (4 oz.)	120	30.2
Quick thaw (Birds Eye)	½ cup (5 oz.)	114	28.7
Unsweetened, solids & liq. (USDA)	½ cup (2.9 oz.)	45	11.2
BLUEBERRY PIE:			
Home recipe (USDA)	⅙ of 9″ pie (5.6 oz.)	382	55.1
(Hostess)	4½-oz. pie	421	53.6
(Tastykake)	4-oz. pie	376	57.8
Frozen:			
(Banquet)	5-oz. serving	366	55.8
(Morton)	⅙ of 24-oz. pie	289	40.3
(Mrs. Smith's)	⅙ of 8″ pie (4.2 oz.)	294	40.0
Tart (Pepperidge Farm)	3-oz. tart	277	34.5
BLUEBERRY PIE FILLING:			
(Comstock)	1 cup (10¾ oz.)	332 ·	82.8
(Lucky Leaf)	8 oz.	256	61.4
BLUEBERRY PRESERVE			
(Smucker's)	1 T.	52	13.3
BLUEBERRY SYRUP			
(Smucker's)	1 T. (.6 oz.)	45	11.6
BLUEBERRY TURNOVER, frozen (Pepperidge Farm)	1 turnover (3.3 oz.)	321	32.0
BLUEFISH (USDA):			
Raw, whole	1 lb. (weighed whole)	271	0.
Raw, meat only	4 oz.	133	0.

(USDA): United States Department of Agriculture
(HEW/FAO): Health, Education and Welfare/Food and Agriculture Organization
* Prepared as Package Directs

Food and Description	Measure or Quantity	Calories	Carbo- hydrates (grams)
Baked or broiled	4.4-oz. piece (3½" x 3" x ½")	199	0.
Fried	5.3-oz. piece (3½" x 3" x ½")	308	7.0
BOCKWURST (USDA)	1 oz.	75	.2
BOLOGNA:			
(Armour Star)	1 oz.	99	0.
(Eckrich) regular	1-oz. slice	94	1.5
(Eckrich) lunch, garlic or pickled	1 oz.	94	1.5
(Hormel) all meat	1 oz.	85	.5
(Hormel) coarse ground	1 oz.	75	.9
(Oscar Mayer) all meat	1-oz. slice	89	.8
(Oscar Mayer) German Brand	.8-oz. slice	55	.4
(Oscar Mayer) Lebanon	.8-oz. slice	46	.9
(Vienna)	1 oz.	67	.7
(Wilson)	1 oz.	87	.5
BONITO, raw (USDA):			
Whole	1 lb. (weighed whole)	442	0.
Meat only	4 oz.	191	0.
BORDEAUX WINE (See also individual regional, vineyard or brand names or **CLARET WINE**):			
Rouge (Cruse) 10½% alcohol	3 fl. oz.	63	
BORSCHT:			
(Manischewitz)	8 oz. (by wt.)	72	17.5
*Concentrate, frozen (Aunt Leah's)	8 fl. oz.	46	
*Concentrate, frozen, diet (Aunt Leah's)	8 fl. oz.	25	
Egg (Mother's)	8 fl. oz.	48	
BOSCO (Best Foods)	1 T. (.7 oz.)	57	12.9
BOSTON BROWN BREAD (See **BREAD**)			
BOSTON CREAM PIE:			
Frozen (Mrs. Smith's)	⅛ of 8" pie (3.3 oz.)	329	51.7
*Mix (Betty Crocker)	⅛ of pie	265	47.9

Food and Description	Measure or Quantity	Calories	Carbohydrates (grams)
BOUILLON CUBE (See individual flavors)			
BOURBON WHISKY, Unflavored (See **DISTILLED LIQUOR**)			
BOURBON WHISKY, PEACH FLAVORED (Old Mr. Boston) 70 proof	1 fl. oz.	100	8.0
BOYSENBERRY: Fresh (See **BLACKBERRY,** fresh)			
Canned, low calorie (S and W) *Nutradiet*	4 oz.	36	9.8
Frozen, sweetened (USDA)	10-oz. pkg.	272	69.2
BOYSENBERRY JELLY (Smucker's)	1 T. (.7 oz.)	50	12.9
BOYSENBERRY PIE, frozen:			
(Banquet)	5-oz. serving	374	55.8
(Morton)	⅙ of 20-oz. pie	249	36.3
BOYSENBERRY PRESERVE:			
Sweetened (Smucker's)	1 T. (.7 oz.)	52	13.3
Low calorie:			
(S and W)	1 T. (.5 oz.)	11	2.5
(Slenderella)	1 T. (.7 oz.)	25	6.4
BRAINS, all animals, raw (USDA)	4 oz.	142	.9
BRAN BREAKFAST CEREAL:			
Plain:			
All-Bran (Kellogg's)	½ cup (1 oz.)	64	19.3
Bran-Buds (Kellogg's)	⅓ cup (1 oz.)	73	20.6
40% bran flakes (Kellogg's)	¾ cup (1 oz.)	70	21.5
40% bran flakes (Post)	¾ cup (1 oz.)	70	21.0
100% bran (Nabisco)	½ cup (1 oz.)	97	18.6

(USDA): United States Department of Agriculture
(HEW/FAO): Health, Education and Welfare/Food and Agriculture Organization
* Prepared as Package Directs

Food and Description	Measure or Quantity	Calories	Carbohydrates (grams)
Raisin bran flakes:			
(Kellogg's)	¾ cup (1⅜ oz.)	101	29.6
(Post)	½ cup (1 oz.)	92	21.0
Cinnamon (Post)	½ cup (1 oz.)	92	21.0
BRANDY, unflavored (See **DISTILLED LIQUOR**)			
BRANDY EXTRACT:			
Pure (Ehlers)	1 tsp.	7	
Imitation (Durkee)	1 tsp. (4 grams)	15	
Imitation (Ehlers)	1 tsp.	18	
Imitation (French's)	1 tsp.	16	
BRANDY, FLAVORED:			
Apricot:			
(Bols) 70 proof	1 fl. oz.	100	7.4
(Garnier) 70 proof	1 fl. oz.	86	7.1
(Hiram Walker) 70 proof	1 fl. oz.	88	7.5
(Leroux) 70 proof	1 fl. oz.	92	8.6
(Old Mr. Boston) 70 proof	1 fl. oz.	100	8.0
(Mr. Boston's) apricot & brandy, 42 proof	1 fl. oz.	75	8.0
Blackberry:			
(Bols) 70 proof	1 fl. oz.	100	7.4
(Garnier) 70 proof	1 fl. oz.	86	7.1
(Hiram Walker) 70 proof	1 fl. oz.	86	7.0
(Leroux) 70 proof	1 fl. oz.	91	8.3
(Leroux) Polish, 70 proof	1 fl. oz.	92	8.6
(Old Mr. Boston) 70 proof	1 fl. oz.	100	8.0
(Mr. Boston's) blackberry & brandy, 42 proof	1 fl. oz.	75	8.0
Cherry:			
(Bols) 70 proof	1 fl. oz.	100	7.4
(Garnier) 70 proof	1 fl. oz.	86	7.1
(Hiram Walker) 70 proof	1 fl. oz.	86	7.0
(Leroux) 70 proof	1 fl. oz.	91	8.3
(Old Mr. Boston) wild cherry, 70 proof	1 fl. oz.	100	8.0
(Mr. Boston's) wild cherry & brandy, 42 proof	1 fl. oz.	75	8.0
Coffee:			
(Garnier) 70 proof	1 fl. oz.	86	7.1
(Old Mr. Boston) 70 proof	1 fl. oz.	74	1.0

Food and Description	Measure or Quantity	Calories	Carbo-hydrates (grams)
(Leroux) coffee & brandy, 70 proof	1 fl. oz.	91	8.3
Ginger:			
(Garnier) 70 proof	1 fl. oz.	74	4.0
(Hiram Walker) 70 proof	1 fl. oz.	72	3.5
(Leroux) 70 proof	1 fl. oz.	76	4.4
(Leroux) sharp, 70 proof	1 fl. oz.	77	4.7
(Old Mr. Boston) 70 proof	1 fl. oz.	74	1.0
(Mr. Boston's) ginger & brandy, 42 proof	1 fl. oz.	75	8.0
Peach:			
(Garnier) 70 proof	1 fl. oz.	86	7.1
(Hiram Walker) 70 proof	1 fl. oz.	87	7.2
(Leroux) 70 proof	1 fl. oz.	93	8.9
(Old Mr. Boston) 70 proof	1 fl. oz.	100	8.0
(Mr. Boston's) peach & brandy, 42 proof	1 fl. oz.	75	8.0
BRATWURST (Oscar Mayer)	1 oz.	94	.4
BRAUNSCHWEIGER:			
(Oscar Mayer)	1 oz.	107	.2
(Wilson)	1 oz.	90	.7
Liver cheese (Oscar Mayer)	1.3-oz. slice	102	.6
BRAZIL NUT (USDA):			
Whole, in shell	1 cup (4.3 oz.)	383	6.4
Shelled	½ cup (2.5 oz.)	458	7.6
Shelled	4 nuts (.6 oz.)	114	1.9
BREAD (listed by type or brand name):			
Banana nut loaf (Van de Kamp's)	14-oz. loaf	1288	
Boston brown (USDA)	1.7-oz. slice (3"x¾")	101	21.9
Cheese, party (Pepperidge Farm)	1 slice (6 grams)	18	2.7
Cinnamon raisin:			
(Pepperidge Farm)	.9-oz. slice	74	13.6
(Thomas')	.8-oz. slice	60	12.2

(USDA): United States Department of Agriculture
(HEW/FAO): Health, Education and Welfare/Food and Agriculture Organization
* Prepared as Package Directs

Food and Description	Measure or Quantity	Calories	Carbo-hydrates (grams)
Corn & molasses			
(Pepperidge Farm)	.9-oz. slice	71	14.3
Cracked-wheat:			
(USDA) 20 slices to 1 lb.	.8-oz. slice	60	12.0
(Pepperidge Farm)	.9-oz. slice	69	13.0
Honey (Wonder)	.8-oz. slice	61	11.1
Date-nut loaf:			
(Mannafood)	.9-oz. slice	71	
(Thomas')	1.1-oz. slice	94	18.5
(Van de Kamp's)	1-lb. 2-oz. loaf	1720	
Dutch Crunch, 1-lb. loaf			
(Van de Kamp's)	.8-oz. slice	63	
Egg sesame, 1-lb. loaf			
(Van de Kamp's)	.8-oz. slice	77	
English muffin loaf, 1-lb. loaf			
(Van de Kamp's)	1-oz. slice	65	4.8
Finn Crisp	1 piece (6 grams)	22	
Flat, Norwegian (Ideal)	1 double wafer	25	5.5
French:			
(USDA) 20 slices to 1 lb.	.8-oz. slice	67	12.7
(Pepperidge Farm)	1" slice (1.1 oz.)	84	15.5
(Wonder)	1-oz. slice	75	13.9
Glutogen Gluten (Thomas')	1 slice (.5 oz.)	35	6.4
Hollywood, dark or light	1 slice	46	10.0
Honey bran, 1-lb. loaf			
(Van de Kamp's)	.7-oz. slice	77	
Honey Wheatberry			
(Pepperidge Farm)	1.1-oz. slice	78	15.4
Italian:			
(USDA) 20 slices to 1 lb.	.8-oz. slice	63	13.0
(Pepperidge Farm)	1" slice (1.2 oz.)	88	16.0
King's Bread (Wasa)	1 slice (3.5 oz.)	365	75.0
Low sodium, 1-lb. loaf			
(Van de Kamp's)	.8-oz. slice	66	
Natural Health (Arnold)	.9-oz. slice	73	10.8
Oatmeal:			
(Arnold)	.8-oz. slice	64	10.9
(Pepperidge Farm)	.9-oz. slice	68	12.4
100% Milk 'n Butter, 1 lb. loaf (Van de Kamp's)	.9-oz. slice	71	
Panettone, wine fruit loaf (Van de Kamp's)	1½ lb.	2167	
Profile, dark (Wonder)	.8-oz. slice	59	10.4
Profile, light (Wonder)	.8-oz. slice	59	10.7
Protogen Protein (Thomas')	.7-oz. slice	46	8.9

Food and Description	Measure or Quantity	Calories	Carbo-hydrates (grams)
Pumpernickel:			
(Arnold) Jewish	1.4-oz. slice	104	18.9
(Levy's)	1.1-oz. slice	70	12.4
Family (Pepperidge Farm)	1.2-oz. slice	79	15.8
Party (Pepperidge Farm)	8-gram slice	20	3.8
(Wonder)	.8-oz. slice	54	11.0
Raisin:			
Cinnamon (See Cinnamon raisin)			
Orange (Arnold)	.9-oz. slice	76	12.6
Tea (Arnold)	.9-oz. slice	76	12.2
Rite Diet (Thomas')	.7-oz. slice	50	9.3
Roman Meal, regular	.8-oz. slice	63	11.2
Rye:			
Beefsteak (Wonder)	.8-oz. slice	59	10.4
Family (Pepperidge Farm)	1.2-oz. slice	81	15.5
Jewish (Arnold)	1.2-oz. slice	94	16.7
Melba thin, Jewish (Arnold)	.6-oz. slice	43	7.8
Party (Pepperidge Farm)	6-gram slice	16	3.0
Seedless (Pepperidge Farm)	1.2-oz. slice	83	15.4
Westchester, with or without caraway seeds (Levy's)	1.1-oz. slice	55	12.1
With or without caraway seeds (Levy's)	1.1-oz. slice	70	12.1
(Wonder)	.8-oz. slice	55	10.5
Salt rising (USDA)	.9-oz. slice	67	13.0
Slender Key (Arnold)	.8-oz. slice	56	10.1
Soft sandwich, 1½-lb. loaf (Arnold)	.8-oz. slice	67	10.6
Toaster cake (See **TOASTER CAKE)**			
Vienna (USDA)	.8-oz. slice	67	12.7
Wheat:			
(Wonder) golden	.8-oz. slice	60	10.7
(Wonder) *Home Pride*	.8-oz. slice	59	10.4
Wheat germ (Pepperidge Farm)	.9-oz. slice	68	12.2

(USDA): United States Department of Agriculture
(HEW/FAO): Health, Education and Welfare/Food and Agriculture Organization
* Prepared as Package Directs

Food and Description	Measure or Quantity	Calories	Carbo- hydrates (grams)
White:			
Prepared with 1–2% non-fat dry milk (USDA)	.8-oz. slice	62	11.6
Prepared with 3–4% non-fat dry milk (USDA)	.8-oz. slice	62	11.6
Prepared with 5–6% non-fat dry milk (USDA)	.8-oz. slice	63	11.5
(Arnold) Melba thin	.5-oz. slice	43	7.1
(Arnold) small family	.8-oz. slice	68	11.0
(Arnold) toasting	1.1-oz. slice	88	14.0
(Pepperidge Farm):			
Large loaf	1-oz. slice	75	13.4
Sandwich	.8-oz. slice	66	11.8
Sliced	.9-oz. slice	74	12.7
Toasting	1.2-oz. slice	91	17.1
Very thin slice	.5-oz. slice	41	7.9
(Thomas')	.9-oz. slice	69	13.5
(Wonder) 1½-lb. loaf:			
32 slices to loaf	¾-oz. slice	55	10.2
26 slices to loaf	.9-oz. slice	68	12.5
22 slices to loaf	1.1-oz. slice	80	14.8
Brick Oven (Arnold)	.8-oz. slice	68	11.0
English Tea Loaf (Pepperidge Farm)	.9-oz. slice	72	12.0
Hearthstone (Arnold) 1 lb. loaf	.9-oz. slice	71	12.0
Whole-wheat:			
Prepared with 2% nonfat dry milk (USDA)	.9-oz. slice	61	11.9
Prepared with 2% nonfat dry milk (USDA)	.8-oz. slice	56	11.0
Prepared with water (USDA)	.9-oz. slice	60	12.3
(Arnold) Melba thin	.6-oz. slice	44	6.7
(Pepperidge Farm)	.9-oz. slice	62	11.8
(Thomas')	.9-oz. slice	64	12.0
(Wonder)	.8-oz. slice	59	11.4
Brick Oven, 1-lb. loaf (Arnold)	.8-oz. slice	65	10.0
BREAD, CANNED:			
Banana nut (Dromedary)	½″ slice (1 oz.)	75	12.4
Brown, plain (B&M)	½″ slice (1.6 oz.)	83	18.2
Brown, with raisins (B&M)	½″ slice (1.6 oz.)	83	17.6
Chocolate nut (Crosse & Blackwell)	½″ slice (1 oz.)	65	14.8

Food and Description	Measure or Quantity	Calories	Carbo-hydrates (grams)
Chocolate nut (Dromedary)	½" slice (1 oz.)	86	14.5
Date & nut (Crosse & Blackwell)	½" slice (1 oz.)	65	12.6
Date & nut (Dromedary)	½" slice (1 oz.)	74	12.8
BREAD CRUMBS:			
(Buitoni)	1 oz.	104	18.5
(Old London)	1 cup (4½ oz.)	468	97.2
Seasoned (Contadina)	1 cup (4.1 oz.)	397	77.6
(Wonder)	1 oz.	108	20.5
BREAD DOUGH, frozen			
(Morton)	1 oz.	82	15.2
***BREAD MIX** (Pillsbury):			
Banana	¹⁄₁₂ of loaf	150	26.0
Cranberry	¹⁄₁₂ of loaf	170	31.0
Date	¹⁄₁₂ of loaf	170	33.0
BREAD PUDDING with raisins, home recipe (USDA)	1 cup (9.3 oz.)	496	75.3
BREAD STICK:			
Cheese (Keebler)	1 piece (3 grams)	10	1.8
Dietetic (Stella D'oro)	1 piece (9 grams)	39	6.3
Garlic (Keebler)	1 piece (3 grams)	11	1.9
Onion (Keebler)	1 piece (3 grams)	10	1.9
Onion (Stella D'oro)	1 piece (.4 oz.)	42	6.8
Regular (Stella D'oro)	1 piece (10 grams)	40	6.6
Salt:			
(USDA)	1 oz.	109	21.3
Vienna type (USDA)	1 oz.	86	16.4
(Keebler)	1 piece (3 grams)	10	1.9
Sesame (Stella D'oro)	1 piece (9 grams)	42	5.7
BREAD STUFFING MIX:			
Dry (USDA)	1 cup (2½ oz.)	263	51.4
*Crumb, type, prepared with water & fat (USDA)	4 oz.	406	40.4
*Crumb type, prepared with water & fat (USDA)	1 cup (5 oz.)	505	50.2

(USDA): United States Department of Agriculture
(HEW/FAO): Health, Education and Welfare/Food and Agriculture
            Organization

* Prepared as Package Directs

Food and Description	Measure or Quantity	Calories	Carbo hydrate (grams)
*Moist type, prepared with water, egg & fat (USDA)	4 oz.	236	22.
*Moist type, prepared with water, egg & fat (USDA)	1 cup (7.2 oz.)	422	40.0
Corn bread (Pepperidge Farm)	8-oz. pkg.	836	167.1
Cube (Pepperidge Farm)	7-oz. pkg.	756	147.0
Herb seasoned (Pepperidge Farm)	8-oz. pkg.	836	178.8
Seasoned (Uncle Ben's) Stuff 'N Stuff:			
Dry	6-oz. pkg.	615	126.3
*Without butter	½ cup (2.9 oz.)	118	24.2
BREADFRUIT, fresh (USDA):			
Whole	1 lb. (weighed untrimmed)	360	91.5
Peeled & trimmed	4 oz. (weighed trimmed)	117	29.7
BRIGHT & EARLY	6 fl. oz. (6.6 oz.)	100	21.6
BROCCOLI:			
Raw, whole (USDA)	1 lb. (weighed untrimmed)	89	16.3
Raw, large leaves removed (USDA)	1 lb. (weighed partially trimmed)	113	20.9
Boiled, ½" pieces, drained (USDA)	½ cup (2.8 oz.)	20	3.9
Boiled, drained (USDA)	1 med. stalk (6.3 oz.)	47	8.1
Frozen:			
Chopped or cut:			
(Birds Eye)	⅓ of 10-oz. pkg.	27	3.6
In cream sauce (Green Giant)	⅓ of 10-oz. pkg.	57	6.4
Spears:			
(Birds Eye)	⅓ of 10-oz. pkg.	26	3.6
Baby spears (Birds Eye)	⅓ of 10-oz. pkg.	26	3.6
& noodle casserole (Green Giant)	⅓ of 10-oz. pkg.	95	9.6
In butter sauce (Green Giant)	⅓ of 10-oz. pkg.	48	5.1

Food and Description	Measure or Quantity	Calories	Carbo- hydrates (grams)
In cheese sauce (Green Giant)	⅓ of 10-oz. pkg.	60	6.4
In Hollandaise sauce (Birds Eye)	⅓ of 10-oz. pkg.	100	3.2
BROTH & SEASONING (See also individual kinds):			
Maggi	1 T. (.6 oz.)	22	.1
Golden (George Washington)	1 packet (4 grams)	5	1.0
Rich Brown (George Washington)	1 packet (4 grams)	5	1.2
BROWNIE (See **COOKIE**)			
BRUSSELS SPROUTS:			
Raw (USDA)	1 lb.	188	34.6
Boiled, 1¼"-1½" dia., drained (USDA)	1 cup (7-8 sprouts, 5.5 oz.)	56	9.9
Frozen:			
Boiled, drained (USDA)	4 oz.	37	7.4
Baby sprouts (Birds Eye)	½ cup (3.3 oz.)	34	5.7
Au gratin, casserole (Green Giant)	⅓ of 10-oz. pkg.	71	8.3
In butter sauce (Green Giant)	⅓ of 10-oz. pkg.	58	5.9
BUBBLE UP, soft drink	6 fl. oz.	73	18.4
BUCKWHEAT:			
Flour (See **FLOUR**)			
Groats:			
(Birkett) *Wolff's Kasha*	1 oz.	108	23.3
(Pocono) whole, brown	1 oz.	104	19.4
(Pocono) whole, white	1 oz.	102	20.1
BUC WHEATS, cereal (General Mills)	1 cup	102	23.4
BUFFALOFISH, raw (USDA):			
Whole	1 lb. (weighed whole)	164	0.
Meat only	4 oz.	128	0.

(USDA): United States Department of Agriculture
(HEW/FAO): Health, Education and Welfare/Food and Agriculture Organization
* Prepared as Package Directs

Food and Description	Measure or Quantity	Calories	Carbo- hydrate (grams
BULGAR (from hard red winter wheat) (USDA):			
Dry	1 lb.	1605	343.
Canned:			
Unseasoned (USDA)	4 oz.	191	39.
Seasoned (USDA)	4 oz.	206	37.
BULLHEAD, raw (USDA):			
Whole	1 lb. (weighed whole)	72	0.
Meat only	4 oz.	95	0.
BULLOCK'S-HEART (See **CUSTARD APPLE**)			
BUN (See **ROLL**)			
BURBOT, raw (USDA):			
Whole	1 lb. (weighed whole)	56	0.
Meat only	4 oz.	93	0.
BURGUNDY WINE (See also individual regional, vineyard, grape or brand names):			
(Gallo) 13% alcohol	3 fl. oz.	52	.
(Gallo) hearty, 14% alcohol	3 fl. oz.	48	1.
(Gold Seal) 12% alcohol	3 fl. oz.	82	.
(Great Western) 12.5% alcohol	3 fl. oz.	69	
(Inglenook) Navalle, 12% alcohol	3 fl. oz. (2.9 oz.)	64	1.
(Inglenook) Vintage, 12% alcohol	3 fl. oz. (2.9 oz.)	59	.
(Italian Swiss Colony) 13% alcohol	3 fl. oz. (2.9 oz.)	61	.
(Italian Swiss Colony-Gold Medal) 12.3% alcohol	3 fl. oz.	63	.
(Louis M. Martini) 12½% alcohol	3 fl. oz.	90	.
(Mogen David) American, 12% alcohol	3 fl. oz.	24	1.8
(Petri) 13% alcohol	3 fl. oz. (2.9 oz.)	63	1.3
(Taylor) 12.5% alcohol	3 fl. oz.	72	Tr.

Food and Description	Measure or Quantity	Calories	Carbo-hydrates (grams)
BURGUNDY WINE, SPARKLING:			
(Barton & Guestier) French red, 12% alcohol	3 fl. oz.	69	2.2
(Chanson) French red	3 fl. oz.	72	3.6
(Gold Seal) 12% alcohol	3 fl. oz.	87	2.6
(Great Western) 12% alcohol	3 fl. oz.	88	5.0
(Lejon) 12% alcohol	3 fl. oz.	67	2.3
(Taylor) 12.5% alcohol	3 fl. oz.	78	1.8
BURRITOS, frozen (Rosarita):			
Bean	8-oz. pkg.	486	
Bean & bacon (Patio)	½-oz. roll	47	4.4
Beef (Patio)	½-oz. roll	48	4.0
Chicken (Patio)	½-oz. roll	50	4.5
BUTTER, salted or unsalted:			
(USDA)	¼ lb. (1 stick, ½ cup)	812	.5
(USDA)	1 T. (⅛ stick, .5 oz.)	100	.1
(Breakstone)	1 T. (.5 oz.)	100	.1
(Sealtest)	1 T. (.5 oz.)	110	.1
Whipped (Breakstone)	1 T. (9 grams)	67	.1
Whipped (Sealtest)	1 T. (9 grams)	68	.1
BUTTER BEAN (See BEAN LIMA)			
***BUTTER BRICKLE CAKE MIX** (Betty Crocker)	1/12 of cake	203	35.9
BUTTER CAKE (Van de Kamp's)	1-lb. loaf	1284	
BUTTERFISH, raw (USDA): Gulf:			
Whole	1 lb. (weighed whole)	220	0.
Meat only	4 oz.	180	0.

(USDA): United States Department of Agriculture
(HEW/FAO): Health, Education and Welfare/Food and Agriculture Organization
* Prepared as Package Directs

Food and Description	Measure or Quantity	Calories	Carbo-hydrates (grams)
Northern:			
Whole	1 lb. (weighed whole)	391	0.
Meat only	4 oz.	192	0.
BUTTER FLAVORING:			
(Durkee)	1 tsp. (4 grams)	3	
Imitation (Ehlers)	1 tsp.	7	
(French's)	1 tsp.	8	
BUTTERMILK (See MILK)			
BUTTERNUT (USDA):			
Whole	1 lb. (weighed in shell)	399	5.3
Shelled	4 oz.	713	9.5
BUTTER OIL or dehydrated butter (USDA)	1 cup (7.2 oz.)	1787	0.
BUTTERSCOTCH MORSELS (Nestlé's)	6-oz. pkg.	900	102.1
BUTTERSCOTCH PIE:			
Home recipe (USDA)	⅛ of 9″ pie (5.4 oz.)	406	58.2
Frozen, cream (Banquet)	2½-oz. serving	187	27.0
BUTTERSCOTCH PIE FILLING MIX:			
*With whole milk, low calorie (D-Zerta)	½ cup (4.5 oz.)	99	9.8
*With nonfat milk, low calorie (D-Zerta)	½ cup (4.5 oz.)	60	10.0
BUTTERSCOTCH PUDDING:			
Canned (Del Monte)	5-oz. can	191	32.6
Canned (Betty Crocker)	½ cup	171	29.2
Canned (Hunt's)	5-oz. can	238	30.3
Chilled (Sealtest)	4 oz.	124	20.6
BUTTERSCOTCH PUDDING MIX:			
Sweetened:			
*Instant (Jell-O)	½ cup (5.3 oz.)	178	30.5
*Instant (My-T-Fine)	½ cup (5 oz.)	175	32.5
*Instant (Royal)	½ cup (5.1 oz.)	176	28.8
*Regular (Jell-O)	½ cup (5.2 oz.)	173	29.3

Food and Description	Measure or Quantity	Calories	Carbo- hydrates (grams)
*Regular (My-T-Fine)	½ cup (5.1 oz.)	190	32.8
Low calorie (D-Zerta)	½ cup (4.6 oz.)	107	12.2
B-V (Wilson)	1 tsp. (¼ oz.)	11	.6

C

CABBAGE:
White (USDA):
Raw:

Whole	1 lb. (weighed untrimmed)	86	19.3
Finely shredded or chopped	1 cup (3.2 oz.)	22	4.9
Coarsely shredded or sliced	1 cup (2.5 oz.)	17	3.8
Wedge	3½"x4½"	24	5.4

Boiled:

Shredded, in small amount of water, short time, drained	½ cup (2.6 oz.)	15	3.1
Wedges, in large amount of water, long time, drained	½ cup (3.2 oz.)	16	3.7
Dehydrated	1 oz.	87	20.9
Red, raw, whole (USDA)	1 lb. (weighed untrimmed)	111	24.7
Red, canned, sweet & sour (Greenwood's)	½ cup (4.8 oz.)	77	16.7
Savory, raw, whole (USDA)	1 lb. (weighed untrimmed)	86	16.5

CABBAGE, CHINESE or CELERY, raw (USDA):

Whole	1 lb. (weighed untrimmed)	62	13.2
1" pieces, leaves with stalk	½ cup (1.3 oz.)	5	1.1

(USDA): United States Department of Agriculture
(HEW/FAO): Health, Education and Welfare/Food and Agriculture
          Organization
* Prepared as Package Directs

Food and Description	Measure or Quantity	Calories	Carbo-hydrates (grams)
CABBAGE ROLLS, stuffed with beef, in tomato sauce, frozen (Holloway House)	1 roll (7 oz.)	184	
CABBAGE, SPOON or **WHITE MUSTARD** (USDA):			
Raw, untrimmed	1 lb.	69	12.5
Boiled, drained	½ cup (3 oz.)	12	2.0
CABERNET SAUVIGNON WINE:			
(Inglenook) Estate, 12% alcohol	3 fl. oz. (2.9 oz.)	58	.3
(Louis M. Martini) 12½% alcohol	3 fl. oz.	90	.2
CACTUS COOLER, soft drink (Canada Dry)	6 fl. oz. (6.4 oz.)	86	21.6
CAKE. Most cakes are listed elsewhere by kind of cake such as **ANGEL FOOD** or **CHOCOLATE** or brand name, such as *YANKEE DOODLES.* (USDA):			
Plain, home recipe:			
Without icing	⅑ of 9″ sq. (3 oz., 3″x3″x1″)	313	48.1
With chocolate icing	3.5-oz. piece (¹⁄₁₆ of 10″ layer cake)	368	59.4
With boiled white icing	⅑ of 9″ sq. (3 oz., 3″x3″x1″)	401	70.6
With uncooked white icing	3.5-oz. piece (¹⁄₁₆ of 10″ layer cake)	367	63.3
White, home recipe:			
Without icing	⅑ of 9″ sq. (3 oz., 3″x3″x1″)	322	46.4
With coconut icing	¹⁄₁₆ of 10″ layer cake (3.5 oz.)	371	60.7
With uncooked white icing	¹⁄₁₆ of 10″ layer cake (3.5 oz.)	375	62.9
Yellow, home recipe:			
Without icing	⅑ of 9″ sq. (3 oz., 3″x3″x1″)	312	50.1
With caramel icing	3.5-oz. piece	362	61.3
With chocolate icing, 2-layer	¹⁄₁₆ of 9″ cake (2.6 oz.)	274	45.3

Food and Description	Measure or Quantity	Calories	Carbo-hydrates (grams)
CAKE DECORATOR, canned, any color (Pillsbury)	1 T.	70	12.0
CAKE FROSTING (See **CAKE ICING & CAKE ICING MIX**)			
CAKE ICING:			
Butterscotch (Betty Crocker)	¹⁄₁₂ of 16.5-oz. can	164	27.8
Caramel, home recipe (USDA)	4 oz.	408	86.8
Cherry (Betty Crocker)	¹⁄₁₂ of 16.5-oz. can	167	28.0
Chocolate, home recipe (USDA)	½ cup (4.9 oz.)	519	93.0
Chocolate (Betty Crocker)	¹⁄₁₂ of 16.5 oz. can	162	25.0
Chocolate fudge (Pillsbury)	¹⁄₁₂ of pkg.	150	29.0
Coconut, home recipe (USDA)	½ cup (2.9 oz.)	302	62.2
Dark Dutch fudge (Betty Crocker)	¹⁄₁₂ of 16.5-oz. can	153	24.7
Double Dutch (Pillsbury)	¹⁄₁₂ of pkg.	150	29.0
Lemon (Betty Crocker)	¹⁄₁₂ of 16.5-oz. can	166	28.0
Milk chocolate (Betty Crocker)	¹⁄₁₂ of 16.5-oz. can	164	27.2
Vanilla (Betty Crocker)	¹⁄₁₂ of 16.5-oz. can	166	28.0
Vanilla (Pillsbury)	¹⁄₁₂ of pkg.	150	29.0
White, home recipe (USDA):			
Boiled	½ cup (1.6 oz.)	149	37.7
Uncooked	4 oz.	426	92.5
CAKE ICING MIX:			
*Banana, creamy (Betty Crocker)	¹⁄₁₂ of cake's icing	139	29.5

(USDA): United States Department of Agriculture
(HEW/FAO): Health, Education and Welfare/Food and Agriculture Organization
* Prepared as Package Directs

Food and Description	Measure or Quantity	Calories	Carbohydrates (grams)
*Butter Brickle, creamy (Betty Crocker)	¹⁄₁₂ of cake's icing	140	29.7
*Caramel (Pillsbury)	¹⁄₁₂ of cake's icing	160	28.0
*Caramel, creamy (Betty Crocker)	¹⁄₁₂ of cake's icing	139	29.6
*Cherry, creamy (Betty Crocker)	¹⁄₁₂ of cake's icing	139	29.3
*Cherry fluff (Betty Crocker)	¹⁄₁₂ of cake's icing	59	16.6
Cherry fudge, creamy (Betty Crocker)	¹⁄₁₂ of cake's icing	132	28.5
*Chocolate, fluffy (Betty Crocker)	¹⁄₁₂ of cake's icing	70	12.8
*Chocolate fudge, creamy (Betty Crocker)	¹⁄₁₂ of cake's icing	134	28.6
*Chocolate fudge (Pillsbury)	¹⁄₁₂ of cake's icing	160	28.0
*Chocolate, light (Pillsbury)	¹⁄₁₂ of cake's icing	150	29.0
*Chocolate malt, creamy (Betty Crocker)	¹⁄₁₂ of cake's icing	136	28.7
*Chocolate, walnut, creamy (Betty Crocker)	¹⁄₁₂ of cake's icing	131	26.6
*Coconut almond (Pillsbury)	¹⁄₁₂ of cake's icing	170	17.0
*Coconut pecan, creamy (Betty Crocker)	¹⁄₁₂ of cake's icing	102	16.6
*Coconut, toasted, creamy (Betty Crocker)	¹⁄₁₂ of cake's icing	141	28.7
*Dark chocolate fudge, creamy (Betty Crocker)	¹⁄₁₂ of cake's icing	130	27.4
*Fudge (Dromedary)	1" x 1" x ½" piece (5 oz.)	55	9.9
*Fudge nugget, creamy (Betty Crocker)	¹⁄₁₂ of cake's icing	133	28.6
*Lemon (Pillsbury)	¹⁄₁₂ of cake's icing	160	28.0
*Lemon, creamy (Betty Crocker)	¹⁄₁₂ of cake's icing	134	28.5
*Lemon, fluff (Betty Crocker)	¹⁄₁₂ of cake's icing	134	28.3
*Orange, creamy (Betty Crocker)	¹⁄₁₂ of cake's icing	58	14.9
*Pineapple, creamy (Betty Crocker)	¹⁄₁₂ of cake's icing	134	28.4
*Sour cream, chocolate fudge, creamy (Betty Crocker)	¹⁄₁₂ of cake's icing	129	27.5
*Sour cream, white (Betty Crocker)	¹⁄₁₂ of cake's icng	130	29.0

Food and Description	Measure or Quantity	Calories	Carbo-hydrates (grams)
*Spice, creamy (Betty Crocker)	1/12 of cake's icing	139	29.2
*Strawberry (Pillsbury)	1/12 of cake's icing	150	27.0
*Vanilla (Pillsbury)	1/12 of cake's icing	160	29.0
*White, creamy (Betty Crocker)	1/12 of cake's icing	140	29.8
*White, fluffy (Betty Crocker)	1/12 of cake's icing	58	14.9
*White, fluffy (Pillsbury)	1/12 of cake's icing	70	17.0

CAKE MIX. Most cake mixes are listed by kind of cake, such as ANGEL FOOD CAKE MIX, CHOCOLATE CAKE MIX, etc.

Food and Description	Measure or Quantity	Calories	Carbo-hydrates (grams)
White:			
Layer (USDA)	1 oz.	123	22.2
*With chocolate icing, 2-layer (USDA)	1/16 of 9" cake (2.5 oz.)	249	44.6
*Layer (Betty Crocker)	1/12 of cake	190	35.5
*Sour cream, layer (Betty Crocker)	1/12 of cake	191	34.1
*(Duncan Hines)	1/12 of cake (2.6 oz.)	190	36.6
*(Pillsbury)	1/12 of cake	200	34.0
*Whipping cream (Pillsbury)	1/12 of cake	230	35.0
*(Swans Down)	1/12 of cake (2.5 oz.)	177	36.2
Yellow:			
(USDA)	1 oz.	124	22.0
*With chocolate icing (USDA)	1/16 of 9" cake (2.6 oz.)	253	43.2
*(Betty Crocker) layer	1/12 of cake	202	35.5
*Butter (Betty Crocker)	1/12 of cake	278	37.0
*Butter (Pillsbury)	1/12 of cake	210	34.0
*(Duncan Hines)	1/12 of cake	202	35.0
*Golden (Duncan Hines)	1/12 of cake (3.3 oz.)	283	37.0

(USDA): United States Department of Agriculture
(HEW/FAO): Health, Education and Welfare/Food and Agriculture Organization
* Prepared as Package Directs

Food and Description	Measure or Quantity	Calories	Carbo- hydrates (grams)
*Golden butter (Duncan Hines)	1 cake	3396	444.0
*Butter flavor (Pillsbury)	1/12 of cake	210	34.0
*(Swans Down)	1/12 of cake (2.5 oz.)	186	36.1
CAMPARI, 45 proof	1 fl. oz. (1.1 oz.)	66	7.1
CANADIAN WHISKY (See **DISTILLED LIQUOR**)			
CANDIED FRUIT (See individual kinds)			
CANDY. The following values of candies from the U.S. Department of Agriculture are representative of the types sold commercially. These values may be useful when individual brands or sizes are not known:			
Almond:			
Chocolate-coated	1 cup (6.3 oz.)	1024	71.3
Chocolate-coated	1 oz.	161	11.2
Sugar-coated or Jordan	1 oz.	129	19.9
Butterscotch	1 oz.	113	26.9
Candy corn	1 oz.	103	25.4
Caramel:			
Plain	1 oz.	113	21.7
Plain with nuts	1 oz.	121	20.0
Chocolate	1 oz.	113	21.7
Chocolate with nuts	1 oz.	121	20.0
Chocolate-flavored roll	1 oz.	112	23.4
Chocolate:			
Bittersweet	1 oz.	135	13.3
Milk:			
Plain	1 oz.	147	16.1
With almonds	1 oz.	151	14.5
With peanuts	1 oz.	154	12.6
Semisweet	1 oz.	144	16.2
Sweet	1 oz.	150	16.4
Chocolate discs, sugar-coated	1 oz.	132	20.6
Coconut center, chocolate-coated	1 oz.	124	20.4
Fondant, plain	1 oz.	103	25.4

Food and Description	Measure or Quantity	Calories	Carbo-hydrates (grams)
Fondant, chocolate-covered	1 oz.	116	23.0
Fudge:			
Chocolate fudge	1 oz.	113	21.3
Chocolate fudge, chocolate-coated	1 oz.	122	20.7
Chocolate fudge with nuts	1 oz.	121	19.6
Chocolate fudge with nuts, chocolate-coated	1 oz.	128	19.1
Vanilla fudge	1 oz.	113	21.2
Vanilla fudge with nuts	1 oz.	120	19.5
With peanuts & caramel, chocolate-coated	1 oz.	130	16.6
Gum drops	1 oz.	98	24.8
Hard	1 oz.	109	27.6
Honeycombed hard candy, with peanut butter, chocolate-covered	1 oz.	131	20.0
Jelly beans	1 oz.	104	26.4
Marshmallows	1 oz.	90	22.8
Mints, uncoated	1 oz.	103	25.4
Nougat & caramel, chocolate-covered	1 oz.	118	20.6
Peanut bar	1 oz.	146	13.4
Peanut brittle	1 oz.	119	23.0
Peanuts, chocolate-covered	1 oz.	159	11.1
Raisins, chocolate-covered	1 oz.	120	20.0
Vanilla creams, chocolate-covered	1 oz.	123	19.9
CANDY, COMMERCIAL (See also **CANDY, DIETETIC**):			
Air Bon (Whitman's)	1 piece	10	
Almonds, chocolate-covered:			
Candy-coated (Hershey's)	1 oz.	142	17.2
(Kraft)	1 piece (3 grams)	14	1.0
Almond, sugar-coated (Blue Diamond)	1 oz.	130	
Almond Cluster:			
(Kraft)	1 piece (.4 oz.)	63	5.0
(Peter Paul)	1¾₁₆-oz. pkg.	171	19.8

(USDA): United States Department of Agriculture
(HEW/FAO): Health, Education and Welfare/Food and Agriculture
    Organization
* Prepared as Package Directs

Food and Description	Measure or Quantity	Calories	Carbo-hydrates (grams)
Almond Joy (Peter Paul)	1 bar (1½ oz.)	198	24.1
Almond Toffee Bar (Kraft)	1-oz. bar	142	17.9
Babies, chocolate flavor (Heide)	1 oz.	101	
Baby Ruth (Curtiss)	1 oz.	135	21.0
Baffle Bar (Cardinet's)	1 bar (1¾ oz.)	189	10.9
Berries (Mason) .	1 oz.	100	
Black-Crows (Mason)	1 oz.	100	
Brazil nuts, chocolate-covered (Kraft)	1 piece (6 grams)	32	1.7
Bridge Mix:			
Almond (Kraft)	1 piece (4 grams)	22	1.6
Caramelette (Kraft)	1 piece (3 grams)	12	1.9
Jelly (Kraft)	1 piece (3 grams)	12	1.9
Malted milk ball (Kraft)	1 piece (2 grams)	11	1.4
Mintette (Kraft)	1 piece (3 grams)	12	1.8
Peanut (Kraft)	1 piece (1 gram)	8	.5
Peanut crunch (Kraft)	1 piece (5 grams)	23	3.4
Raisin (Kraft)	1 piece (1 gram)	5	.8
(Nabisco)	1 piece (2 grams)	8	1.4
Butterfinger (Curtiss)	1 oz.	134	21.0
Butternut (Hollywood)	1 bar (1¼ oz.)	168	20.6
Butterscotch Skimmers (Nabisco)	1 piece (6 grams)	25	5.7
Candy Corn:			
(Brach's)	1 piece (2 grams)	7	1.8
(Heide)	1 oz.	101	
Caramel:			
(Curtiss)	1 oz.	119	24.1
Caramelette (Kraft)	1 piece (3 grams)	12	1.9
Chocolate (Kraft)	1 piece (8 grams)	33	6.2
Chocolate, bar (Kraft)	1 piece (6 grams)	26	4.9
Chocolate-covered (Brach's)	1 piece (10 grams)	41	7.4
Coconut (Kraft)	1 piece (8 grams)	32	5.5
Milk Duds (Holloway)	1 oz.	111	
Milk Maid (Brach's)	1 piece (9 grams)	34	6.3
Vanilla, bar (Kraft)	1 piece (6 grams)	26	4.9
Vanilla, plain (Kraft)	1 piece (8 grams)	33	6.2
Vanilla, chocolate-covered (Kraft)	1 piece (9 grams)	39	6.2
Vanilla, *Twisteroo* (Kraft)	1 piece (6 grams)	25	4.7
Caravelle (Peter Paul)	1½-oz. bar	190	28.5
Carmallow (Queen Anne)	1 piece	83	
Cashew cluster (Kraft)	1 piece (.4 oz.)	58	4.9

Food and Description	Measure or Quantity	Calories	Carbohydrates (grams)
Charleston Chew:			
Bar	¾-oz. bar	90	16.2
Bite-size	1 piece (7 grams)	30	5.4
Cherry, chocolate-covered:			
(Brach's)	1 piece (.6 oz.)	66	13.2
Dark (Nabisco)	1 piece (.6 oz.)	67	13.0
Milk (Nabisco)	1 piece (.6 oz.)	66	13.1
Cherry-A-Let (Hoffman)	1 piece	215	
Chewees (Curtiss)	1 oz.	116	24.1
Chocolate bar:			
Milk chocolate:			
(Ghirardelli)	1.1-oz. bar	169	18.9
(Hershey's)	1¼-oz. bar	218	22.6
(Hershey's)	¼-oz. miniature	39	4.0
(Nestlés)	1 oz.	148	13.1
Mint chocolate			
(Ghirardelli)	1.1-oz. bar	171	18.7
Semisweet (Ghirardelli)	1 sq. (1 oz.)	151	16.7
Semisweet (Nestlé's)	1 oz.	141	17.3
Special dark (Hershey's)	1.4-oz. bar	38	4.4
Chocolate bar with almonds:			
(Ghirardelli)	1.1-oz. bar	173	17.6
(Hershey's)	1.3-oz. bar	205	18.8
(Hershey's)	.5-oz.	79	7.3
(Nestlé's)	1 oz.	149	15.3
Chocolate blocks, milk:			
(Ghirardelli)	1 sq. (1 oz.)	147	16.2
(Hershey's)	1 oz.	145	17.8
Chocolate Crisp Bar:			
(Ghirardelli)	1-oz. bar	161	17.6
(Kraft)	1 oz.	132	18.6
Chocolate Crunch Bar			
(Nestlé's)	1 oz.	140	17.8
Chocolate Parfait			
(Pearson's)	1 piece	34	
Choc-Shop (Hoffman)	1 piece	241	
Chuckles	1 oz.	92	23.0
Chunky	1 oz.	131	
Circlets (Curtiss)	1 oz.	108	26.1
Circus Peanuts (Brach's)	1 piece (7 grams)	27	6.4

(USDA): United States Department of Agriculture
(HEW/FAO): Health, Education and Welfare/Food and Agriculture
Organization
* Prepared as Package Directs

Food and Description	Measure or Quantity	Calories	Carbo-hydrates (grams)
Cluster:			
Crispy (Nabisco)	1 piece (.6 oz.)	65	14.0
Peanut, chocolate-covered:			
(Brach's)	1 piece (.5 oz.)	79	7.0
(Hoffman)	1 cluster	204	
(Kraft)	1 piece (.4 oz.)	59	4.1
Royal Clusters (Nabisco)	1 piece (.6 oz.)	78	7.5
Coco-Mello (Nabisco)	1 piece (.7 oz.)	91	13.8
Coconut:			
Bar (Curtiss)	1 oz.	126	21.0
Bar (Nabisco) *Welch's*	1 piece (1.1 oz.)	132	21.8
Bon Bons (Brach's)	1 piece (.6 oz.)	70	12.6
Cream egg (Hershey's)	1 oz.	142	20.4
Neapolitan (Brach's)	1 piece (.4 oz.)	48	8.0
Squares (Nabisco)	1 piece (.5 oz.)	64	12.3
Coffee-ets (Saylor's)	1 piece	13	
Coffee Nips (Pearson's)	1 piece	26	
Cup-O-Gold (Hoffman)	1 piece	210	
Dots (Mason)	1 oz.	100	
Eggs (Nabisco) *Chuckles*	1 piece (2 grams)	10	2.3
Fiddle Faddle	1½-oz. packet	177	34.7
5th Avenue Bar (Luden's):			
5¢ size	1 bar	71	
10¢ size	1 bar	129	
15¢ size	1 bar	179	
Frappe (Welch's)	1 piece (1.1 oz.)	132	23.5
Fruit 'n Nut chocolate bar (Nestlé's)	1 oz.	140	16.5
Fudge:			
Bar (Nabisco) *Welch's*	1 piece (1.1 oz.)	144	20.5
Fudgies, bar (Kraft)	1 piece (7 grams)	27	5.0
Nut, bar (Nabisco)	1 piece (.5 oz.)	71	10.2
Good & Fruity	1 oz.	106	26.3
Good & Plenty	1 oz.	100	24.8
Hard candy:			
(Bonomo)	1 oz.	112	
(H-B)	1 piece	12	2.9
(Peerless Maid)	1 piece	22	5.6
Butterscotch:			
(Reed's)	1 piece	17	
Disks (Brach's)	1 piece (6 grams)	23	5.7
Cinnamon (Reed's)	1 piece	17	
Lemon drops (Brach's)	1 piece (4 grams)	15	3.8
Peppermint (Reed's)	1 piece	17	
Pops, assorted (Brach's)	1 piece (5 grams)	19	4.8

Food and Description	Measure or Quantity	Calories	Carbo-hydrates (grams)
Root beer (Reed's)	1 piece	17	
Sherbit (F&F)	1 piece	9	2.2
Sour balls (Brach's)	1 piece (6 grams)	22	5.7
Spearmint (Reed's)	1 piece	17	
Stix Bars (Jolly Rancher)	1 oz.	102	25.5
Stix Kisses (Jolly Rancher)	1 piece	27	7.0
Stix Pak (Jolly Rancher)	1 piece	18	4.0
Wintergreen (Reed's)	1 piece	17	
Hershey-Ets, candy-coated	1.1-oz. pkg.	154	23.1
Hollywood	1½-oz. bar	185	28.9
Jelly (See also individual flavors and brand names in this section):			
Beans:			
(Brach's)	1 piece (3 grams)	11	2.8
(Heide)	1 oz.	90	
Big Ben Jellies (Brach's)	1 piece (8 grams)	26	6.8
Iced Jelly Cones (Brach's)	1 piece (4 grams)	15	3.4
Nougats (Brach's)	1 piece (.4 oz.)	43	10.0
Rings (Nabisco) *Chuckles*	1 piece (.4 oz.)	37	9.0
Jube Jels (Brach's)	1 piece (3 grams)	11	2.7
Jujubes, assorted (Nabisco)	1 piece	13	3.3
Jujyfruits (Heide)	1 oz.	94	
Kisses, milk chocolate (Hershey's)	1 piece (5 grams)	26	2.7
Krackel Bar (Hershey's)	1.4-oz. bar	212	23.3
Licorice:			
(Nabisco) *Chuckles*	1 piece (.4 oz.)	36	9.0
Diamond Drops (Heide)	1 oz.	94	
Pastilles (Heide)	1 oz.	96	
(Switzer) red or black	1 oz.	100	24.0
Twist (American Licorice Co.):			
Black	1 piece	27	6.4
Red	1 piece	33	7.3
Life Savers (Beech-Nut):			
Drop	1 piece (3 grams)	10	2.4
Mint	1 piece (2 grams)	7	1.7
Lozenges, mint or winter-green (Brach's)	1 piece (3 grams)	11	2.9

(USDA): United States Department of Agriculture
(HEW/FAO): Health, Education and Welfare/Food and Agriculture Organization
* Prepared as Package Directs

Food and Description	Measure or Quantity	Calories	Carbo-hydrates (grams)
Mallo Cup (Boyer):			
5¢ size	¾-oz. cup	104	14.8
10¢ size	1¼-oz. cup	173	24.6
15¢ size	1⅝-oz. cup	225	32.5
Malted Milk Balls, milk chocolate-covered (Brach's)	1 piece (2 grams)	9	1.6
Malted Milk Crunch (Welch's)	1 piece (2 grams)	9	.9
Maple Nut Goodies (Brach's)	1 piece (6 grams)	29	4.0
Mars Almond Bar (M&M/Mars)	1 oz.	130	16.9
Marshmallow:			
(Campfire)	1 oz.	111	24.9
Chocolate (Kraft)	1 piece (7 grams)	24	5.4
Coconut (Kraft)	1 piece (.4 oz.)	40	7.5
Eggs (Nabisco) *Chuckles*	1 piece (10 grams)	38	9.3
Flavored, regular (Kraft)	1 piece (7 grams)	23	5.8
Flavored, miniature (Kraft)	1 piece (<1 gram)	2	.5
Royal Marshmallow (Curtiss)	1 oz.	90	22.0
White, miniature (Kraft)	1 piece (<1 gram)	2	.5
White, regular (Kraft)	1 piece (7 grams)	23	5.8
Mary Jane (Miller):			
1¢ size	1 piece (.3 oz.)	31	5.6
5¢ size	1 piece (1.2 oz.)	125	21.8
Milk Shake (Hollywood)	1¼ oz.	150	26.8
Milky Way, milk or dark chocolate (M&M/Mars)	1 oz.	120	17.7
Mint or peppermint:			
Afterdinner (Richardson):			
Butter	1 oz.	109	27.0
Colored, pastel	1 oz.	109	28.0
Jelly center	1 oz.	104	26.0
Midget	1 oz.	109	27.0
Striped	1 oz.	109	28.0
Buttermint (Kraft)	1 piece (2 grams)	8	2.0
Chocolate-covered bar (Brach's)	1 piece (.6 oz.)	74	13.8
Chocolate-covered (Richardson)	1 oz.	106	27.0
Dessert (Brach's)	1 piece (<1 gram)	4	.9
Encore (Kraft)	1 piece (2 grams)	6	1.7
Jamaica Mints (Nabisco)	1 piece (6 grams)	24	5.8
Liberty Mints (Nabisco)	1 piece (6 grams)	24	5.8

Food and Description	Measure or Quantity	Calories	Carbo-hydrates (grams)
Merri-mints (Delson)	1 piece	30	
Mini-mint (Kraft)	1 piece (3 grams)	12	1.9
Mint Parfait (Pearson's)	1 piece	34	
Party (Kraft)	1 piece (2 grams)	8	2.0
Pattie, chocolate-covered:			
(Brach's)	1 piece (.4 oz.)	50	9.2
(Hoffman)	1 piece	120	
Junior Mint Pattie			
(Nabisco)	1 piece (2 grams)	10	2.0
Mason Mints	1 oz.	200	
Peppermint pattie			
(Nabisco)	1 piece (.5 oz.)	64	12.5
Sherbit, pressed mints			
(F & F)	1 piece	7	1.8
Starlight Mints (Brach's)	1 piece (5 grams)	19	4.8
Swedish (Brach's)	1 piece (2 grams)	8	1.9
Thin (Delson)	1 piece	45	
Thin (Nabisco)	1 piece (.4 oz.)	42	8.1
Wafers (Nabisco)	1 piece (2 grams)	10	1.0
Mounds (Peter Paul)	1 9/10-oz. pkg.	236	31.1
M&M's (M&M/Mars):			
Chocolate	1 oz.	140	18.1
Peanut	1 oz.	140	16.8
Mr. Goodbar (Hershey's)	1 8/10-oz. bar	283	20.2
Necco:			
Canada Mints	1 piece	13	
Necco Mints	1 piece	7	
Wintergreen	1 piece	13	
North Pole (F&F)	1 bar (1⅜ oz.)	150	31.0
Nougat centers (Nabisco)			
Chuckles	1 piece (4 grams)	17	4.2
Nutty Crunch (Nabisco)	1 piece (½ oz.)	71	10.2
$100,000 Bar (Nestlé's)	1 oz.	121	18.9
Orange Slices (Brach's)	1 piece (.6 oz.)	55	14.4
Orange slices (Nabisco)			
Chuckles	1 piece (8 grams)	29	7.2
Payday (Hollywood)	1¼ oz.	154	22.3
Peaks (Mason)	1 oz.	175	
Peanut:			
Chocolate-covered:			

(USDA): United States Department of Agriculture
(HEW/FAO): Health, Education and Welfare/Food and Agriculture Organization
* Prepared as Package Directs

Food and Description	Measure or Quantity	Calories	Carbohydrates (grams)
(BB)	1 oz.	158	6.5
(Brach's)	1 piece (2 grams)	11	1.1
(Hershey's) candy-coated	1 oz.	139	17.9
(Kraft)	1 piece (2 grams)	12	.9
(Nabisco)	1 piece (4 grams)	24	1.6
(Tom Houston)	1 oz.	157	10.9
French Burnt (Brach's)	1 piece (1 gram)	5	.6
Peanut Brittle:			
(Bonomo)	1 oz.	132	
(Kraft)	1 oz.	126	19.8
Coconut (Kraft)	1 oz.	125	21.7
Jumbo Peanut Block Bar (Planters)	1⅜-oz. bar	191	19.2
Peanut Butter Cup:			
(Boyer):			
5¢ size	¾-oz. cup	130	10.8
10¢ size	1¼-oz. cup	216	17.9
15¢ size	1⅝-oz. cup	281	23.6
(Reese's) 1 to pkg.	1.2-oz. cup	177	18.1
Smoothie (Boyer):			
5¢ size	¾-oz. cup	135	10.8
10¢ size	1¼-oz. cup	224	17.9
15¢ size	1⅝-oz. cup	292	23.6
Peanut Butter Egg (Reese's)	1 oz.	133	12.4
Peanut Plank (Tom Houston)	1½-oz. bar	202	21.1
P-Nut Butter Crunch (Pearson's)	1 piece	35	
Pom Poms (Nabisco)	1 piece (3 grams)	14	2.3
Poppycock	1 oz.	147	22.0
Raisin, chocolate-covered:			
(Brach's)	1 piece (1 gram)	4	.7
(Ghirardelli)	1.1-oz. bar	160	19.4
(Nabisco)	1 piece (<1 gram)	4	.6
Raisinets (B&B)	5¢ box	140	15.4
Rally (Hershey's)	1.4-oz. bar	202	21.1
Red Hot Dollars (Heide)	1 oz.	94	
Saf-T-Pops (Curtiss)	1 oz.	108	26.1
Snickers (M&M/Mars)	1 oz.	130	15.0
Spearmint Leaves (Brach's)	1 piece (7 grams)	23	5.9
Spearmint Leaves (Nabisco) *Chuckles*	1 piece (8 grams)	27	6.6
Spicettes (Brach's)	1 piece (3 grams)	10	2.5

Food and Description	Measure or Quantity	Calories	Carbo-hydrates (grams)
Sprigs, sweet chocolate (Hershey's)	1 oz.	136	18.3
Sprint, chocolate wafer bar (M&M/Mars)	1 oz.	150	16.2
Stark Wafer Roll	1¼-oz. piece	132	32.9
Stars, chocolate:			
(Brach's)	1 piece (3 grams)	16	1.7
(Nabisco)	1 piece (3 grams)	15	1.6
Sugar Babies (Nabisco)	1 piece (2 grams)	6	1.3
Sugar Daddy (Nabisco):			
Giant sucker	1 piece (1 lb.)	1809	398.6
Junior sucker	1 piece (.4 oz.)	50	11.1
Junior sucker, chocolate-flavored	1 piece (.4 oz.)	51	10.6
Nugget	1 piece (7 grams)	27	6.0
Sucker, caramel	1 piece (1.1 oz.)	121	26.4
Sugar Mama (Nabisco)	1 piece (.8 oz.)	101	18.6
Sugar Wafer (F&F)	1¼-oz. pkg.	180	26.0
Taffy:			
Salt water (Brach's)	1 piece (8 grams)	31	6.8
Turkish (Bonomo):			
Bar	1⅛ oz.	115	29.3
Bite-size	1 piece	19	4.6
Miniatures	1 piece	21	5.6
Nibbles, chocolate-covered	1 piece	9	1.7
Pop	1 piece	45	11.3
Roll	1¢ size	21	5.6
3 Musketeers Bar (M&M/Mars)	1 oz.	120	19.6
Toffee:			
Assorted (Brach's)	1 piece (7 grams)	28	5.2
Chocolate (Kraft)	1 piece (7 grams)	27	5.1
Coffee (Kraft)	1 piece (7 grams)	28	5.2
Rum butter (Kraft)	1 piece (7 grams)	28	5.2
Vanilla (Kraft)	1 piece (7 grams)	28	5.2
Tootsie Roll:			
Regular:			
1¢ size or midgee	1 piece (.23 oz.)	27	5.0
2¢ size	1 piece (.37 oz.)	43	8.1

(USDA): United States Department of Agriculture
(HEW/FAO): Health, Education and Welfare/Food and Agriculture Organization
* Prepared as Package Directs

Food and Description	Measure or Quantity	Calories	Carbohydrates (grams)
5¢ size	1 piece (1 oz.)	116	21.5
10¢ size	1 piece (1.75 oz.)	202	37.7
Vending-machine size	1 piece (.18 oz.)	21	3.9
Pop, 2 for 5¢ size	1 piece (.5 oz.)	55	13.2
Pop, 5¢ size	1 piece (1 oz.)	110	26.4
Pop-drop	1 piece (5 grams)	18	4.4
Triple Decker Bar (Nestlé's)	1 oz.	148	16.8
Twizzlers (Y&S):			
Chocolate	1 oz.	102	22.0
Grape	1 oz.	96	23.0
Licorice bars	1¾ oz.	183	42.0
Strawberry	1¾ oz.	178	24.0
U-No (Cardinet's)	1 bar (⅞ oz.)	161	9.3
Virginia Nut Roll (Queen Anne)	10¢ size	250	
Walnut Hill (F&F)	1 bar (1⅜ oz.)	177	29.0
Wetem & Wearem (Heide)	1 oz.	94	
Whirligigs (Nabisco)	1 piece (6 grams)	26	5.1
CANDY, DIETETIC:			
Chocolate, assorted:			
Milk (Estee)	1 piece (8 grams)	49	3.3
Slimtreats	1 piece (2 grams)	13	1.3
Chocolate bar with almonds:			
(Estee)	¾-oz. bar	125	9.6
(Estee)	3-oz. bar	497	38.2
(Estee) *ST*	⅝-oz. bar	106	8.0
Chocolate bar, bittersweet:			
(Estee)	¾-oz. bar	124	10.4
(Estee)	3-oz. bar	496	41.6
Chocolate bar, coconut			
(Estee)	¾-oz. bar	129	9.4
Chocolate bar, crunch:			
(Estee)	⅝-oz. bar	101	8.3
(Estee)	2½-oz. bar	41	33.4
Chocolate bar, fruit-nut			
(Estee)	3-oz. bar	493	37.4
Chocolate bar, milk:			
(Estee)	¾-oz. bar	128	9.4
(Estee)	3-oz. bar	509	37.4
(Estee) *ST*	⅝-oz. bar	100	8.3
Chocolate bar, peppermint			
(Estee)	¾-oz. bar	126	10.2
Chocolate bar, white			
(Estee)	3-oz. bar	473	40.0
Creams, assorted (Estee)	1 piece (8 grams)	49	3.4

Food and Description	Measure or Quantity	Calories	Carbo-hydrates (grams)
Cream, peppermint (Estee)	1 piece (8 grams)	49	3.4
Gum drops:			
Assorted (Estee)	1 piece (3 grams)	11	2.8
Fruit (Estee)	1 piece (2 grams)	3	.3
Licorice (Estee)	1 piece (2 grams)	2	.6
Hard candy:			
Coffee (Estee)	1 piece (3 grams)	12	2.8
Licorice (Estee)	1 piece (3 grams)	11	2.8
Peppermint (Estee)	1 piece (3 grams)	11	2.8
Slimtreats	1 piece (3 grams)	9	2.5
Mint:			
Butterscotch (Estee)	1 piece	4	1.0
Chocolate (Estee)	1 piece	4	1.0
Fruit flavors (Estee)	1 piece	4	1.0
Peppermint (Estee)	1 piece	4	1.0
Spearmint (Estee)	1 piece	4	1.0
Thin (Dia-Mel)	1 piece (6 grams)	22	1.5
Wintermint (Estee)	1 piece	4	1.0
Nut, chocolate-covered (Estee)	1 piece (8 grams)	47	3.2
Peanut, chocolate-covered (Estee)	1 piece (1 gram)	7	.5
Peanut butter cup (Estee)	1 cup (8 grams)	45	2.5
Petit fours (Estee)	1 piece (8 grams)	48	2.5
Raisin, chocolate-covered (Estee)	1 piece (1 gram)	5	.6
TV mix (Estee)	1 piece (2 grams)	9	.7
CANE SYRUP (USDA)	1 T. (.7 oz.)	55	14.3
CANTALOUPE, fresh:			
Whole, medium (USDA)	1 lb. (weighed with skin & cavity contents)	68	17.0
Whole (USDA)	½ med. melon, 5″ dia. (13.6 oz.)	58	14.4
Cubed (USDA)	½ cup (2.9 oz.)	24	6.1
CAPE GOOSEBERRY (See **GROUND-CHERRY**)			
CAPERS (Crosse & Blackwell)	1 T. (.6 oz.)	6	1.0

(USDA): United States Department of Agriculture
(HEW/FAO): Health, Education and Welfare/Food and Agriculture Organization
* Prepared as Package Directs

Food and Description	Measure or Quantity	Calories	Carbo-hydrates (grams)
CAPICOLA or CAPACOLA SAUSAGE (USDA)	1 oz.	141	0.
CAP'N CRUNCH, cereal:			
Crunchberries (Quaker)	¾ cup (1 oz.)	119	23.8
Peanut butter (Quaker)	¾ cup (1 oz.)	128	21.3
Regular (Quaker)	¾ cup (1 oz.)	123	22.8
Vanilla (Quaker)	¾ cup (1 oz.)	116	23.8
CAPPELLA WINE (Italian Swiss Colony) 13% alcohol	3 fl. oz. (2.9 oz.)	64	1.5
CARAMBOLA, raw (USDA):			
Whole	1 lb. (weighed whole)	149	34.1
Flesh only	4 oz.	40	9.1
CARAMEL CAKE, home recipe (USDA):			
Without icing	⅛ of 9" sq. (2 oz.)	331	46.2
With caramel icing	2-oz. serving	215	33.5
CARAMEL CAKE MIX:			
*(Duncan Hines)	¹⁄₁₂ of cake (2.7 oz.)	202	35.0
*Pudding (Betty Crocker)	⅛ of cake	225	44.4
*CARAMEL NUT PUDDING, instant (Royal)	½ cup (5.1 oz.)	194	3.3
CARAWAY SEED (Data supplied by General Mills)	1 oz.	72	12.3
CARISSA or NATAL PLUM, raw:			
Whole (USDA)	1 lb. (weighed whole)	273	62.4
Flesh only (USDA)	4 oz.	79	18.1
CARNATION INSTANT BREAKFAST:			
Chocolate fudge	1 pkg. (1.3 oz.)	128	22.2
Coffee	1 pkg. (1.3 oz.)	128	24.2
Vanilla	1 pkg. (1.2 oz.)	128	24.4
CAROB FLOUR (See **FLOUR**)			

Food and Description	Measure or Quantity	Calories	Carbo- hydrates (grams)
CAROUSEL WINE (Gold Seal):			
Pink or white, 13–14% alcohol	3 fl. oz. (3.3 oz.)	125	9.8
Red, 13–14% alcohol	3 fl. oz. (3.2 oz.)	104	5.2
CARP, raw (USDA):			
Whole	1 lb. (weighed whole)	156	0.
Meat only	4 oz.	130	0.
CARROT:			
Raw (USDA):			
Whole	1 lb. (weighed with full tops)	112	26.0
Partially trimmed	1 lb. (weighed without tops, with skins)	156	36.1
Trimmed	5½" x 1" carrot (1.8 oz.)	21	4.8
Trimmed	25 thin strips (1.8 oz.)	21	4.8
Chunks	½ cup (2.4 oz.)	29	6.7
Diced	½ cup (2.5 oz.)	30	7.0
Grated or shredded	½ cup (1.9 oz.)	23	5.3
Slices	½ cup (2.2 oz.)	27	6.2
Strips*	½ cup (2 oz.)	24	5.6
Boiled (USDA):			
Chunks, drained	½ cup (2.8 oz.)	25	5.8
Diced, drained	½ cup (2.4 oz.)	22	5.0
Slices, drained	½ cup (2.6 oz.)	24	5.4
Canned, regular pack:			
Diced, solids & liq. (USDA)	½ cup (4.3 oz.)	34	8.0
Drained (Butter Kernel)	½ cup	29	7.0
Drained (Del Monte)	½ cup (2.8 oz.)	23	5.0
Small (Le Sueur)	⅓ of 15-oz. can	31	7.2
Solids & liq. (Stokely-Van Camp)	½ cup (4 oz.)	32	7.4
Canned, dietetic pack:			
Low sodium, solids & liq. (USDA)	4 oz.	25	5.7

(USDA): United States Department of Agriculture
(HEW/FAO): Health, Education and Welfare/Food and Agriculture Organization
* Prepared as Package Directs

Food and Description	Measure or Quantity	Calories	Carbo-hydrates (grams)
Low sodium, drained solids (USDA)	½ cup (2.8 oz.)	20	4.5
Diced, solids & liq. (Blue Boy)	4 oz.	48	5.9
Slices (S and W) *Nutradiet*	4 oz.	25	5.7
Dehydrated (USDA)	1 oz.	97	23.0
Frozen, with brown sugar glaze (Birds Eye)	½ cup (3.3 oz.)	87	16.8
CASABA MELON, fresh (USDA):			
Whole	1 lb. (weighed whole)	61	14.7
Flesh only	4 oz.	31	7.4
CASHEW NUT:			
(USDA)	1 oz.	159	8.3
(USDA)	½ cup (2.5 oz.)	393	20.5
(USDA)	5 large or 8 med.	60	3.1
Freshnut	1 oz.	169	7.3
(Tom Houston)	15 nuts (1.1 oz.)	168	8.8
Dry roasted (Flavor House)	1 oz.	172	6.0
Dry roasted (Planters)	1 oz.	171	7.9
Dry roasted (Skippy)	1 oz.	164	8.2
Oil roasted (Planters)	15¢ bag (.9 oz.)	159	7.0
Oil roasted (Skippy)	1 oz.	177	8.1
CATAWBA WINE:			
(Great Western) pink, 13% alcohol	3 fl. oz.	111	11.0
(Mogen David) New York State, 12% alcohol	3 fl. oz.	75	11.6
CATFISH, freshwater, raw, fillet (USDA)	4 oz.	117	0.
CATSUP:			
Regular pack:			
(USDA)	1 T. (.6 oz.)	19	4.6
(USDA)	½ cup (5 oz.)	149	35.8
(Bama)	1 T. (.6 oz.)	19	4.8
(Del Monte)	1 T. (.7 oz.)	20	5.2
(Heinz)	1 T.	16	3.8
(Hunt's)	1 T. (.6 oz.)	18	5.8
(Nalley's)	1 oz.	31	6.9
(Smucker's)	1 T. (.6 oz.)	19	4.6

Food and Description	Measure or Quantity	Calories	Carbo- hydrates (grams)
Dietetic pack:			
(USDA)	1 T. (.6 oz.)	19	4.6
(Tillie Lewis)	1 T. (.7 oz.)	8	1.8
CAULIFLOWER:			
Raw (USDA):			
Whole	1 lb. (weighed untrimmed)	48	9.2
Flowerbuds	½ cup (1.8 oz.)	14	2.6
Slices	½ cup (1.5 oz.)	11	2.2
Boiled, flowerbuds, drained (USDA)	½ cup (2.2 oz.)	14	2.5
Frozen:			
Not thawed (USDA)	10-oz. pkg.	62	12.2
Boiled, drained (USDA)	⅓ pkg. (3.3 oz.)	21	3.2
(Birds Eye)	⅓ of 10-oz. pkg.	21	3.2
Au gratin (Stouffer's)	⅓ of 10-oz. pkg.	113	6.0
Cut, in butter sauce (Green Giant)	⅓ of 10-oz. pkg.	44	4.3
Hungarian, sour cream (Green Giant)	⅓ of 10-oz. pkg.	70	7.7
In cheese sauce (Green Giant)	⅓ of 10-oz. pkg.	63	6.6
CAULIFLOWER, SWEET PICKLED (Smucker's)	1 bud (.5 oz.)	24	5.5
CAVIAR, STURGEON (USDA):			
Pressed	1 oz.	90	1.4
Whole eggs	1 T. (.6 oz.)	42	.5
CELERIAC ROOT, raw (USDA):			
Whole	1 lb. (weighed unpared)	156	33.2
Pared	4 oz.	45	9.6
CELERY, all varieties (USDA):			
Fresh:			
Whole	1 lb. (weighed untrimmed)	58	13.3

(USDA): United States Department of Agriculture
(HEW/FAO): Health, Education and Welfare/Food and Agriculture
⠀⠀⠀⠀⠀⠀⠀⠀⠀⠀⠀Organization
* Prepared as Package Directs

Food and Description	Measure or Quantity	Calories	Carbo-hydrates (grams)
1 large outer stalk	8″ x 1½″ at root end (1.4 oz.)	7	1.6
Diced, chopped or cut in chunks	½ cup (2.1 oz.)	10	2.3
Slices	½ cup (1.8 oz.)	9	2.1
Boiled, drained solids:			
Diced or cut in chunks	½ cup (2.7 oz.)	11	2.4
Slices	½ cup (3 oz.)	12	2.6
CELERY CABBAGE (See **CABBAGE, CHINESE**)			
CELERY SEASONING (French's)	1 tsp. (5 grams)	2	.1
CELERY SOUP, Cream of:			
Condensed (USDA)	8 oz. (by wt.)	163	16.8
*Prepared with equal volume water (USDA)	1 cup (8.5 oz.)	86	8.9
*Prepared with equal volume milk (USDA)	1 cup (8.4 oz.)	169	15.2
*(Campbell)	1 cup	75	7.3
*(Heinz)	1 cup (8½ oz.)	101	9.0
CEREAL BREAKFAST FOODS (See kind of cereal such as **CORN FLAKES** or brand name such as *KIX*)			
CERTS (Warner-Lambert)	1 piece	6	1.5
CERVELAT (USDA):			
Dry	1 oz.	128	.5
Soft	1 oz.	87	.5
CHABLIS WINE:			
(Barton & Guestier) 12% alcohol	3 fl. oz.	60	.1
(Chanson) St. Vincent, 11½% alcohol	3 fl. oz.	81	6.3
(Cruse) 11% alcohol	3 fl. oz.	66	
(Gallo) 12% alcohol	3 fl. oz.	50	.9
(Gallo) pink, 13% alcohol	3 fl. oz.	61	3.0
(Gold Seal) 12% alcohol	3 fl. oz.	82	.4
(Great Western) 12.5% alcohol	3 fl. oz.	69	1.7
(Great Western) Diamond, 12.5% alcohol	3 fl. oz.	66	

Food and Description	Measure or Quantity	Calories	Carbo-hydrates (grams)
(Inglenook) Navalle, 12% alcohol	3 fl. oz.	59	.5
(Inglenook) Vintage, 12% alcohol	3 fl. oz. (2.9 oz.)	56	.2
(Italian Swiss Colony) Gold, 12% alcohol	3 fl. oz. (2.9 oz.)	66	3.0
(Italian Swiss Colony) pink, 12% alcohol	3 fl. oz. (2.9 oz.)	67	3.2
(Louis M. Martini) 12½% alcohol	3 fl. oz.	90	.2
CHAMPAGNE:			
(Bollinger)	3 fl. oz.	72	3.6
(Gold Seal) brut, 12% alcohol	3 fl. oz.	85	1.4
(Gold Seal) brut *C.F.*, 12% alcohol	3 fl. oz.	82	.7
(Gold Seal) pink, extra dry, 12% alcohol	3 fl. oz.	87	2.6
(Great Western) 12.5% alcohol	3 fl. oz.	84	5.0
(Great Western) brut, 12.5% alcohol	3 fl. oz.	75	3.2
(Great Western) extra dry, 12.5% alcohol	3 fl. oz.	78	4.5
(Great Western) pink, 12.5% alcohol	3 fl. oz.	81	4.7
(Great Western) special reserve, 12.5% alcohol	3 fl. oz.	78	3.8
(Lejon) 12% alcohol	3 fl. oz. (2.9 oz.)	66	2.5
(Mogen David) American Concord red, 12% alcohol	3 fl. oz.	90	8.9
(Mogen David) American dry, 12% alcohol	3 fl. oz.	36	4.4
(Mumm's) Cordon Rouge brut, 12% alcohol	3 fl. oz.	65	1.4
(Mumm's) extra dry, 12% alcohol	3 fl. oz.	82	5.6
(Taylor) brut, 12.5% alcohol	3 fl. oz.	75	1.4
(Taylor) dry, 12.5% alcohol	3 fl. oz.	78	2.0

(USDA): United States Department of Agriculture
(HEW/FAO): Health, Education and Welfare/Food and Agriculture Organization
* Prepared as Package Directs

Food and Description	Measure or Quantity	Calories	Carbo-hydrates (grams)
(Taylor) pink, 12.5% alcohol	3 fl. oz.	81	2.9
(Veuve Clicquot) 12.5% alcohol	3 fl. oz.	78	.6
CHARD, Swiss (USDA):			
Raw, whole	1 lb. (weighed untrimmed)	104	19.2
Raw, trimmed	4 oz.	28	5.2
Boiled, drained solids	½ cup (3.4 oz.)	17	3.2
CHARLOTTE RUSSE, with ladyfingers, whipped cream filling, home recipe (USDA)	4 oz.	324	38.0
CHATEAU LA GARDE CLARET, French red Bordeaux (Chanson) 11½% alcohol	3 fl. oz.	60	6.3
CHATEAUNEUF-DU-PAPE, French red Rhone: (Barton & Guestier) 13.5% alcohol	3 fl. oz.	70	.5
(Chanson) 13% alcohol	3 fl. oz.	90	6.3
(Cruse) 12% alcohol	3 fl. oz.	72	
CHATEAU OLIVIER BLANC, French white Graves (Chanson) 11½% alcohol	3 fl. oz.	60	6.3
CHATEAU OLIVIER ROUGE, French red Graves (Chanson) 11½% alcohol	3 fl. oz.	60	6.3
CHATEAU PONTET CANET (Cruse) 12% alcohol	3 fl. oz.	72	
CHATEAU RAUSAN SEGLA, French red Bordeaux (Chanson) 11½% alcohol	3 fl. oz.	60	6.3
CHATEAU ST. GERMAIN, French red Bordeaux (Chanson) 11½% alcohol	3 fl. oz.	60	6.3
CHATEAU VOIGNY, French Sauternes (Chanson) 13% alcohol	3 fl. oz.	96	7.5

Food and Description	Measure or Quantity	Calories	Carbo-hydrates (grams)
CHAYOTE, raw (USDA):			
Whole	1 lb. (weighed unpared)	108	27.4
Pared	4 oz.	32	8.1
***CHEDDAR CHEESE SOUP**			
(Campbell)	1 cup	141	9.7
CHEERIOS, cereal (General Mills)	1¼ cups (1 oz.)	112	20.2
CHEESE:			
American or cheddar:			
Natural:			
(USDA)	1″ cube (.6 oz.)	68	.4
Diced (USDA)	1 cup (4.6 oz.)	521	2.8
Grated or shredded (USDA)	1 cup (3.9 oz.)	442	2.3
Grated or shredded (USDA)	1 T. (7 grams)	27	.1
(Kraft)	1 oz.	113	.6
Cheddar (Sealtest)	1 oz.	115	.6
Sharp cheddar, *Wispride*	1 T. (.5 oz.)	50	1.5
Process:			
(USDA)	1″ cube (.6 oz.)	67	.3
*(Borden)	¾-oz. slice	83	1.2
(Borden) *Miracle Melt*	1 T. (.5 oz.)	38	.6
(Breakstone)	1 oz.	105	.5
(Kraft) loaf or slice	1 oz.	105	.5
(Sealtest)	1 oz.	105	.5
Vera Sharp (Borden)	1 oz.	104	.6
Dried, sharp cheddar (Information supplied by General Mills)	1 oz.	171	1.7
American Blue, process (Borden) *Miracle Melt*	1 T. (.5 oz.)	38	.5
Asiago (Frigo)	1 oz.	113	.6
Bleu or blue:			
(USDA) natural	1″ cube (.6 oz.)	63	.3
(Borden) Blufort	1¼-oz. pkg.	131	.7
(Borden) Danish	1 oz.	105	.6

(USDA): United States Department of Agriculture
(HEW/FAO): Health, Education and Welfare/Food and Agriculture Organization
* Prepared as Package Directs

Food and Description	Measure or Quantity	Calories	Carbo- hydrates (grams)
(Borden) Flora Danica	1 oz.	105	.6
(Foremost Blue Moon)	1 T.	52	Tr.
(Frigo)	1 oz.	99	.5
(Kraft) natural	1 oz.	99	.5
(Stella)	1 oz.	112	.6
Wispride	1 T. (.5 oz.)	49	1.6
Bondost, natural (Kraft)	1 oz.	103	.4
Brick:			
Natural (USDA)	1 oz.	105	.5
Natural (Kraft)	1 oz.	103	.3
Process, slices (Kraft)	1 oz.	101	.4
Camembert, domestic:			
Natural (USDA)	1 oz.	85	.5
(Borden)	1 oz.	86	.5
Natural (Kraft)	1 oz.	85	.5
Caraway, natural (Kraft)	1 oz.	111	.6
Chantelle, natural (Kraft)	1 oz.	90	.3
Cheddar (See American)			
Colby, natural (Kraft)	1 oz.	111	.6
Cottage:			
Creamed, unflavored:			
(USDA) large or small curd	1 T. (.5 oz.)	16	.4
(Alta-Dena) made with raw, nonfat milk	1 cup	232	
(Axelrod's)	8-oz. container	218	3.5
(Borden)	8-oz. container	240	6.6
Lite Line, low fat (Borden)	1 cup	189	7.0
California (Breakstone)	8-oz. container	216	4.8
Tangy small curd (Breakstone)	8-oz. container	216	4.8
Tiny soft curd (Breakstone)	8-oz. container	216	4.8
(Dean)	8-oz. container	218	5.4
(Foremost Blue Moon)	1 oz.	30	.4
(Kraft)	1 oz.	27	.9
(Sealtest)	1 cup (7.9 oz.)	213	4.7
Light n' Lively, low fat (Sealtest)	1 cup (7.9 oz.)	155	5.6
Low fat, 2% fat (Sealtest)	1 cup (7.9 oz.)	193	7.4
Creamed, flavored:			
Chive (Breakstone)	8-oz. container	216	4.8
Chive (Sealtest)	1 cup (7.9 oz.)	211	4.7

Food and Description	Measure or Quantity	Calories	Carbo-hydrates (grams)
Chive-pepper (Sealtest)	1 cup (8 oz.)	206	5.4
Peach, low fat (Breakstone)	8-oz. container	232	24.9
Peach-pineapple (Sealtest)	1 cup (7.9 oz.)	228	17.9
Pineapple, low fat (Breakstone)	8-oz. container	268	34.2
Pineapple (Breakstone)	1 T. (.6 oz.)	19	2.4
Pineapple (Sealtest)	1 cup (7.9 oz.)	222	16.1
Spring Garden Salad (Sealtest)	1 cup (7.9 oz.)	208	6.7
Uncreamed:			
(Borden)	1 cup	200	6.2
(Dean)	8-oz. container	191	3.6
(Kraft)	1 oz.	26	.6
(Sealtest)	1 cup (7.9 oz.)	179	1.6
Pot style (Borden)	8-oz. container	195	6.1
Pot style (Breakstone)	1 T. (.6 oz.)	12	.3
Skim milk, no salt added (Breakstone)	8-oz. container	182	1.6
Country Charm (Fisher)	1 oz.	89	.4
Cream Cheese:			
Plain, unwhipped:			
(Borden)	1 oz.	101	1.5
(Breakstone)	1 oz.	98	.6
(Breakstone)	1 T. (.5 oz.)	49	.3
(Kraft) *Hostess*	1 oz.	98	.6
Philadelphia (Kraft)	1 oz.	104	.9
(Sealtest)	1 oz.	98	.6
Imitation, *Philadelphia* (Kraft)	1 oz.	52	1.9
Plain, whipped (Breakstone):			
Temp-Tee	1 oz.	98	.6
Temp-Tee	1 T. (9 grams)	32	.2
Flavored, unwhipped:			
Chive (Borden)	1 oz.	96	.6
Chive (Kraft) *Hostess*	1 oz.	84	.8
Chive (Kraft) *Philadelphia*	1 oz.	84	.8

(USDA): United States Department of Agriculture
(HEW/FAO): Health, Education and Welfare/Food and Agriculture Organization
* Prepared as Package Directs

Food and Description	Measure or Quantity	Calories	Carbohydrates (grams)
Olive-pimento (Kraft) Hostess			
Pimento (Borden)	1 oz.	76	.6
Pimento (Kraft) Philadelphia	1 oz.	85	.7
Roquefort (Kraft) Hostess	1 oz.	80	.7
Flavored, whipped (Kraft):			
Catalina	1 oz.	94	1.1
With bacon & horseradish	1 oz.	96	.7
With blue cheese	1 oz.	97	1.2
With chive	1 oz.	92	1.0
With onion	1 oz.	93	1.5
With pimento	1 oz.	91	1.2
With salami	1 oz.	88	1.2
With smoked salmon	1 oz.	90	1.7
Edam (House of Gold)	1 oz.	105	.3
Edam, natural (Kraft)	1 oz.	104	.3
Farmer, midget (Breakstone)	1 oz.	40	.6
Farmer (Dean)	1 oz.	46	.7
Fontina, natural (Kraft)	1 oz.	113	.6
Fontina (Stella)	1 oz.	112	.6
Frankenmuth, natural (Kraft)	1 oz.	113	.7
Gjetost, natural (Kraft)	1 oz.	134	13.0
Gorgonzola (Foremost Blue Moon)	1 oz.	110	Tr.
Gorgonzola, natural (Kraft)	1 oz.	111	.4
Gouda (Borden) Dutch Maid	1 oz.	86	.5
Gouda, baby (Foremost Blue Moon)	1 oz.	120	Tr.
Gouda, natural (Kraft)	1 oz.	107	.5
Gruyère, process (Borden)	1 oz.	93	1.4
Gruyère, natural (Kraft)	1 oz.	110	.6
Gruyère, Swiss Knight	1 oz.	101	.5
Jack-dry, natural (Kraft)	1 oz.	101	.4
Jack-fresh, natural (Kraft)	1 oz.	95	.4
Kisses, mild (Borden)	1 piece (6 grams)	18	.5
Kisses, tangy (Borden)	1 piece (6 grams)	19	.5
Lagerkase, natural (Kraft)	1 oz.	107	.3
Leyden, natural (Kraft)	1 oz.	80	.7

Food and Description	Measure or Quantity	Calories	Carbo-hydrates (grams)
Liederkranz (Borden)	1 oz.	86	.4
Limburger, natural (Kraft)	1 oz.	98	.6
MacLaren's, process, cold pack (Kraft)	1 oz.	109	.6
Monterey Jack (Borden)	1 oz.	103	.6
Monterey Jack (Frigo)	1 oz.	103	.4
Monterey Jack, natural (Kraft)	1 oz.	102	.4
Mozzarella:			
(Borden)	1 oz.	96	.8
(Frigo)	1 oz.	79	.3
Natural, low moisture, part skim (Kraft)	1 oz.	84	.3
Natural, low moisture, part skim, pizza (Kraft)	1 oz.	79	.3
Shredded (Kraft)	1 oz.	79	.3
Muenster, natural (Borden)	1 oz.	85	.7
Muenster, natural (Kraft)	1 oz.	100	.3
Muenster, process, slices (Kraft)	1 oz.	102	.6
Neufchâtel:			
Process (Borden)	1 oz.	73	6.5
Loaf (Kraft)	1 oz.	69	.7
Natural (Kraft)			
Calorie-Wise	1 oz.	70	.7
Nuworld, natural (Kraft)	1 oz.	103	.7
Old English, process, loaf or slices (Kraft)	1 oz.	105	.5
Parmesan:			
Natural:			
(USDA)	1 oz.	111	.8
(Frigo)	1 oz.	107	.8
(Kraft)	1 oz.	107	.8
(Stella)	1 oz.	103	.9
Grated:			
(USDA) loosely packed	1 cup (3.7 oz.)	494	3.6
(USDA) loosely packed	1 T. (7 grams)	31	.2
(Borden)	1 oz.	143	8.8
(Buitoni)	1 oz.	118	.8

(USDA): United States Department of Agriculture
(HEW/FAO): Health, Education and Welfare/Food and Agriculture Organization
* Prepared as Package Directs

Food and Description	Measure or Quantity	Calories	Carbo- hydrates (grams)
(Frigo)	1 T. (6 grams)	27	.2
(Kraft)	1 oz.	127	1.0
Shredded (Kraft)	1 oz.	114	.9
Parmesan & Romano, grated:			
(Borden)	1 oz.	135	2.2
(Kraft)	1 oz.	130	1.0
Pepato (Frigo)	1 oz.	110	.8
Pimento American, process:			
(USDA)	1 oz.	105	.5
(Borden)	1 oz.	104	.5
Loaf or slices (Kraft)	1 oz.	103	.4
Pizza:			
(Borden)	1 oz.	85	.8
(Frigo)	1 oz.	73	.3
(Kraft)	1 oz.	73	.3
Port du Salut (Foremost Blue Moon)	1 oz.	100	Tr.
Port du Salut, natural (Kraft)	1 oz.	100	.3
Primost, natural (Kraft)	1 oz.	134	13.0
Provolone (Borden)	1 oz.	93	1.0
Provolone (Frigo)	1 oz.	99	.5
Provolone, natural (Kraft)	1 oz.	99	.5
Ricotta cheese (Sierra)	1 oz.	50	1.3
Romano:			
Natural:			
(Borden) Italian pecorino	1 oz.	114	.8
(Frigo)	1 oz.	110	.8
(Stella)	1 oz.	106	.6
Grated:			
(Buitoni)	1 oz.	123	1.1
(Frigo)	1 T. (6 grams)	29	.2
(Kraft)	1 oz.	134	1.0
Shredded (Kraft)	1 oz.	121	.9
Romano & Parmesan, plain (Kraft)	1 oz.	133	1.0
Roquefort, natural:			
(Borden) Napolean	1 oz.	107	.6
(Kraft)	1 oz.	105	.5
Sage, natural (Kraft)	1 oz.	113	.6
Sap Sago, natural (Kraft)	1 oz.	76	1.7
Sardo Romano, natural (Kraft)	1 oz.	109	.8
Scamorze (Frigo)	1 oz.	79	.3

Food and Description	Measure or Quantity	Calories	Carbo-hydrates (grams)
Scamorze, natural (Kraft)	1 oz.	100	.3
Swiss, domestic:			
Natural:			
(Foremost Blue Moon)	1 oz.	105	1.0
(Kraft)	1 oz.	104	.5
(Sealtest)	1 oz.	105	.5
Process:			
(Borden)	¾-oz. slice	72	.8
Loaf (Kraft)	1 oz.	92	.5
Slices (Kraft)	1 oz.	95	.6
With Muenster (Kraft)	1 oz.	98	.6
Swiss, imported, natural:			
(Borden) Finland	1 oz.	104	.5
(Borden) Switzerland	1 oz.	104	.5
Washed curd, natural (Kraft)	1 oz.	107	.6
CHEESE CAKE, frozen (Mrs. Smith's)	⅛ of 8" cake (4 oz.)	214	23.3
CHEESE CAKE MIX:			
*(Jell-O)	⅛ of cake including crust (3.3 oz.)	255	31.4
*(Royal) *No-Bake*	⅛ of 9" cake including crust (3.2 oz.)	278	31.9
CHEESE DIP (See DIP)			
CHEESE FONDUE:			
Home recipe (USDA)	4 oz.	301	11.3
(Borden)	6-oz. serving	354	15.3
CHEESE FOOD, process:			
American:			
(USDA)	1 oz.	92	2.0
(Borden)	1" x 1" x 1" piece (.8 oz.)	71	2.5
Grated (Borden)	1 oz.	129	8.4

(USDA): United States Department of Agriculture
(HEW/FAO): Health, Education and Welfare/Food and Agriculture Organization
* Prepared as Package Directs

Food and Description	Measure or Quantity	Calories	Carbo-hydrates (grams)
Grated, used in			
Kraft Dinner	1 oz.	129	8.4
Slices (Kraft)	1 oz.	94	2.4
Cheez 'n bacon (Kraft)	¾-oz. slice	76	.8
Links (Kraft) *Handi-Snack*:			
Bacon	1 oz.	93	2.2
Jalapeno	1 oz.	92	2.2
Nippy	1 oz.	92	2.2
Smokelle	1 oz.	93	2.2
Swiss	1 oz.	90	1.4
Loaf:			
Munst-ett (Kraft)	1 oz.	100	1.7
Pizzalone (Kraft)	1 oz.	99	.5
Super blend (Kraft)	1 oz.	92	1.6
Pimento (Borden)	1 oz.	91	2.0
Salami, slices (Kraft)	1 oz.	94	2.6
Swiss (Borden) cold pack	.7-oz. slice	62	1.1
Swiss, slices (Kraft)	1 oz.	92	2.3
CHEESE PIE:			
(Tastykake)	4 oz. pie	357	51.2
Frozen, pineapple:			
(Mrs. Smith's)	⅛ of 8″ pie (4 oz.)	273	36.4
(Mrs. Smith's)	⅛ of 10″ pie (5.4 oz.)	341	45.4
CHEESE PUFF, hors d'oeuvres, frozen (Durkee)	1 piece (.5 oz.)	.59	2.9
CHEESE SOUFFLE:			
Home recipe (USDA)	¼ of 7″ soufflé (3.9 oz.)	240	6.8
Frozen (Stouffer's)	12-oz. pkg.	730	35.0
CHEESE SPREAD:			
American, process:			
(USDA)	1 T. (.5 oz.)	40	1.1
(Borden)	.7 oz.	63	1.6
(Kraft) *Swankyswig*	1 oz.	77	1.7
(Nabisco) *Snack Mate*	1 tsp. (5 grams)	15	.4
Bacon (Borden) cheese 'n bacon	1 oz.	72	1.8
Cheddar (Nabisco) *Snack Mate*	1 tsp. (5 grams)	15	.4
Cheez Whiz, process (Kraft)	1 oz.	76	1.7
Count Down (Fisher)	1 oz.	42	2.8

Food and Description	Measure or Quantity	Calories	Carbo- hydrates (grams)
Garlic, process (Borden)	1 oz.	72	1.8
Garlic, process (Kraft) *Swankyswig*	1 oz.	86	1.8
Imitation, *Chef's Delight*	1 oz.	41	3.4
Imitation (Kraft) *Calorie-Wise*	1 oz.	48	3.6
Jalapeño (Kraft) *Cheez Whiz*	1 oz.	76	1.9
Limburger (Kraft)	1 oz.	69	.4
Neufchâtel:			
Bacon & horseradish (Kraft) *Party Snacks*	1 oz.	74	.7
Chipped beef (Kraft) *Party Snacks*	1 oz.	67	1.2
Chive (Kraft) *Party Snacks*	1 oz.	69	.8
Clam (Kraft) *Party Snacks*	1 oz.	67	.8
Onion (Kraft) *Party Snacks*	1 oz.	66	1.6
Pimento (Borden)	1 T. (.5 oz.)	36	1.8
Pineapple (Borden)	1 T. (.5 oz.)	36	1.8
Old English (Kraft) *Swankyswig*	1 oz.	96	.6
Onion flavor, French (Nabisco) *Snack Mate*	1 tsp. (5 grams)	15	.4
Pimento:			
(Borden) *Country Store*	1 T. (.5 oz.)	36	1.7
(Kraft) *Cheez Whiz*	1 oz.	76	1.7
(Kraft) *Squeez-A-Snak*	1 oz.	86	.6
(Nabisco) *Snack Mate*	1 tsp. (5 oz.)	15	.4
(Sealtest)	1 oz.	77	1.7
Sharp (Kraft) *Squeez-A-Snak*	1 oz.	85	.6
Sharpie, process (Kraft)	1 oz.	90	.5
Smoke (Kraft) *Squeez-A-Snak*	1 oz.	83	4.8
Smokelle Swankyswig, process (Kraft)	1 oz.	90	.5
Smokey cheese (Borden)	1 oz.	72	1.8

(USDA): United States Department of Agriculture
(HEW/FAO): Health, Education and Welfare/Food and Agriculture Organization
* Prepared as Package Directs

Food and Description	Measure or Quantity	Calories	Carbo-hydrates (grams)
Velva Kreme (Borden)	1 oz.	94	1.1
Velveeta, process (Kraft)	1 oz.	84	2.6
CHEESE STRAW:			
(USDA)	5″ x ⅜″ x ⅜″ piece (6 grams)	27	2.1
(Durkee)	1 piece (8 grams)	29	1.2
CHELOIS WINE (Great Western) 12.5% alcohol	3 fl. oz.	72	2.2
CHENIN BLANC WINE:			
(Inglenook) Estate, 12% alcohol	3 fl. oz. (2.9 oz.)	60	1.3
(Louis M. Martini) dry, 12½% alcohol	3 fl. oz.	90	.2
CHERIMOYA, raw (USDA):			
Whole	1 lb. (weighed with skin & seeds)	247	63.1
Flesh only	4 oz.	107	27.2
CHERI SUISSE, Swiss liqueur (Leroux) 60 proof	1 fl. oz.	90	10.2
CHERRY:			
Sour:			
Fresh (USDA):			
Whole	1 lb. (weighed with stems)	213	52.5
Whole	1 lb. (weighed without stems)	242	59.7
Pitted	½ cup (2.7 oz.)	45	11.0
Canned, syrup pack, pitted (USDA):			
Light syrup	4 oz. (with liq.)	84	21.2
Heavy syrup	½ cup (with liq.)	116	29.5
Extra heavy syrup	4 oz. (with liq.)	127	32.4
Canned, water pack, pitted, solids & liq.:			
(USDA)	½ cup (4.3 oz.)	52	13.1
(Stokely-Van Camp)	½ cup	49	12.2
Frozen, pitted (USDA):			
Sweetened	½ cup (4.6 oz.)	146	36.1
Unsweetened	4 oz.	62	15.2
Sweet:			
Fresh (USDA):			
Whole	1 lb. (weighed		

Food and Description	Measure or Quantity	Calories	Carbo-hydrates (grams)
	with stems)	286	71.0
Whole, with stems	½ cup (2.3 oz.)	41	10.2
Pitted	½ cup (2.9 oz.)	57	14.3
Canned, syrup pack, pitted (USDA):			
Light syrup	4 oz. (with liq.)	74	18.7
Heavy syrup	½ cup (with liq., 4.2 oz.)	96	24.2
Extra heavy syrup	4 oz. (with liq.)	113	29.0
Canned, heavy syrup, with pits, dark (Del Monte)	½ cup (4.3 oz.)	92	23.0
Canned, heavy syrup, with pits, Royal Anne (Del Monte)	½ cup (with liq., 4.6 oz.)	109	28.1
Canned, water or dietetic pack, pitted:			
Solids & liq. (Blue Boy)	4 oz.	52	10.4
Royal Anne:			
Solids & liq. (Diet Delight)	½ cup (4.4 oz.)	65	15.0
Unsweetened (S and W) *Nutradiet*	14 whole cherries (3.5 oz.)	47	10.8
Canned (Tillie Lewis) with pits	½ of 8-oz. can	54	12.8
Frozen, quick thaw (Birds Eye)	½ cup (5 oz.)	122	30.8
CHERRY, BLACK, SOFT DRINK:			
Sweetened:			
(Canada Dry)	6 fl. oz.	96	24.0
(Dr. Brown's)	6 fl. oz.	81	20.1
(Hoffman)	6 fl. oz.	87	21.9
(Key Food)	6 fl. oz.	81	20.1
(Kirsch)	6 fl. oz.	88	22.1
(Shasta)	6 fl. oz.	88	22.2
(Waldbaum)	6 fl. oz.	81	20.1
Unsweetened or low calorie:			
(Canada Dry)	6 fl. oz.	11	.2

(USDA): United States Department of Agriculture
(HEW/FAO): Health, Education and Welfare/Food and Agriculture Organization
* Prepared as Package Directs

Food and Description	Measure or Quantity	Calories	Carbo- hydrates (grams)
(Dr. Brown's) *Slim-Ray*	6 fl. oz.	2	.4
(Hoffman)	6 fl. oz.	2	.4
(No-Cal)	6 fl. oz.	2	0.
(Shasta)	6 fl. oz.	1	.1
CHERRY BRANDY			
(DeKuyper) 70 proof	1 fl. oz. (1.1 oz.)	85	6.9
CHERRY CAKE MIX:			
*(Duncan Hines)	1/12 of cake (2.6 oz.)	193	34.8
*Chip (Betty Crocker)	1/12 of cake	198	37.6
CHERRY, CANDIED			
(Liberty)	1 oz.	93	22.6
CHERRY CAKE, shortcake, frozen (Mrs. Smith's)	1/8 of 9" cake (5.7 oz.)	394	55.0
CHERRY DRINK:			
(Hi-C)	6 fl. oz.(6.3 oz.)	90	21.8
(Wagner)	6 fl. oz.	83	20.7
*Mix (Wyler's)	6 fl. oz.	64	15.8
CHERRY EXTRACT:			
Imitation (Ehlers)	1 tsp.	8	
Imitation (French's)	1 tsp.	16	
CHERRY HEERING, Danish liqueur, 49 proof	1 fl. oz.	80	10.0
CHERRY JELLY:			
Sweetened (Smucker's)	1 T. (.7 oz.)	50	12.7
Low calorie:			
(Slenderella)	1 T. (.7 oz.)	26	6.8
(Smucker's)	1 T.	6	1.4
CHERRY KARISE, liqueur (Leroux) 49 proof	1 fl. oz.	71	7.6
CHERRY KIJAFA, Danish wine, 17.5% alcohol	3 fl. oz.	148	15.3
CHERRY LIQUEUR:			
(Bols) 60 proof	1 fl. oz.	96	8.9
(DeKuyper) 50 proof	1 fl. oz. (1.1 oz.)	75	8.5
(Hiram Walker) 60 proof	1 fl. oz.	82	8.2
(Leroux) 60 proof	1 fl. oz.	80	7.6

Food and Description	Measure or Quantity	Calories	Carbo-hydrates (grams)
CHERRY, MARASCHINO			
(Liberty)	1 average cherry	8	1.9
CHERRY PIE:			
Home recipe, 2 crusts			
(USDA)	⅙ of 9" pie (5.6 oz.)	412	60.7
(Drake's)	2-oz. pie	203	25.3
(Hostess)	4½-oz. pie	427	54.9
Cherry-apple (Tastykake)	4-oz. pie	373	56.8
Frozen:			
(Banquet)	5-oz. serving	352	50.2
(Morton)	⅙ of 24-oz. pie	342	39.6
(Mrs. Smith's)	⅙ of 8" pie (4.2 oz.)	309	43.3
Tart (Pepperidge Farm)	3-oz. pie	277	34.3
CHERRY PIE FILLING:			
(Comstock)	1 cup (10¾ oz.)	334	84.6
(Lucky Leaf)	8 oz.	242	58.2
(Wilderness)	21-oz. can	720	168.3
CHERRY PRESERVE:			
Sweetened (Bama)	1 T. (.7 oz.)	54	13.5
Low calorie (Dia-Mel)	1 T.	6	1.4
Low calorie (Louis Sherry)	1 T. (.5 oz.)	6	1.5
CHERRY SOFT DRINK,			
Sweetened:			
(Canada Dry)	6 fl. oz.	96	24.0
Fanta	6 fl. oz.	85	21.9
(Mission)	6 fl. oz.	94	23.0
(Nedick's)	6 fl. oz.	81	20.1
(Yoo-Hoo) high-protein	6 fl. oz. (6.4 oz.)	100	18.9
(Yukon Club)	6 fl. oz.	86	21.5
CHERRY SYRUP, dietetic			
(No-Cal)	1 tsp. (5 grams)	1	0.
CHERRY TURNOVER, frozen			
(Pepperidge Farm)	1 turnover (3.3 oz.)	342	30.3

(USDA): United States Department of Agriculture
(HEW/FAO): Health, Education and Welfare/Food and Agriculture Organization
* Prepared as Package Directs

Food and Description	Measure or Quantity	Calories	Carbohydrates (grams)
CHERRY WINE (Mogen David) 12% alcohol	3 fl. oz.	126	16.9
CHERVIL, raw (USDA)	1 oz.	16	3.3
CHESTNUT (USDA):			
Fresh, in shell	1 lb. (weighed in shell)	713	154.7
Fresh, shelled	4 oz.	220	47.7
Dried, in shell	1 lb. (weighed in shell)	1402	292.4
Dried, shelled	4 oz.	428	89.1
CHESTNUT FLOUR (See FLOUR, CHESTNUT)			
CHEWING GUM:			
Sweetened:			
(USDA)	1 piece (3 grams)	10	2.9
Bazooka, bubble, 1¢ size	1 piece	18	4.5
Bazooka, bubble, 5¢ size	1 piece	85	21.2
Beechies	1 tablet (2 grams)	6	1.6
Beech-Nut	1 stick (3 grams)	10	2.3
Beemans	1 stick	9	2.3
Black Jack	1 stick	9	2.3
Chiclets	5¢ pkg.	65	
Chiclets, tiny size	1 piece	6	1.1
Cinnamint	1 stick	10	2.3
Clove	1 stick	9	2.3
Dentyne	1 piece	4	1.2
Doublemint	1 stick (3 grams)	8	2.3
Fruit Punch	1 stick	10	2.3
Juicy Fruit	1 stick (3 grams)	9	2.4
Peppermint (Clark)	1 piece	10	2.3
Sour (Warner-Lambert)	1 stick	10	
Sour lemon (Clark)	1 stick	10	2.3
Spearmint (Wrigley's)	1 stick (3 grams)	8	2.2
Teaberry	1 stick	10	2.3
Unsweetened or dietetic:			
All flavors (Clark)	1 stick	7	1.7
All flavors (Estee)	1 section (1 gram)	4	.9
Bazooka, bubble, sugarless	1 piece	16	Tr.
Bubble (Estee)	1 piece (1 gram)	4	.9
*Care*Free* (Beech-Nut)	1 stick (3 grams)	7	Tr.
(Harvey's)	1 stick	4	1.0
Peppermint (Amurol)	1 stick	5	1.8

Food and Description	Measure or Quantity	Calories	Carbohydrates (grams)
CHIANTI WINE:			
(Antinori):			
Classico, 12½% alcohol	3 fl. oz.	87	6.3
1955, 12½% alcohol	3 fl. oz.	87	6.3
Vintage, 12½% alcohol	3 fl. oz.	87	6.3
Brolio Classico, 13% alcohol	3 fl. oz.	66	.3
(Gancia) Classico, 12½% alcohol	3 fl. oz.	75	
(Italian Swiss Colony) 13% alcohol	3 fl. oz. (2.9 oz.)	83	2.9
(Louis M. Martini) 12½% alcohol	3 fl. oz.	90	.2
CHICKEN (See also **CHICKEN, CANNED**)			
(USDA):			
Broiler, cooked, meat only	4 oz.	154	0.
Capon, raw, with bone	1 lb. (weighed ready-to-cook)	937	0.
Fryer:			
Raw:			
Ready-to-cook	1 lb. (weighed ready-to-cook)	382	0.
Breast	1 lb. (weighed with bone)	394	0.
Leg or drumstick	1 lb. (weighed with bone)	313	0.
Thigh	1 lb. (weighed with bone)	435	0.
Fried. A 2½-pound chicken (weighed before cooking with bone) will give you:			
Back	1 back (2.2 oz.)	139	2.7
Breast	½ breast (3⅓ oz.)	154	1.1
Leg or drumstick	1 leg (2 oz.)	87	.4
Neck	1 neck (2.1 oz.)	121	1.9
Rib	1 rib (.7 oz.)	42	.8
Thigh	1 thigh (2¼ oz.)	118	1.2
Wing	1 wing (1¾ oz.)	78	.8
Fried skin	1 oz.	119	2.6

(USDA): United States Department of Agriculture
(HEW/FAO): Health, Education and Welfare/Food and Agriculture Organization
* Prepared as Package Directs

Food and Description	Measure or Quantity	Calories	Carbohydrates (grams)
Hen and cock:			
Raw	1 lb. (weighed ready-to-cook)	987	0.
Stewed:			
Meat only	4 oz.	236	0.
Chopped	½ cup (2.5 oz.)	150	0.
Diced	½ cup (2.4 oz.)	139	0.
Ground	½ cup (2 oz.)	116	0.
Roaster:			
Raw	1 lb. (weighed ready-to-cook)	791	0.
Roasted:			
Dark meat without skin	4 oz.	209	0.
Light meat without skin	4 oz.	206	0.
CHICKEN A-LA KING:			
Home recipe (USDA)	1 cup (8.6 oz.)	468	12.2
Canned (College Inn)	5-oz. serving	150	4.0
Canned (Richardson & Robbins)	1 cup (7.9 oz.)	272	14.4
Canned (Swanson)	1 cup	260	12.8
Frozen (Banquet) cookin' bag	5 oz.	140	9.0
CHICKEN BOUILLON/ BROTH, cube or powder (See also **CHICKEN SOUP**):			
(Croyden House)	1 tsp. (5 grams)	12	2.5
(Herb-Ox)	1 cube (4 grams)	6	.6
(Herb-Ox)	1 packet (5 grams)	12	1.9
*(Knorr Swiss)	6 fl. oz.	13	
(Maggi)	1 cube or 1 tsp.	8	1.1
(Steero)	1 cube (4 grams)	6	.4
(Wyler's)	1 cube	6	.7
(Wyler's) instant	1 envelope (4 grams)	8	.9
(Wyler's) no salt added	1 cube (4 grams)	11	1.6
CHICKEN CACCIATORE			
(Hormel)	1-lb. can	386	8.2
CHICKEN, CANNED:			
Boned:			
(USDA)	½ cup (3 oz.)	168	0.
(College Inn)	4 oz.	299	0.
(Lynden Farms) solids & liq.	5-oz. jar	229	0.

Food and Description	Measure or Quantity	Calories	Carbo-hydrates (grams)
(Swanson) with broth	5-oz. can	223	0.
Whole (Lynden Farms)	52-oz. can	1170	0.
CHICKEN, CREAMED, frozen (Stouffer's)	11½-oz. pkg.	613	16.2
CHICKEN DINNER:			
Canned:			
Dumplings (College Inn)	5-oz. serving	170	12.0
Noodle (Heinz)	8½-oz. can	186	18.9
Noodle (Lynden Farms)	14-oz. jar	413	31.8
Noodle with vegetables (Lynden Farms)	15-oz. can	434	38.2
Frozen:			
(Weight Watchers)	10-oz. luncheon	284	6.3
Boneless chicken (Swanson) *Hungry Man*	19-oz. dinner	746	63.7
Chicken & dumplings:			
Buffet (Banquet)	2-lb. pkg.	1306	110.8
(Tom Thumb)	3-lb. 8-oz. tray	1920	112.6
Chicken liver & onions (Weight Watchers)	11½-oz. luncheon	234	3.9
Creole (Weight Watchers)	12-oz. luncheon	211	10.2
& dumplings:			
(Morton)	11-oz. dinner	356	28.1
(Morton)	16-oz. dinner	699	77.2
& noodles:			
(Banquet)	12-oz. dinner	374	50.7
(Morton)	10¼-oz. dinner	392	52.2
Fried:			
(Banquet)	12-oz. dinner	530	48.4
(Morton)	11-oz. dinner	449	40.6
(Swanson)	11½-oz. dinner	600	46.6
(Swanson) 3-course	15-oz. dinner	639	62.6

CHICKEN & DUMPLINGS
(See **CHICKEN DINNER**)

(USDA): United States Department of Agriculture
(HEW/FAO): Health, Education and Welfare/Food and Agriculture
Organization
* Prepared as Package Directs

Food and Description	Measure or Quantity	Calories	Carbo-hydrates (grams)
CHICKEN FRICASSEE:			
Home recipe (USDA)	1 cup (8.5 oz.)	386	7.7
Canned (College Inn)	1 cup	234	14.8
Canned (Richardson & Robbins)	1 cup (7.9 oz.)	256	15.1
CHICKEN, FRIED, frozen, with whipped potato (Swanson)	7-oz. pkg.	412	27.0
CHICKEN, GIZZARD (USDA):			
Raw	2 oz.	64	.4
Simmered	2 oz.	84	.4
CHICKEN LIVER (See LIVER)			
CHICKEN LIVER, CHOPPED (Mrs. Kornberg's)	6-oz. pkg.	260	
CHICKEN LIVER PUFF, hors d'oeuvres, frozen (Durkee)	1 piece (.5 oz.)	48	3.1
CHICKEN & NOODLES:			
Home recipe (USDA)	1 cup (8.5 oz.)	367	25.7
Canned (College Inn)	5-oz. serving	170	17.0
Frozen (Banquet) buffet	2-lb. pkg.	735	61.2
Frozen, escalloped (Stouffer's)	11½-oz. pkg.	589	35.9
CHICKEN PIE:			
Baked, home recipe (USDA)	8 oz. (4¼" dia.)	533	41.5
Frozen:			
(Banquet)	8-oz. pie	427	39.0
(Morton)	8-oz. pie	445	34.0
(Stouffer's)	10-oz. pie	722	44.2
(Swanson)	8-oz. pie	445	40.0
(Swanson) deep dish	16-oz. pie	708	55.5
CHICKEN PUFF, hors d'oeuvres, frozen (Durkee)	1 piece (.5 oz.)	49	3.0
CHICKEN RAVIOLI (Lynden Farms)	14½-oz. can	452	74.0
CHICKEN SOUP, canned:			
(Campbell) *Chunky*	1 cup	155	15.8
*Barley (Manischewitz)	8 oz. (by wt.)	83	12.3

Food and Description	Measure or Quantity	Calories	Carbo-hydrates (grams)
Broth:			
*(Campbell)	1 cup	53	.9
*(Claybourne) dietetic	8 oz.	9	0.
(College Inn)	1 cup	30	.1
(Lynden Farms)	1 cup (8 oz.)	14	0.
(Richardson & Robbins)	1 cup (8.1 oz.)	32	1.6
(Swanson)	1 cup	31	.2
With rice (Richardson & Robbins)	1 cup (8.1 oz.)	48	5.0
Consommé:			
Condensed (USDA)	8 oz. (by wt.)	41	3.4
*Prepared with equal volume water (USDA)	1 cup (8.5 oz.)	22	1.9
Cream of:			
Condensed (USDA)	8 oz. (by wt.)	179	15.2
*Prepared with equal volume milk (USDA)	1 cup (8.6 oz.)	179	14.5
*Prepared with equal volume water (USDA)	1 cup (8.5 oz.)	94	7.9
*(Campbell)	1 cup	87	7.2
*(Heinz)	1 cup (8.5 oz.)	93	8.3
(Heinz) *Great American*	1 cup (8.5 oz.)	108	9.0
*& Dumplings (Campbell)	1 cup	95	4.8
Gumbo:			
Condensed (USDA)	8 oz. (by wt.)	104	13.8
*Prepared with equal volume water (USDA)	1 cup (8.5 oz.)	55	7.4
*(Campbell)	1 cup	55	8.3
Creole (Heinz) *Great American*	1 cup (8¾ oz.)	96	15.0
& Noodle:			
Condensed (USDA)	8 oz. (by wt.)	120	15.0
*Prepared with equal volume water (USDA)	1 cup (8.5 oz.)	65	8.2
*(Campbell)	1 cup	62	8.2
Noodle-O's (Campbell)	1 cup	67	9.0
*(Heinz)	1 cup (8.5 oz.)	75	9.5
*(Manischewitz)	1 cup (8.1 oz.)	46	4.2
(Tillie Lewis) dietetic	1 cup (8 oz.)	53	6.8
With dumplings (Heinz) *Great American*	1 cup (8.5 oz.)	89	8.9

(USDA): United States Department of Agriculture
(HEW/FAO): Health, Education and Welfare/Food and Agriculture
  Organization

* Prepared as Package Directs

Food and Description	Measure or Quantity	Calories	Carbohydrates (grams)
*With stars (Campbell)	1 cup	57	6.9
*With stars (Heinz)	1 cup (8.5 oz.)	66	7.9
& Rice:			
Condensed (USDA)	8 oz. (by wt.)	89	10.7
*Prepared with equal volume water (USDA)	1 cup (8.5 oz.)	48	5.8
*(Campbell)	1 cup	49	5.6
*(Heinz)	1 cup (8.5 oz.)	61	6.7
*(Manischewitz)	8 oz. (by wt.)	47	5.3
With mushrooms (Heinz) *Great American*	1 cup (8.5 oz.)	96	11.6
Vegetable:			
Condensed (USDA)	8 oz. (by wt.)	141	17.5
*Prepared with equal volume water (USDA)	1 cup (8.6 oz.)	76	9.6
*(Campbell)	1 cup	68	8.6
*(Heinz)	1 cup (8.5 oz.)	85	9.3
*(Manischewitz)	1 cup	55	7.8
*With Kasha (Manischewitz)	1 cup	41	5.4
CHICKEN SOUP MIX:			
Cream of (Lipton) *Cup-a-Soup*	1 pkg. (.8 oz.)	95	9.7
Cream of (Wyler's)	1 pkg. (.8 oz.)	93	14.7
& Noodle:			
*(Lipton)	1 cup	53	7.2
(Lipton) *Cup-a-Soup*	1 pkg. (.4 oz.)	38	5.9
& Rice:			
*(Lipton)	1 cup (8 oz.)	62	8.0
*(Wyler's)	6 fl. oz.	49	8.6
*Vegetable (Lipton)	1 cup	74	10.4
Vegetable (Lipton) *Cup-a-Soup*	1 pkg. (.5 oz.)	41	7.2
*Vegetable (Wyler's)	6 fl. oz.	28	4.0
CHICKEN SPREAD:			
(Swanson)	5-oz. can	283	2.0
(Underwood)	1 T. (.5 oz.)	31	.5
CHICKEN STEW:			
Canned:			
(B&M)	1 cup (7.9 oz.)	128	15.3
(Swanson)	1 cup	166	16.3
With dumplings (Heinz)	8½-oz. can	202	22.1
CHICKEN STOCK BASE			
(French's)	1 tsp. (3 grams)	8	1.2

Food and Description	Measure or Quantity	Calories	Carbo-hydrates (grams)
CHICKEN TAMALE PIE, canned (Lynden Farms)	½ tamale pie with sauce (3.8 oz.)	143	12.0
CHICK-PEAS or GARBANZOS, dry (USDA)	1 cup (7.1 oz.)	720	122.0
CHICKORY GREENS, raw (USDA):			
Untrimmed	½ lb. (weighed untrimmed)	37	7.0
Trimmed	4 oz.	23	4.3
CHICORY, WITLOOF, Belgian or French endive, raw, bleached head (USDA):			
Untrimmed	½ lb. (weighed untrimmed)	30	6.4
Trimmed, cut	½ cup (.9 oz.)	4	.8
CHILI or CHILI CON CARNE:			
Canned, beans only, spiced (Gebhardt)	1 cup	184	
Canned, with beans:			
(USDA)	1 cup (8.8 oz.)	332	30.5
(Armour Star)	15½-oz. can	692	59.3
(Austex)	15½-oz. can (1¾ cups)	584	53.6
(Chef Boy-Ar-Dee)	¼ of 30-oz. can	307	24.1
(Heinz)	8¾-oz. can	352	28.2
(Hormel)	½ of 15-oz. can	320	23.5
(Hormel)	8-oz. can	275	17.5
(Libby's)	8 oz.	293	33.6
(Morton House)	1 cup (8 oz.)	367	31.3
(Nalley's) mild or hot	8 oz.	345	26.8
(Rosarita)	8 oz.	376	27.2
(Rutherford)	8 oz.	379	
(Silver Skillet)	8 oz.	334	19.5
(Swanson)	1 cup	270	21.8
(Van Camp)	1 cup (8 oz.)	304	28.0
(Wilson)	½ of 15½-oz. can	315	26.4

(USDA): United States Department of Agriculture
(HEW/FAO): Health, Education and Welfare/Food and Agriculture Organization
* Prepared as Package Directs

Food and Description	Measure or Quantity	Calories	Carbo-hydrates (grams)
Canned, without beans:			
(USDA)	1 cup (9 oz.)	510	14.8
(Armour Star)	15½-oz. can	835	25.5
(Austex)	15-oz. can (1¾ cups)	851	24.7
(Bunker Hill)	10¼-oz. can	657	
(Chef Boy-Ar-Dee)	½ of 15¼-oz. can	328	14.0
(Hormel)	½ of 15-oz. can	340	7.6
(Libby's)	8 oz.	399	12.0
(Morton House)	15-oz. can	1065	
(Nalley's)	8 oz.	311	12.9
(Rutherford)	8 oz.	447	
(Van Camp)	1 cup	460	13.2
(Wilson)	½ of 15½-oz. can	420	12.7
Frozen, with beans (Banquet)	8-oz. bag	310	21.5
CHILI BEEF SOUP, canned:			
*(Campbell)	1 cup	149	20.8
*(Heinz)	1 cup (8¾ oz.)	161	21.2
(Heinz) *Great American*	1 cup (8¾ oz.)	179	22.0
CHILI CON CARNE MIX:			
*With meat & beans (Durkee)	3½ cups (2¼-oz. dry pkg.)	1720	94.0
*Without meat & beans (Durkee)	1¼ cups (2¼-oz. dry pkg.)	196	44.6
CHILI CON CARNE SPREAD:			
With beans (Oscar Mayer)	1 oz.	62	3.3
Without beans (Oscar Mayer)	1 oz.	78	2.5
*CHILI DOG SAUCE MIX (McCormick)	.9-oz. serving	18	4.0
CHILI POWDER, with added seasonings (USDA)	1 T. (.5 oz.)	51	8.5
CHILI SAUCE:			
(USDA)	1 T. (.5 oz.)	16	3.7
(Del Monte)	1 T. (.5 oz.)	18	4.6
(Heinz)	1 T. (.6 oz.)	19	4.9
(Hunt's)	1 T. (.6 oz.)	21	4.9
CHILI SEASONING MIX:			
Chili-O (French's)	1¾-oz. pkg.	123	23.8
(Lawry's)	1.6-oz. pkg	137	23.6

Food and Description	Measure or Quantity	Calories	Carbo- hydrates (grams)
CHINESE DATE (See **JUJUBE**)			
CHINESE DINNER, frozen:			
Beef chop suey (Chun King)	11-oz. dinner	310	46.0
Chicken chow mein (Banquet)	12-oz. dinner	282	38.8
CHIPS (See **CRACKERS** for **CORN CHIPS** and **POTATO CHIPS**)			
CHITTERLINGS, canned (Hormel)	1-lb. 2-oz. can	832	.5
CHIVES, raw (USDA)	½ lb.	64	13.2
CHOCOLATE, BAKING:			
Bitter or unsweetened:			
(Baker's)	1 oz. (1 sq.)	136	7.7
Pre-melted, *Choco-Bake*	1-oz. packet	172	10.2
(Hershey's)	1 oz.	183	6.3
Sweetened:			
Chips, semisweet (Baker's)	¼ cup (1½ oz.)	191	28.5
Chips, semisweet (Ghirardelli)	⅓ cup (2 oz.)	299	35.6
Chips, milk (Hershey's)	¼ cup (1.5 oz.)	234	25.1
Chips, semisweet (Hershey's)	¼ cup (1.5 oz.)	227	26.5
Chips, mini, semisweet (Hershey's)	¼ cup (1.5 oz.)	227	26.5
German sweet (Baker's)	1 oz. (4½ sq.)	141	16.9
Morsels, milk (Nestlé's)	1 oz.	152	18.0
Morsels, semisweet Nestlé's)	1 oz.	137	18.1
Semisweet (Baker's)	1 oz. (1 sq.)	132	16.2
CHOCOLATE CAKE:			
Home recipe (USDA):			
Without icing	3 oz.	311	44.2
With chocolate icing	⅟₁₆ of 10″ cake (4.2 oz.)	443	67.0

(USDA): United States Department of Agriculture
(HEW/FAO): Health, Education and Welfare/Food and Agriculture Organization
* Prepared as Package Directs

Food and Description	Measure or Quantity	Calories	Carbo-hydrates (grams)
With uncooked white icing	1/16 of 10″ cake (4.2 oz.)	443	71.0
Frozen:			
Frosted (Sara Lee)	1 oz.	102	16.0
Fudge layer (Pepperidge Farm)	1/8 of cake (3 oz.)	315	43.4
German chocolate:			
(Morton)	1 serving (2.2 oz.)	230	28.0
(Sara Lee)	1 oz.	91	12.0
Golden (Pepperidge Farm)	1/8 of cake (3 oz.)	320	43.6
CHOCOLATE CAKE MIX (See also **FUDGE CAKE MIX**):			
Chocolate malt (USDA)	1 oz.	116	22.4
*Chocolate malt, uncooked white icing (USDA)	4 oz.	392	75.5
*Chocolate malt (Betty Crocker)	1/12 of cake	200	35.8
*Chocolate pudding (Betty Crocker)	1/6 of cake	221	44.0
*Deep chocolate (Duncan Hines)	1/12 of cake (2.7 oz.)	201	34.2
*Double Dutch (Pillsbury)	1/12 of cake	210	33.0
*German chocolate (Betty Crocker)	1/12 of cake	200	35.9
*German chocolate (Pillsbury)	1/12 of cake	210	34.0
*German chocolate, Streusel (Pillsbury)	1/12 of cake	350	52.0
*German chocolate (Swans Down)	1/12 of cake	187	35.8
*Macaroon (Pillsbury) *Bundt*	1/12 of cake	360	52.0
*Milk chocolate (Betty Crocker)	1/12 of cake	199	35.0
*Streusel (Pillsbury)	1/12 of cake	340	52.0
*Swiss chocolate (Duncan Hines)	1/12 of cake (2.7 oz.)	201	34.2

Food and Description	Measure or Quantity	Calories	Carbo- hydrates (grams)
CHOCOLATE CANDY (See CANDY)			
CHOCOLATE DRINK, canned (Borden)	9½-fl.-oz. can	232	32.1
CHOCOLATE DRINK MIX:			
Dutch, instant (Borden)	2 heaping tsps. (¾ oz.)	87	18.9
Hot (USDA)	1 cup (4.9 oz.)	545	102.7
Hot (USDA)	1 oz.	111	21.0
Instant (Ghirardelli)	1 T. (.4 oz.)	48	10.5
Quik	2 heaping tsps.	56	14.4
CHOCOLATE EXTRACT, imitation (Durkee)	1 tsp. (3 grams)	7	
CHOCOLATE, GROUND (Ghirardelli)	¼ cup (1.3 oz.)	163	30.4
CHOCOLATE, HOT, home recipe (USDA)	1 cup (8.8 oz.)	238	26.0
CHOCOLATE ICE CREAM (See also individual brands):			
(Borden) 9.5% fat	¼ pt. (2.3 oz.)	126	16.9
(Meadow Gold) 10% fat	¼ pt.	128	16.5
(Sealtest)	¼ pt. (2.3 oz.)	136	17.3
French (Prestige)	¼ pt. (2.6 oz.)	182	18.0
CHOCOLATE PIE:			
Chiffon, home recipe (USDA)	⅛ of 9″ pie (4.9 oz.)	459	61.2
Meringue, home recipe (USDA)	⅛ of 9″ pie (4.9 oz.)	353	46.9
Nut (Tastykake)	4½-oz. pie	451	64.3
Frozen:			
Cream:			
(Banquet)	2½-oz. serving	202	28.5

(USDA): United States Department of Agriculture
(HEW/FAO): Health, Education and Welfare/Food and Agriculture Organization
* Prepared as Package Directs

Food and Description	Measure or Quantity	Calories	Carbo- hydrates (grams)
(Mrs. Smith's)	⅛ of 8″ pie (2.8 oz.)	247	33.3
Meringue (Mrs. Smith's)	⅛ of 10″ pie (5.2 oz.)	514	61.2
Tart (Pepperidge Farm)	3-oz. pie tart	306	35.2
Velvet nut (Kraft)	⅛ of 16¾-oz. pie	303	30.4
CHOCOLATE PUDDING, Sweetened:			
home recipe with starch base (USDA)	½ cup (4.6 oz.)	192	33.4
Canned:			
(Betty Crocker)	½ cup	175	29.8
(Hunt's)	5-oz. can	239	30.5
(My-T-Fine) *Rich 'N Ready*	5-oz. can	191	32.9
(Thank You)	½ cup	175	29.2
Dark 'N' Sweet (Royal) *Creamerino*	5-oz. container	250	39.0
Fudge (Betty Crocker)	½ cup	175	30.0
Fudge (Del Monte)	5-oz. can	198	32.4
Fudge (Hunt's)	5-oz. can	229	28.9
Fudge (My-T-Fine) *Rich 'N Ready*	5-oz. can	186	34.3
Milk chocolate (Del Monte)	5-oz. can	202	33.6
Milk chocolate (Royal) *Creamerino*	5-oz. container	244	38.3
Chilled (Sanna) dark chocolate	4½-oz. container	191	28.6
Chilled (Sealtest)	4 oz.	136	22.8
Chilled (Breakstone) dark chocolate	5-oz. container	256	35.5
CHOCOLATE PUDDING or PIE FILLING MIX: Sweetened:			
Regular:			
*(Jell-O)	½ cup (5.2 oz.)	174	29.5
*(My-T-Fine)	½ cup	187	31.3
*(Royal)	½ cup (5.1 oz.)	196	31.7
*(Royal) *Dark 'N' Sweet*	½ cup (5.1 oz.)	195	30.7
*Almond (My-T-Fine)	½ cup	196	31.2
*Fudge (Jell-O)	½ cup (5.2 oz.)	174	29.5
*Fudge (My-T-Fine)	½ cup (5 oz.)	190	31.2

Food and Description	Measure or Quantity	Calories	Carbo-hydrates (grams)
*Milk chocolate (Jell-O)	½ cup (5.2 oz.)	174	29.5
*Tapioca (Royal)	½ cup (5.1 oz.)	185	29.2
Instant:			
*(Jell-O)	½ cup (5.4 oz.)	190	33.4
*(Royal)	½ cup (5.1 oz.)	194	31.8
*(Royal) *Dark 'N' Sweet*	½ cup (5.1 oz.)	194	31.7
*Fudge (Jell-O)	½ cup (5.4 oz.)	190	33.4
*Low calorie (D-Zerta)	½ cup (4.6 oz.)	102	11.0
CHOCOLATE RENNET CUSTARD MIX (Junket):			
Powder:			
Dry	1 oz.	116	25.2
*With sugar	4 oz.	113	14.9
Tablet:			
Dry	1 tablet	1	.2
*With sugar	4 oz.	101	13.4
CHOCOLATE SOFT DRINK:			
Sweetened:			
(Canada Dry)	6 fl. oz.	79	19.8
(Cott) cream	6 fl. oz.	92	22.0
(Hoffman) *Cocoa Cooler*	6 fl. oz.	89	22.3
(Hoffman) cream	6 fl. oz.	87	21.9
(Mission) cream	6 fl. oz.	92	22.0
(Yoo Hoo) high protein	6 fl. oz. (6.4 oz.)	100	18.9
(Yukon Club) cream	6 fl. oz.	87	21.9
Low calorie:			
(Canada Dry)	6 fl. oz.	9	.7
(Cott)	6 fl. oz.	2	.2
(Hoffman)	6 fl. oz.	1	.2
(Mission)	6 fl. oz.	2	.2
(No-Cal)	6 fl. oz.	3	0.
(Shasta)	6 fl. oz.	1	.2
CHOCOLATE SYRUP:			
Sweetened:			
Fudge (USDA)	1 T. (.7 oz.)	63	10.3
Thin type (USDA)	1 T. (.7 oz.)	47	11.9
(Hershey's)	1 T. (.6 oz.)	44	9.6

(USDA): United States Department of Agriculture
(HEW/FAO): Health, Education and Welfare/Food and Agriculture Organization
* Prepared as Package Directs

Food and Description	Measure or Quantity	Calories	Carbo-hydrates (grams)
(Smucker's)	1 T. (.6 oz.)	51	11.2
Low calorie (Slim-ette)			
Choco-top	1 T. (.5 oz.)	9	1.6
CHOP SUEY:			
Home recipe, with meat			
(USDA)	1 cup (8.8 oz.)	300	12.8
Canned:			
With meat (USDA)	1 cup (8.8 oz.)	155	10.5
Chicken (Hung's)	8 oz.	120	12.3
Meatless (Hung's)	8 oz.	112	11.2
Pork (Mow Sang)	20-oz. can	167	14.0
Frozen, beef (Banquet)	7-oz. bag	121	9.5
Frozen, dinner (Banquet)	12-oz. dinner	282	38.8
Mix (Durkee)	1⅝-oz. pkg.	128	18.6
CHOW CHOW:			
Sour (USDA)	1 oz.	8	1.2
Sweet (USDA)	1 oz.	33	7.7
(Crosse & Blackwell)	1 T. (.6 oz.)	6	1.0
CHOW MEIN:			
Home recipe, chicken,			
without noodles(USDA)	8 oz.	231	9.1
Canned:			
Without noodles (USDA)	8 oz.	86	16.2
Beef (Chun King)	1 cup	150	11.0
Beef (La Choy)	1 cup	77	4.0
Chicken:			
(Chun King)	1 cup	100	11.2
(Hung's)	8 oz.	104	10.4
(La Choy)	1 cup	74	5.0
(La Choy) bi-pack	1 cup	118	8.0
Meatless:			
(Chun King)	1 cup	83	9.4
(Hung's)	8 oz.	96	8.8
Pork (Chun King)			
Divider-Pak	7-oz. serving (¼ can)	160	11.0
Frozen:			
Beef (Chun King)	½ of 15-oz. pkg.	90	10.0
Chicken (Banquet)	7-oz. bag	123	10.8
Chicken with rice			
(Swanson)	8½-oz. pkg.	188	24.3
Shrimp (Chun King)	½ of 15-oz. pkg.	190	14.0
Shrimp (Temple)	1 cup	132	15.0

Food and Description	Measure or Quantity	Calories	Carbohydrates (grams)
Vegetable (Temple)	1 cup	68	12.0
Mix (Durkee)	1⅝-oz. pkg.	128	18.6

CHOW MEIN NOODLES (See NOODLES, CHOW MEIN)

CHUB, raw (USDA):

Whole	1 lb. (weighed whole)	217	0.
Meat only	4 oz.	164	0.

CHUTNEY, *Major Grey's* (Crosse & Blackwell) | 1 T. (.8 oz.) | 53 | 13.1 |

CIDER (See APPLE CIDER)

CINNAMON, GROUND (Information supplied by General Mills Laboratory) | 1 oz. | 114 | 25.1 |

CINNAMON STICKS, frozen (Aunt Jemima) | 3 pieces (1¾ oz.) | 145 | 21.3 |

CITRON, CANDIED (Liberty) | 1 oz. | 93 | 22.6 |

CITRUS COOLER (Hi-C) | 6 fl. oz. (6.3 oz.) | 90 | 21.7 |

CITRUS SALAD, canned (See GRAPEFRUIT & ORANGE SECTIONS)

CITRUS SOFT DRINK:
low calorie:

Flair, sugar-free	6 fl. oz.	1	.2
(No-Cal)	6 fl. oz.	2	0.

CLACKERS, cereal (General Mills) | 1 cup (1 oz.) | 111 | 22.1 |

CLAM:
Raw, hard or round:

Meat & liq. (USDA)	1 lb. (weighed in shell)	71	6.1

(USDA): United States Department of Agriculture
(HEW/FAO): Health, Education and Welfare/Food and Agriculture Organization
* Prepared as Package Directs

Food and Description	Measure or Quantity	Calories	Carbohydrates (grams)
Meat only (USDA)	1 cup (8 oz.)	182	13.4
Raw, soft, meat & liq. (USDA)	1 lb. (weighed in shell)	142	5.3
Raw, soft, meat only (USDA)	1 cup (8 oz.)	186	3.0
Canned, all kinds:			
Solids & liq. (Bumble Bee)	4½-oz. can	66	3.6
Chopped & minced, solids & liq. (Doxsee)	4 oz.	59	3.2
Chopped & liq. (Doxsee)	4 oz.	66	
Chopped, meat only (Doxsee)	4 oz.	111	2.1
Chopped (Snow)	4 oz.	68	2.4
Creamed, with mushrooms (Snow)	4 oz.	127	7.7
Minced (Snow)	4 oz.	68	2.4
Steamed, meat & broth (Doxsee)	1 pt. 8 fl. oz.	152	
Steamed, meat only (Doxsee)	1 pt. 8 fl. oz.	66	
Whole (Doxsee)	4 oz.	62	
CLAM CAKE, frozen, thins (Mrs. Paul's)	2½-oz. cake	147	16.0
CLAM CHOWDER:			
Manhattan, canned:			
*(Campbell)	1 cup	72	10.5
(Campbell) *Chunky*	1 cup	120	16.9
(Crosse & Blackwell)	6½ oz. (½ can)	61	12.9
*(Doxsee)	1 cup (8.6 oz.)	112	17.7
(Heinz) *Great American*	1 cup (8½ oz.)	111	14.2
(Snow)	8 oz.	85	7.8
New England:			
Canned:			
*(Campbell)	1 cup	157	16.4
(Crosse & Blackwell)	6½ oz. (½ can)	101	10.3
*(Doxsee)	1 cup (8.6 oz.)	214	27.0
(Snow)	½ of 15-oz. can	129	18.3
Mix (Lipton) *Cup-a-Soup*	.8-oz. pkg.	102	12.2
CLAM COCKTAIL (Sau-Sea)	4 oz.	80	19.1
CLAM FRITTERS, home recipe (USDA)	1.4-oz. fritter (2" x 1¾")	124	12.4

COCOA [121]

Food and Description	Measure or Quantity	Calories	Carbo-hydrates (grams)
CLAM JUICE/LIQUOR, canned:			
(USDA)	1 cup (8.3 oz.)	45	5.0
(Doxsee)	8 oz.	43	
(Snow)	8 oz.	31	1.6
CLAM SOUP MIX (Wyler's)	.8-oz. pkg.	112	13.6
CLAM STEW, frozen (Snow)	8 oz.	198	12.9
CLAM STICKS, frozen (Mrs. Paul's)	.8-oz. piece	46	5.9
CLAMATO COCKTAIL (Mott's)	4 oz.	43	9.1
CLARET WINE:			
(Gold Seal) 12% alcohol	3 fl. oz.	82	.4
(Inglenook) Navalle, 12% alcohol	3 fl. oz.	60	.3
(Louis M. Martini) 12.5% alcohol	3 fl. oz.	90	.2
(Taylor) 12.5% alcohol	3 fl. oz.	72	Tr.
CLARISTINE LIQUEUR (Leroux) 86 proof	1 fl. oz.	114	10.8
CLORETS:			
Chewing gum	1 piece	6	1.3
Mint	1 piece	6	1.6
CLUB SODA SOFT DRINK, any brand, regular or dietetic	6 fl. oz.	0	0.
COCKTAIL HOST COCKTAIL, liquid mix (Holland House)	1½ fl. oz.	70	18.0
COCOA, dry:			
Low fat (USDA)	1 T. (5 grams)	10	3.1
Medium-low fat (USDA)	1 T. (5 grams)	12	2.9
Medium-high fat (USDA)	1 T. (5 grams)	14	2.8
High fat (USDA)	1 T.	16	2.6

(USDA): United States Department of Agriculture
(HEW/FAO): Health, Education and Welfare/Food and Agriculture Organization
* Prepared as Package Directs

Food and Description	*Measure or Quantity*	*Calories*	*Carbohydrates (grams)*
Unsweetened (Droste)	1 T. (7 grams)	21	2.9
Unsweetened (Hershey's)	½ cup (1.5 oz.)	185	19.8
Unsweetened (Hershey's)	1 T. (5 grams)	22	2.4
COCOA, HOME RECIPE (USDA)	1 cup (8.8 oz.)	242	27.2
***COCOA KRISPIES*, cereal** (Kellogg's)	1 cup (1 oz.)	111	24.8
COCOA MIX:			
(Kraft)	1 oz.	105	21.3
*(Kraft)	1 cup	129	26.5
(Nestlé's) *Ever Ready*	3 heaping tsps. (.8 oz)	105	19.6
Hot (Hershey's)	1-oz. packet	116	21.2
Hot (Nestlé's)	1-oz. packet	101	22.1
Instant (Hershey's)	3 T. (¾ oz.)	84	19.0
Instant, milk chocolate (Carnation)	1-oz. pkg.	120	20.5
Instant, *Swiss Miss*	1 oz.	103	20.0
***COCOA PEBBLES*, cereal** (Post)	⅞ cup (1 oz.)	111	25.0
***COCOA PUFFS*, cereal** (General Mills)	1 cup (1 oz.)	109	25.2
COCONUT:			
Fresh (USDA):			
Whole	1 lb. (weighed in shell)	816	22.2
Meat only	4 oz.	392	10.7
Meat only	2" x 2" x ½" piece (1.6 oz.)	156	4.2
Grated or shredded, loosely packed	½ cup (1.4 oz.)	225	6.1
Dried, canned or packaged:			
Angel Flake (Baker's)	¼ cup (.7 oz.)	89	7.4
Chocolate (Durkee)	¼ cup (.6 oz.)	88	7.8
Cookie (Baker's)	¼ cup (1 oz.)	140	11.6
Crunchies (Baker's)	¼ cup (1.1 oz.)	176	10.3
Lemon or orange (Durkee)	¼ cup (.6 oz.)	90	7.7
Premium shred (Baker's)	¼ cup (.8 oz.)	105	9.1
COCONUT CAKE, frozen (Pepperidge Farm)	⅙ of cake (3 oz.)	323	46.0

Food and Description	Measure or Quantity	Calories	Carbo-hydrates (grams)
*COCONUT CAKE MIX			
(Duncan Hines)	½₂ of cake (2.7 oz.)	200	35.0
COCONUT PIE:			
Cream:			
(Tastykake)	4-oz. pie	467	48.4
Frozen:			
(Banquet)	2½ oz.	209	24.2
(Morton)	¼ of 16-oz. pie	206	27.8
(Mrs. Smith's)	⅛ of 8" pie (2.8 oz.)	233	31.7
Tart (Pepperidge Farm)	3-oz. pie tart	310	29.0
Custard:			
Home recipe (USDA)	⅛ of 9" pie (5.4 oz.)	357	37.8
Frozen:			
Baked (USDA)	5 oz.	354	41.9
Unbaked (USDA)	5 oz.	291	38.5
(Banquet)	5 oz.	294	39.8
(Morton)	⅛ of 22-oz. pie	224	30.5
(Mrs. Smith's)	⅛ of 8" pie (4 oz.)	265	31.7
Meringue (Mrs. Smith's)	⅛ of 10" pie (5.2 oz.)	438	48.8
COCONUT PIE FILLING MIX (Also see COCONUT PUDDING MIX):			
Custard & pie, dry (USDA)	1 oz.	133	20.0
*Custard, prepared with egg yolk or milk (USDA)	5 oz. (including crust)	288	41.3
COCONUT PUDDING MIX:			
*Cream, regular (Jell-O)	½ cup (5.2 oz.)	175	25.8
*Cream, instant (Jell-O)	½ cup (5.3 oz.)	188	29.0
*Toasted, instant (Royal)	½ cup (5.1 oz.)	184	27.3
COCONUT SOFT DRINK			
(Yoo-Hoo) high protein	6 fl. oz. (6.4 oz.)	100	18.9

(USDA): United States Department of Agriculture
(HEW/FAO): Health, Education and Welfare/Food and Agriculture Organization
* Prepared as Package Directs

Food and Description	Measure or Quantity	Calories	Carbohydrates (grams)
COCO WHEATS, cereal	3 T. (1.3 oz.)	132	27.2
COD:			
Raw, whole (USDA)	1 lb. (weighed whole)	110	0.
Raw, meat only (USDA)	4 oz.	88	0.
Broiled (USDA)	4 oz.	193	0.
Canned (USDA)	4 oz.	96	0.
Dehydrated, lightly salted (USDA)	4 oz.	425	0.
Dried, salted (USDA)	5½″ x 1½″ x ½″ (2.8 oz.)	104	0.
Frozen (Gorton)	⅓ of 1-lb. pkg.	117	0.
Frozen (Ship Ahoy)	⅓ of 1-lb. pkg.	112	0.
COFFEE:			
Max-Pax	¾ cup	2	.5
*Regular (Maxwell House)	¾ cup	2	.4
*Regular (Yuban)	¾ cup	2	.4
Instant:			
Dry (USDA)	1 rounded tsp. (2 grams)	3	.9
*(USDA)	1 cup (8.4 oz.)	3	.9
(Borden)	1 rounded tsp. (2 grams)	5	.9
*(Chase & Sanborn)	5 fl. oz.	1	Tr.
Kava (Borden)	1 tsp. (1 gram)	3	.5
*(Maxwell House)	¾ cup	4	.9
Nescafé	1 slightly rounded tsp. (2 grams)	4	.7
*(Yuban)	¾ cup	4	.9
Decaffeinated:			
Decaf	1 tsp. (2 grams)	4	.6
Sanka, regular	¾ cup	2	.4
Freeze-dried:			
Maxim	¾ cup	4	.9
Taster's Choice	1 slightly rounded tsp. (2 grams)	4	.7
COFFEE CAKE:			
(Drake's) junior	1 pkg. (1.1 oz.)	126	18.4
(Drake's) large	11-oz. cake	1195	181.9
(Drake's) small	2.4-oz. cake	280	40.3
Almond Danish with icing (Pillsbury)	1 roll	140	20.0

Food and Description	Measure or Quantity	Calories	Carbohydrates (grams)
Blueberry ring (Sara Lee)	1 oz.	108	15.0
Butterfly (Mrs. Smith's)	1 piece (2¾ oz.)	299	38.0
Butter horn (Van de Kamp's)	1 piece (2.2 oz.)	287	
Cherry (Mrs. Smith's)	1 piece (2¾ oz.)	238	25.0
Cinnamon with icing (Pillsbury)	1 roll	115	18.0
Cinnamon twist (Pepperidge Farm)	⅛ of cake (1.8 oz.)	156	21.3
Cinnamon, 1-lb. loaf (Van de Kamp's)	1 slice (.8 oz.)	85	
Danish pastry, without fruit or nuts (USDA)	1" x 4¼" dia. (2.3 oz.)	274	29.6
Danish (Mrs. Smith's) tray pack	1 piece (1¾ oz.)	190	23.0
Danish, apple (Morton)	1 cake (13.5 oz.)	1130	166.6
Danish, apple (Sara Lee)	1 oz.	84	11.0
Danish, caramel (Pillsbury)	1 roll	155	20.5
Danish, cherry (Sara Lee)	1 oz.	75	11.0
Lemon ring (Drake's)	13-oz. ring	1028	217.3
Melt-A-Way (Morton)	13-oz. cake	1511	184.8
Pecan (Pepperidge Farm)	1 piece (1.7 oz.)	195	20.5
COFFEE CAKE MIX:			
Dry (USDA)	1 oz.	122	21.9
*Prepared with egg & milk (USDA)	2 oz.	183	29.7
*(Aunt Jemima)	⅛ of cake (1.9 oz.)	186	30.7
COFFEE-MATE, cream substitute	1 tsp. (1.9 oz.)	11	1.0
COFFEE-RICH, cream substitute	1 tsp. (5 grams)	8	.7
COFFEE SOFT DRINK, low calorie (No-Cal)	6 fl. oz.	3	<.1
COFFEE SOUTHERN, liqueur	1 fl. oz.	79	8.8

(USDA): United States Department of Agriculture
(HEW/FAO): Health, Education and Welfare/Food and Agriculture Organization
* Prepared as Package Directs

Food and Description	Measure or Quantity	Calories	Carbo- hydrates (grams)
COGNAC (See **DISTILLED LIQUOR**)			
COLA SOFT DRINK:			
Sweetened:			
(Canada Dry) Jamaica	6 fl. oz.	79	19.8
(Clicquot Club)	6 fl. oz.	83	20.0
Coca-Cola	6 fl. oz.	73	18.5
(Cott)	6 fl. oz.	83	20.0
(Dr. Brown's)	6 fl. oz.	81	20.1
(Hoffman)	6 fl. oz.	81	20.1
(Key Food)	6 fl. oz.	77	19.4
(Kirsch)	6 fl. oz.	80	20.1
(Mission)	6 fl. oz.	83	20.0
Mr. Cola	6 fl. oz.	79	20.3
Pepsi-Cola	6 fl. oz. (6.6 oz.)	78	19.7
RC with a twist (Royal Crown)	6 fl. oz. (6.5 oz.)	74	20.5
(Royal Crown)	6 fl. oz. (6.5 oz.)	78	19.5
(Salute)	6 fl. oz.	74	18.8
(Shasta)	6 fl. oz.	76	19.4
Cherry (Shasta)	6 fl. oz.	76	19.4
Low calorie:			
(Canada Dry)	6 fl. oz.	3	.6
Diet Pepsi-Cola	6 fl. oz.	<1	<.1
Diet Rite	6 fl. oz.	<1	Tr.
(Dr. Brown's)	6 fl. oz.	1	.2
(No-Cal)	6 fl. oz.	<1	<.1
RC Cola	6 fl. oz.	<1	Tr.
(Shasta)	6 fl. oz.	<1	<.1
Cherry (Shasta)	6 fl. oz.	<1	<.1
Tab	6 fl. oz.	<1	<.1
COLA SYRUP, dietetic (No-Cal)	1 tsp. (5 grams)	<1	Tr.
COLD DUCK WINE (Great Western)	3 fl. oz.	93	
COLESLAW, not drained (USDA):			
Prepared with commercial French dressing	4 oz.	108	8.6
Prepared with homemade French dressing	4 oz.	146	5.8
Prepared with mayonnaise	4 oz.	163	5.4

Food and Description	Measure or Quantity	Calories	Carbo-hydrates (grams)
Prepared with mayonnaise-type salad dressing	1 cup (4.2 oz.)	118	8.5
COLLARDS:			
Raw (USDA):			
Leaves including stems	1 lb.	181	32.7
Leaves only	½ lb.	70	11.6
Boiled, drained (USDA):			
Leaves, cooked in large amount water	½ cup (3.4 oz.)	29	4.6
Leaves & stems, cooked in small amount water	½ cup (3.4 oz.)	31	4.8
Frozen:			
Not thawed (USDA)	10-oz. pkg.	91	16.4
Boiled, chopped, drained (USDA)	½ cup (3 oz.)	26	4.8
Chopped (Birds Eye)	⅓ of 10-oz. pkg.	29	4.5
COLLINS MIX (Bar-Tender's)	1 serving (⅝ oz.)	70	17.4
COLLINS MIXER, SOFT DRINK (See **TOM COLLINS SOFT DRINK**)			
CONCENTRATE, cereal (Kellogg's)	⅓ cup (1 oz.)	108	14.8
CONCORD WINE:			
(Gold Seal) 13–14% alcohol	3 fl. oz. (3.3 oz.)	125	9.8
(Mogen David) 12% alcohol	3 fl. oz.	120	16.0
Red (Pleasant Valley) 12.5% alcohol	3 fl. oz.	90	
CONSOMMÉ MADRILENE, canned, clear or red (Crosse & Blackwell)	6½ oz. (½ can)	33	2.4
COOKIE. The following are listed by type or brand name:			
Almond crescent (Nabisco)	1 piece (7 grams)	34	5.0
Almond toast, Mandel (Stella D'oro)	1 piece (.5 oz.)	49	9.6

(USDA): United States Department of Agriculture
(HEW/FAO): Health, Education and Welfare/Food and Agriculture Organization
* Prepared as Package Directs

Food and Description	Measure or Quantity	Calories	Carbo-hydrates (grams)
Angelica Goodies (Stella D'oro)	1 piece (.8 oz.)	100	14.6
Angel puffs, dietetic (Stella D'oro)	1 piece	17	1.4
Anginetti (Stella D'oro)	1 piece (5 grams)	28	2.4
Animal cracker:			
(USDA)	1 oz.	122	22.7
(Nabisco) *Barnum's*	1 piece (3 grams)	12	2.0
(Sunshine) regular	1 piece (2 grams)	10	1.7
(Sunshine) iced	1 piece (5 grams)	26	3.7
Anisette sponge (Stella D'oro)	1 piece (.5 oz.)	39	10.0
Anisette toast (Stella D'oro)	1 piece (.4 oz.)	39	7.8
Applesauce (Sunshine)	1 piece (.6 oz.)	86	11.9
Arrowroot (Sunshine)	1 piece (4 grams)	16	3.0
Apple strudel (Nabisco)	1 piece (.4 oz.)	48	6.8
Assortments:			
(USDA)	1 oz.	136	20.1
(Stella D'oro) *Lady Stella Assortment*	1 piece (8 grams)	37	5.0
(Sunshine) *Lady Joan*	1 piece (9 grams)	42	5.8
(Sunshine) *Lady Joan,* iced	1 piece (.4 oz.)	47	6.1
Aunt Sally, iced (Sunshine)	1 piece (.8 oz.)	96	19.7
Bana-Bee (Nab)	1 pkg. (1¾ oz.)	253	31.4
Big Treat (Sunshine)	1 piece (1.3 oz.)	153	26.6
Bordeaux (Pepperidge Farm)	1 piece (8 grams)	36	5.1
Breakfast Treats (Stella D'oro)	1 piece (.8 oz.)	99	15.0
Brown edge wafers (Nabisco)	1 piece (6 grams)	28	4.1
Brownie:			
(Drake's) junior	⅔-oz. cake	80	10.0
(Tastykake)	1 pkg. (2¼ oz.)	242	34.0
Chocolate nut (Pepperidge Farm)	1 piece (.4 oz.)	54	6.3
Peanut butter (Tastykake)	1 pkg. (1¾ oz.)	239	32.0
Pecan fudge (Keebler)	1 pkg. (1.8 oz.)	230	27.9
Pecan fudge, bulk (Keebler)	.9-oz. square	115	13.9
Frozen, with nuts & chocolate icing (USDA)	1 oz.	119	17.2

Food and Description	Measure or Quantity	Calories	Carbo- hydrates (grams)
Brussels (Pepperidge Farm)	1 piece (8 grams)	42	4.6
Butter:			
(Nabisco)	1 piece (5 grams)	23	3.6
(Sunshine)	1 piece (5 grams)	23	3.5
Buttercup (Keebler)	1 piece (5 grams)	24	3.6
Butterscotch Fudgies (Tastykake)	1 pkg. (1¾ oz.)	251	35.0
Capri (Pepperidge Farm)	1 piece (.6 oz.)	82	9.7
Caramel peanut logs (Nabisco) *Hey Days*	1 piece (.8 oz.)	122	13.4
Cardiff (Pepperidge Farm)	1 piece (4 grams)	18	2.5
Cherry Coolers (Sunshine)	1 piece (6 grams)	29	4.5
Chinese almond (Stella D'oro)	1 piece (1.2 oz.)	178	21.5
Chocolate & chocolate- covered:			
(USDA)	1 oz.	126	20.3
Como (Stella D'oro)	1 piece (1.1 oz.)	155	16.8
Chocolate creme (Wise)	1 piece (7 grams)	32	4.9
Peanut bars (Nabisco) *Ideal*	1 piece (.6 oz.)	94	10.3
Pinwheel cakes (Nabisco)	1 piece (1.1 oz.)	139	20.9
Snaps (Nabisco)	1 piece (4 grams)	18	2.7
Snaps (Sunshine)	1 piece (3 grams)	14	2.4
Wafers (Nabisco) *Famous*	1 piece (6 grams)	28	4.7
Chocolate chip:			
(USDA)	1 oz.	134	19.8
(Drake's)	1 piece (.5 oz.)	74	9.9
(Keebler)	1 piece (.6 oz.)	80	11.0
(Nabisco)	1 piece (7 grams)	33	4.5
(Nabisco) *Chips Ahoy*	1 piece (.4 oz.)	51	7.5
(Nabisco) *Family Favorites*	1 piece (7 grams)	33	4.5
Snaps (Nabisco)	1 piece (4 grams)	21	3.4
(Pepperidge Farm)	1 piece (.4 oz.)	52	6.2
(Sunshine) *Chip-A-Roos*	1 piece (.4 oz.)	63	7.7
(Tastykake) *Choc-O-Chip*	1¾-oz. pkg. (.4 pieces)	283	34.8
Cinnamon crisp (Keebler)	1 piece (4 grams)	17	2.7

(USDA): United States Department of Agriculture
(HEW/FAO): Health, Education and Welfare/Food and Agriculture Organization
* Prepared as Package Directs

Food and Description	Measure or Quantity	Calories	Carbo-hydrates (grams)
Cinnamon, spice, vanilla sandwich (Nab) *Crinkles*	1⅝-oz. pkg. (6 pieces)	228	33.4
Cinnamon sugar (Pepperidge Farm)	1 piece (.4 oz.)	52	7.0
Cinnamon toast (Sunshine)	1 piece (3 grams)	13	2.3
Coconut:			
Bars (Nabisco)	1 piece (9 grams)	45	6.3
Bars (Sunshine)	1 piece (.4 oz.)	47	6.2
Chocolate chip (Nabisco)	1 piece (.5 oz.)	77	9.0
Chocolate chip (Sunshine)	1 piece (.6 oz.)	80	9.7
Chocolate drop (Keebler)	1 piece (.5 oz.)	75	8.5
Coconut Kiss (Tastykake)	1¾-oz. pkg. (4 pieces)	318	33.2
Family Favorites (Nabisco)	1 piece (3 grams)	16	2.2
Jumble (Drake's)	1 piece (.4 oz.)	52	7.4
Commodore (Keebler)	1 piece (.5 oz.)	· 65	10.1
Como Delight (Stella D'oro)	1 piece (1.1 oz.)	153	18.3
Cowboys and Indians (Nabisco)	1 piece (2 grams)	10	1.8
Cream Lunch (Sunshine)	1 piece (.4 oz.)	45	7.3
Creme Wafer Stick (Dutch Twin)	1 piece (7 grams)	36	5.9
Creme Wafer Stick (Nabisco)	1 piece (9 grams)	50	5.9
Cup Custard (Sunshine):			
Chocolate	1 piece (.5 oz.)	70	9.3
Vanilla	1 piece (.5 oz.)	71	9.3
Devil's food cake:			
(Nab)	1¼-oz. pkg. (2 pieces)	135	26.8
(Nabisco)	1 piece (.5 oz.)	49	9.8
(Sunshine)	1 piece (.5 oz.)	55	10.9
Dixie Vanilla (Sunshine)	1 piece (.5 oz.)	60	13.1
Dresden (Pepperidge Farm)	1 piece (.6 oz.)	· 83	10.0
Egg Jumbo (Stella D'oro)	1 piece (.4 oz.)	40	7.6
Fig bar:			
(USDA)	1 oz.	101	21.4
(Keebler)	1 piece (.7 oz.)	71	14.4
(Nab) *Fig Newton*	2-oz. pkg. (2 pieces)	208	40.4

Food and Description	Measure or Quantity	Calories	Carbo-hydrates (grams)
(Nabisco) *Fig Newton*	1 piece (.6 oz.)	57	11.2
(Sunshine)	1 piece (.4 oz.)	45	9.2
Fortune (Chun King)	1 piece	31	4.6
Fruit, iced (Nabisco)	1 piece (.6 oz.)	71	13.5
Fudge:			
(Sunshine)	1 piece (.5 oz.)	72	9.4
Chip (Pepperidge Farm)	1 piece (.4 oz.)	51	6.7
Fudge Stripes (Keebler)	1 piece (.4 oz.)	57	7.5
Gingersnap:			
(USDA)	1 oz.	119	22.6
(USDA) crumbs	1 cup (4.1 oz.)	483	91.8
(Keebler)	1 piece (6 grams)	24	4.3
(Nabisco) old-fashioned	1 piece (7 grams)	29	5.4
(Sunshine)	1 piece (6 grams)	24	4.4
Zu Zu (Nabisco)	1 piece (4 grams)	16	3.1
Golden Bars (Stella D'oro)	1 piece (1 oz.)	123	16.0
Golden Fruit (Sunshine)	1 piece (.7 oz.)	61	14.4
Graham Cracker (See **CRACKERS,** Graham)			
Hermit bar, frosted (Tastykake)	1 pkg. (2 oz.)	321	60.8
Home Plate (Keebler)	1 piece (.5 oz.)	58	9.9
Hostest With The Mostest (Stella D'oro)	1 piece (8 grams)	39	5.2
Hydrox (Sunshine):			
Regular or mint	1 piece (.4 oz.)	48	7.1
Vanilla	1 piece (.4 oz.)	50	7.1
Jan Hagel (Keebler)	1 piece (10 grams)	44	6.7
Keebies (Keebler)	1 piece (.4 oz.)	51	7.1
Ladyfingers (USDA)	.4-oz. ladyfinger (3¼" x 1⅜" x 1⅛")	40	7.1
Lemon:			
(Sunshine)	1 piece (.5 oz.)	76	9.8
Jumble rings (Nabisco)	1 piece (.5 oz.)	68	11.0
Lemon Coolers (Sunshine)	1 piece (6 grams)	29	4.5
Nut crunch (Pepperidge Farm)	1 piece (.4 oz.)	57	6.4
Snaps (Nabisco)	1 piece (4 grams)	17	3.1
Lido (Pepperidge Farm)	1 piece (.6 oz.)	91	10.0

(USDA): United States Department of Agriculture
(HEW/FAO): Health, Education and Welfare/Food and Agriculture Organization
* Prepared as Package Directs

Food and Description	Measure or Quantity	Calories	Carbo-hydrates (grams)
Lisbon (Pepperidge Farm)	1 piece (5 grams)	28	3.3
Macaroon:			
(USDA)	1 oz.	135	18.7
Almond (Tastykake)	2-oz. pkg. (2 pieces)	336	35.1
Coconut (Nabisco)			
Bake Shop	1 piece (.7 oz.)	87	12.1
Coconut (Van de Kamp's)	1 piece (.7 oz.)	89	
Sandwich (Nabisco)	1 piece (.5 oz.)	71	9.5
Margherite, chocolate (Stella D'oro)	1 piece (.6 oz.)	73	10.6
Margherite, vanilla (Stella D'oro)	1 piece (.6 oz.)	73	10.5
Marquisette (Pepperidge Farm)	1 piece (8 grams)	45	5.0
Marshmallow:			
(USDA)	1 oz.	116	20.5
Fancy Crests (Nabisco)	1 piece (.5 oz.)	53	10.4
Mallowmars (Nabisco)	1 piece (.5 oz.)	60	8.7
Mallo Puff (Sunshine)	1 piece (.6 oz.)	63	12.2
Minarets (Nabisco)	1 piece (10 grams)	46	5.7
Puffs (Nabisco)	1 piece (.7 oz.)	94	12.8
Sandwich (Nabisco)	1 piece (8 grams)	32	5.7
Twirls (Nabisco)	1 piece (1.1 oz.)	133	21.9
Milano (Pepperidge Farm)	1 piece (.4 oz.)	62	7.2
Milano, mint (Pepperidge Farm)	1 piece (.5 oz.)	76	8.4
Mint sandwich (Nabisco)			
Mystic	1 piece (.6 oz.)	88	10.6
Molasses (USDA)	1 oz.	120	21.5
Molasses & Spice (Sunshine)	1 piece (.6 oz.)	67	11.9
Naples (Pepperidge Farm)	1 piece (6 grams)	33	3.7
Nassau (Pepperidge Farm)	1 piece (.6 oz.)	83	9.2
Oatmeal:			
(Drake's)	1 piece (.5 oz.)	69	10.1
(Keebler) old-fashioned	1 piece (.6 oz.)	79	11.7
(Nabisco)	1 piece (.6 oz.)	82	12.3
(Nabisco) *Family Favorites*	1 piece (5 grams)	24	3.8
(Sunshine)	1 piece (.4 oz.)	58	8.9
(Van de Kamp's)	1 piece (.6 oz.)	59	
Iced (Sunshine)	1 piece (.5 oz.)	69	11.6
Irish (Pepperidge Farm)	1 piece (.4 oz.)	50	7.1
Peanut butter (Sunshine)	1 piece (.6 oz.)	79	10.5
Raisin (USDA)	1 oz.	128	20.8

Food and Description	Measure or Quantity	Calories	Carbo- hydrates (grams)
Raisin (Nabisco)			
Bake Shop	1 piece (.6 oz.)	77	11.5
Raisin (Pepperidge Farm)	1 piece (.4 oz.)	55	7.5
Raisin bar (Tastykake)	1 pkg. (2¼ oz.)	298	47.6
Whole wheat (Drake's)	1 piece (.5 oz.)	75	11.4
Old Country Treats			
(Stella D'oro)	1 piece (.5 oz.)	64	7.1
Orleans (Pepperidge Farm)	1 piece (6 grams)	30	3.5
Peach-apricot pastry			
(Stella D'oro)	1 piece (.8 oz.)	99	15.0
Peanut & peanut butter:			
(USDA)	1 oz.	134	19.0
Bars, cocoa-covered			
(Nabisco) *Crowns*	1 piece (.6 oz.)	92	10.0
Caramel logs (Nabisco)			
Heydays	1 piece (.8 oz.)	122	13.4
Creme patties (Nab)	3 pieces (½-oz. pkg.)	74	8.4
Creme patties (Nab)	6 pieces (1-oz. pkg.)	148	16.8
Creme patties (Nabisco)	1 piece (7 grams)	34	3.9
Creme patties, cocoa-covered (Nabisco)			
Fancy	1 piece (.4 oz.)	60	6.4
Patties (Sunshine)	1 piece (7 grams)	33	4.2
Sandwich (Nabisco)			
Nutter Butter	1 piece (.5 oz.)	69	9.2
Pecan Sandies (Keebler)	1 piece (.6 oz.)	85	9.2
Penguins (Keebler)	1 piece (.8 oz.)	111	14.0
Pfefferneuse, spice drop			
(Stella D'oro)	1 piece	40	
Pirouette (Pepperidge Farm):			
Chocolate laced	1 piece (7 grams)	38	4.5
Lemon or original	1 piece (7 grams)	37	4.4
Pitter Patter (Keebler)	1 piece (.6 oz.)	84	10.9
Pizzelle, Carolines			
(Stella D'oro)	1 piece (.4 oz.)	49	6.7
Raisin:			
(USDA)	1 oz.	107	22.9

(USDA): United States Department of Agriculture
(HEW/FAO): Health, Education and Welfare/Food and Agriculture Organization
* Prepared as Package Directs

Food and Description	Measure or Quantity	Calories	Carbo-hydrates (grams)
Fruit biscuit (Nabisco)	1 piece (.5 oz.)	58	12.3
Rich 'n Chips (Keebler)	1 piece (.5 oz.)	73	8.9
Rochelle (Pepperidge Farm)	1 piece (.6 oz.)	81	9.6
Sandwich, creme:			
(USDA)	1 oz.	140	19.6
(Tom Houston)	1 piece (.5 oz.)	74	8.4
Cameo (Nabisco)	1 piece (.5 oz.)	68	10.5
Chocolate chip (Nabisco)	1 piece (.5 oz.)	73	9.1
Chocolate fudge:			
(Keebler)	1 piece (.7 oz.)	99	13.0
Assorted (Nabisco)			
Cookie Break	1 piece (.4 oz.)	52	7.0
Chocolate (Nabisco)			
Cookie Break	1 piece (.4 oz.)	53	7.1
Orbit (Sunshine)	1 piece (.4 oz.)	51	7.0
Oreo (Nab)	4 pieces (1-oz. pkg.)	140	20.1
Oreo (Nab)	6 pieces (1⅝-oz. pkg.)	228	32.7
Oreo (Nab)	6 pieces (2⅛-oz. pkg.)	298	42.8
Oreo (Nabisco)	1 piece (.4 oz.)	51	7.3
Oreo & Swiss (Nab)	6 pieces (1⅝-oz. pkg.)	230	31.4
Oreo & Swiss (Nab)	6 pieces (2¼-oz. pkg.)	319	43.6
Oreo & Swiss, assortment (Nabisco)	1 piece (.4 oz.)	51	7.0
Pride (Nabisco)	1 piece (.4 oz.)	55	7.3
Social Tea (Nabisco)	1 piece (.4 oz.)	51	7.2
Swiss (Nab)	4 pieces (1-oz. pkg.)	144	18.2
Swiss (Nab)	6 pieces (1¾-oz. pkg.)	252	31.9
Swiss (Nabisco)	1 piece (.4 oz.)	52	6.6
Vanilla (Keebler)	1 piece (.6 oz.)	82	11.1
Vanilla (Nabisco)	1 piece (.4 oz.)	52	7.0
Vienna Finger (Sunshine)	1 piece (.5 oz.)	71	10.5
Sesame, Regina (Stella D'oro)	1 piece (.4 oz.)	51	6.9
Shortbread or shortcake:			
(USDA)	1 oz.	141	18.5
(USDA)	1¾" square (8 grams)	40	5.2
(Nabisco) *Dandy*	1 piece (.4 oz.)	46	7.7

Food and Description	Measure or Quantity	Calories	Carbo-hydrates (grams)
(Pepperidge Farm)	1 piece (.5 oz.)	72	8.3
Cherry nut (Van de Kamp's)	1 piece (.4 oz.)	59	
Lorna Doone (Nab)	4 pieces (1-oz. pkg.)	138	19.0
Lorna Doone (Nab)	6 pieces (1½-oz. pkg.)	207	28.5
Lorna Doone (Nabisco)	1 piece (8 grams)	37	5.1
Pecan (Nabisco)	1 piece (.5 oz.)	80	9.0
Scotties (Sunshine)	1 piece (8 grams)	39	5.0
Striped (Nabisco)	1 piece (10 grams)	50	6.8
Vanilla (Tastykake)	6 pieces (2¼-oz. pkg.)	352	43.8
Social Tea Biscuit (Nabisco)	1 piece (5 grams)	21	3.5
Spiced wafers (Nabisco)	1 piece (10 grams)	41	7.4
Sprinkles (Sunshine)	1 piece (.6 oz.)	57	11.4
Sugar cookie:			
(Keebler) old-fashioned	1 piece (.6 oz.)	78	12.4
(Pepperidge Farm)	1 piece (.4 oz.)	51	7.0
(Sunshine)	1 piece (.6 oz.)	86	11.9
(Van de Kamp's)	1 piece (.6 oz.)	79	
Brown (Nabisco) *Family Favorite*	1 piece (5 grams)	25	3.0
Brown (Pepperidge Farm)	1 piece (.4 oz.)	48	6.9
Rings (Nabisco)	1 piece (.5 oz.)	69	10.7
Sugar wafer:			
(USDA)	1 oz.	137	20.8
(Nab) *Biscos*	3 pieces (⅞-oz. pkg.)	128	17.5
(Nabisco) *Biscos*	1 piece (4 grams)	19	2.5
(Sunshine)	1 piece (9 grams)	43	6.6
Assorted (Dutch Twin)	1 piece (7 grams)	34	4.7
Krisp Kreem (Keebler)	1 piece (6 grams)	31	3.7
Lemon (Sunshine)	1 piece (9 grams)	44	6.5
Swedish Kreme (Keebler)	1 piece (5.7 oz.)	98	12.2
Tahiti (Pepperidge Farm)	1 piece (.5 oz.)	84	8.6
Toy (Sunshine)	1 piece (3 grams)	13	2.1
Vanilla creme (Wise)	1 piece (7 grams)	33	5.0
Vanilla snap (Nabisco)	1 piece (3 grams)	13	2.3

(USDA): United States Department of Agriculture
(HEW/FAO): Health, Education and Welfare/Food and Agriculture Organization
* Prepared as Package Directs

Food and Description	Measure or Quantity	Calories	Carbo-hydrates (grams)
Vanilla wafer:			
(USDA)	1 oz.	131	21.1
(Keebler)	1 piece (4 grams)	19	2.6
(Nabisco) *Nilla*	1 piece (4 grams)	18	2.9
(Sunshine) small	1 piece (3 grams)	15	2.2
Venice (Pepperidge Farm)	1 piece (.4 oz.)	57	6.3
Waffle creme (Dutch Twin)	1 piece (9 grams)	44	6.1
Waffle creme (Nabisco) *Biscos*	1 piece (8 grams)	42	6.0
Yum Yums (Sunshine)	1 piece (.5 oz.)	83	10.4
COOKIE, DIETETIC:			
Angel puffs (Stella D'oro)	1 piece (3 grams)	17	1.5
Apple pastry (Stella D'oro)	1 piece (.8 oz.)	94	13.6
Assorted (Estee)	1 piece (5 grams)	26	3.0
Bittersweet chocolate wafer (Estee)	1 piece (.7 oz.)	115	10.0
Chocolate chip (Dia-Mel)	1 piece (9 grams)	40	5.8
Chocolate chip (Estee)	1 piece (7 grams)	32	4.6
Chocolate wafer (Estee)	1 piece (5 grams)	27	2.4
Fig pastry (Stella D'oro)	1 piece (.9 oz.)	100	15.5
Fruit wafer (Estee)	1 piece (5 grams)	27	2.7
Have-A-Heart (Stella D'oro)	1 piece (.7 oz.)	97	11.3
Kichel (Stella D'oro)	1 piece (1 gram)	8	.7
Milk chocolate wafer (Estee)	1 piece (.7 oz.)	110	10.0
Oatmeal raisin (Estee)	1 piece (7 grams)	34	4.5
Peach-apricot pastry (Stella D'oro)	1 piece (.8 oz.)	104	15.2
Prune pastry (Stella D'oro)	1 piece (.8 oz.)	92	14.3
Royal Nuggets (Stella D'oro)	1 piece (<1 gram)	2	.1
Sandwich (Estee)	1 piece (.4 oz.)	57	7.2
Vanilla wafer (Estee)	1 piece (5 grams)	28	2.6
COOKIE DOUGH,			
Refrigerated:			
Unbaked, plain (USDA)	1 oz.	127	16.7
Baked, plain (USDA)	1 oz.	141	18.4
(Pillsbury):			
Almond, cherry	1 piece	47	6.3
Apple cinnamon	1 piece	53	7.3
Brownie, fudge	2" sq.	140	22.0
Butterscotch nut	1 piece	53	6.7
Chocolate, Swiss-style	1 piece	53	7.0
Chocolate chip	1 piece	57	7.7
Cinnamon sugar	1 piece	50	7.3
Oatmeal & chocolate chip	1 piece	57	7.3

Food and Description	Measure or Quantity	Calories	Carbo-hydrates (grams)
Oatmeal raisin	1 piece	60	9.0
Peanut butter	1 piece	53	6.3
Peanut butter & chocolate chip	1 piece	50	5.7
Sugar	1 piece	53	7.0
COOKIE, HOME RECIPE:			
Brownie with nuts (USDA)	1¾" x 1¾" x ⅞"	97	10.2
Chocolate chip (USDA)	1 oz.	146	17.0
Sugar, soft, thick (USDA)	1 oz.	126	19.3
COOKIE MIX:			
*Apple, Fruit 'N Crunch Bar (Pillsbury)	2" sq.	140	18.0
*Blueberry, Fruit 'N Crunch Bar (Pillsbury)	2" sq.	140	18.0
Brownie:			
*Butterscotch (Betty Crocker)	1½" sq.	59	9.6
*"Cake like," family size (Duncan Hines)	½4 of pan (1.2 oz.)	148	20.1
*"Cake like," regular size (Duncan Hines)	⅟16 of pan (1.2 oz.)	152	20.7
*Fudge (Betty Crocker)	1½" sq.	58	9.6
*Fudge, supreme (Betty Crocker)	1½" sq.	59	9.9
*Fudge, chewy, family size (Duncan Hines)	½4 of pan (1.1 oz.)	142	19.8
*Fudge, chewy, regular size (Duncan Hines)	⅟16 of pan (1.2 oz.)	147	20.5
*Fudge (Pillsbury)	1½" sq.	60	9.5
*German chocolate (Betty Crocker)	1½" sq.	70	12.0
*Walnut (Betty Crocker)	1½" sq.	63	9.5
*Walnut (Pillsbury)	1½" sq.	65	10.0
*Cherry, Fruit 'N Crunch Bar (Pillsbury)	2" sq.	150	21.0

(USDA): United States Department of Agriculture
(HEW/FAO): Health, Education and Welfare/Food and Agriculture
          Organization
* Prepared as Package Directs

Food and Description	Measure or Quantity	Calories	Carbo-hydrates (grams)
Chocolate mint (Nestlé's)	1 oz.	133	20.1
*Date bar (Betty Crocker)	2″ x 1″ bar	58	8.8
*Macaroon, coconut (Betty Crocker)	1 macaroon (1¾″)	73	10.2
Lemon (Nestlé's)	1 oz.	132	20.1
*Peach, Fruit 'N Crunch Bar (Pillsbury)	2″ sq.	140	19.0
*Pecan bar (Pillsbury)	2″ x 1¼″ piece	95	10.5
*Strawberry, Fruit 'N Crunch Bar (Pillsbury)	2″ sq.	140	19.0
Sugar (Nestlé's)	1 oz.	132	20.1
*Toll House with morsels (Nestlé's)	1 piece (.4 oz.)	52	7.2
*Toll House without morsels (Nestlé's)	1 piece (8 grams)	42	5.7
Vienna Dream bar (Betty Crocker)	2″ x 1⅓″	87	10.3

COOKING FATS (See **FATS**)

COOL 'N CREAMY (Birds Eye) — ½ cup (4.4 oz.) — 172 — 27.7

CORDIAL (See individual kinds of liqueur by flavor or brand name)

CORDON D' ALSACE, Alsatian wine, 12% alcohol (Willm) — 3 fl. oz. — 66 — 3.6

CORDON DE BORDEAUX, French Bordeaux, red or white (Chanson) 11½% alcohol — 3 fl. oz. — 60 — 6.3

CORDON DE BOURGOGNE, French white Burgundy, (Chanson) 11½% alcohol — 3 fl. oz. — 81 — 6.3

CORDON DU RHONE, French red Rhone wine, (Chanson) 12% alcohol — 3 fl. oz. — 84 — 6.3

Food and Description	Measure or Quantity	Calories	Carbo-hydrates (grams)
CORN:			
Fresh, white or yellow (USDA):			
Raw, untrimmed, on cob	1 lb. (weighed in husk)	157	36.1
Raw, trimmed, on cob	1 lb. (husk removed)	240	55.1
Boiled, kernels, cut from cob, drained	1 cup (5.9 oz.)	138	31.2
Boiled, whole	4.9-oz. ear (5″ x 1¾″)	70	16.2
Canned, regular pack:			
Golden or yellow, whole kernel:			
Solids & liq., vacuum pack (USDA)	½ cup (3.7 oz.)	88	21.7
Solids & liq., wet pack (USDA)	½ cup (4.5 oz.)	84	20.1
Drained solids, wet pack (USDA)	½ cup (3 oz.)	72	17.0
Drained solids (Butter Kernel)	½ cup (4.1 oz.)	75	18.0
Solids & liq.:			
(Del Monte) vacuum pack	½ cup (3.7 oz.)	91	19.6
(Green Giant)	½ of 8.5-oz. can	80	16.3
(Stokely-Van Camp)	½ cup (4.5 oz.)	74	17.6
Niblets, vacuum pack	⅓ of 12-oz. can	95	19.8
With red & green sweet pepper (Del Monte)	½ cup (3.7 oz.)	88	19.3
White, whole kernel:			
Solids & liq., wet pack (USDA)	½ cup (4.5 oz.)	84	20.1
Drained solids, wet pack (USDA)	½ cup (2.8 oz.)	67	15.8
Drained liq., wet pack (USDA)	4 oz.	29	7.8
Vacuum pack (Green Giant)	⅓ of 12-oz. can	100	20.4

(USDA): United States Department of Agriculture
(HEW/FAO): Health, Education and Welfare/Food and Agriculture Organization
* Prepared as Package Directs

Food and Description	Measure or Quantity	Calories	Carbo-hydrates (grams)
Canned, white or yellow, whole kernel, dietetic pack:			
Solids & liq., wet pack (USDA)	4 oz.	65	15.4
Drained solids (USDA)	4 oz.	86	20.4
Drained liq. (USDA)	4 oz. (by wt.)	19	4.9
Solids & liq. (Blue Boy)	4 oz.	78	16.0
Solids & liq. (Diet Delight)	½ cup (4.4 oz.)	70	16.9
(S and W) *Nutradiet*	4 oz.	59	12.2
Canned, cream style, white or yellow, regular pack:			
Solids & liq. (USDA)	½ cup (4.4 oz.)	102	25.0
(Butter Kernel)	½ cup (4.1 oz.)	92	22.5
Golden (Del Monte)	½ cup (4.4 oz.)	112	25.0
Golden (Green Giant)	½ of 8.5-oz. can	107	23.4
(Libby's)	½ cup (4.1 oz.)	82	20.7
White or golden (Stokely-Van Camp)	½ cup (4.1 oz.)	94	23.0
Canned, cream style, dietetic pack:			
Solids & liq. (USDA)	4 oz.	93	21.0
Solids & liq. (Blue Boy)	4 oz.	105	20.6
(S and W) *Nutradiet*	4 oz.	95	20.1
Frozen:			
On the cob:			
Not thawed (USDA)	4 oz.	111	25.6
Boiled, drained (USDA)	4 oz.	107	24.5
(Birds Eye)	1 ear (3.5 oz.)	98	21.7
Niblet Ears	1 ear (4.9 oz.)	167	35.6
Kernel, cut off cob:			
Not thawed (USDA)	4 oz.	93	22.3
Boiled, drained solids (USDA)	½ cup (3.2 oz.)	72	17.1
(Birds Eye)	½ cup (3.3 oz.)	77	17.8
Sweet, white (Birds Eye)	½ cup (3.3 oz.)	77	17.9
(Green Giant)	⅓ of 10-oz. pkg.	74	15.7
Cream style (Green Giant)	⅓ of 10-oz. pkg.	74	15.7
In butter sauce:			
(Green Giant) white	⅓ of 10-oz. pkg.	112	19.1
Mexicorn	⅓ of 10-oz. pkg.	97	16.0
Niblets	⅓ of 10-oz. pkg.	90	14.9
Scalloped (Green Giant)	⅓ of 10-oz. pkg.	132	16.1
With peas & tomatoes (Birds Eye)	½ cup (3.3 oz.)	67	15.0

Food and Description	Measure or Quantity	Calories	Carbo-hydrates (grams)
CORNBREAD:			
Corn pone, home recipe, prepared with white, whole-ground cornmeal (USDA)	4 oz.	231	41.1
Corn sticks, frozen (Aunt Jemima)	3 pieces (1¾ oz.)	145	22.3
Johnnycake, home recipe, prepared with yellow, degermed cornmeal (USDA)	4 oz.	303	51.6
Southern-style, home recipe, prepared with degermed cornmeal (USDA)	2½″ x 2½″ x 1⅝″ piece	254	39.3
Southern-style, home recipe, prepared with whole-ground cornmeal (USDA)	4 oz.	235	33.0
Spoon bread, home recipe, prepared with white whole-ground cornmeal (USDA)	4 oz.	221	19.2
(Pillsbury) Hungry Jack	1 piece	95	12.5
Sweet (Pillsbury) Hungry Jack	1 piece	100	13.0
CORNBREAD MIX:			
Dry (USDA)	1 oz.	122	20.1
*Prepared with egg & milk (USDA)	2⅜″ muffin (1.4 oz.)	93	13.2
(Albers)	1 oz.	109	19.6
*(Aunt Jemima)	⅙ of cornbread (2.4 oz.)	228	34.9
*(Dromedary)	2″ x 2″ piece (1.4 oz.)	125	18.5
*(Pillsbury) *Ballard*	½ of recipe	160	26.0
CORN CHEX, cereal	1¼ cups (1 oz.)	111	24.0
CORN CHIPS (See **CRACKERS**)			

(USDA): United States Department of Agriculture
(HEW/FAO): Health, Education and Welfare/Food and Agriculture Organization
* Prepared as Package Directs

Food and Description	Measure or Quantity	Calories	Carbohydrates (grams)
CORN CHOWDER, New England (Snow)	8 oz.	159	19.6
CORNED BEEF:			
Uncooked, boneless, medium fat (USDA)	1 lb.	1329	0.
Cooked, boneless, medium fat (USDA)	4 oz.	422	0.
Canned:			
(Armour Star)	4 oz.	322	0.
(Hormel) *Dinty Moore*	4 oz.	253	0.
Brisket (Wilson)			
Tender Made	4 oz.	180	1.0
Packaged (Oscar Mayer)	1 slice (5 grams)	7	.1
Packaged (Vienna)	1 oz.	68	.1
CORNED BEEF HASH, canned:			
(Armour Star)	15½-oz. can	831	36.0
(Austex)	15-oz. can	769	45.5
(Hormel) *Mary Kitchen*	7½ oz.	400	21.0
(Libby's)	4 oz.	192	14.3
(Libby's) home-style	4 oz.	226	13.2
(Nalley's)	4 oz.	179	9.1
(Silver Skillet)	4 oz.	217	10.9
(Van Camp)	½ cup (4.1 oz.)	208	12.3
(Wilson)	15½-oz. can	792	31.6
CORNED BEEF HASH DINNER, frozen (Banquet)	10-oz. dinner	372	42.6
CORNED BEEF SPREAD (Underwood)	1 T. (.5 oz.)	27	.1
CORN FLAKES, cereal:			
(USDA)	1 cup (1 oz.)	112	24.7
Crushed (USDA)	1 cup (2.5 oz.)	270	59.7
Frosted (USDA)	1 cup (1.4 oz.)	154	36.5
Country (General Mills)	1¼ cups (1 oz.)	111	24.3
(Kellogg's)	1⅓ cups (1 oz.)	106	24.2
(Ralston Purina)	1 cup (1 oz.)	109	24.2
(Van Brode)	1 oz.	106	24.2
CORN FRITTER:			
Home recipe (USDA)	4 oz.	428	45.0
Frozen (Mrs. Paul's)	8-oz. pkg.	562	82.2

Food and Description	Measure or Quantity	Calories	Carbo-hydrates (grams)
CORN GRITS (See **HOMINY**)			
CORNMEAL, WHITE or YELLOW:			
Dry:			
Bolted (USDA)	1 cup (4.3 oz.)	442	90.9
Bolted (Aunt Jemima/ Quaker)	1 cup (4 oz.)	408	84.8
Degermed:			
(USDA)	1 cup (4.9 oz.)	502	108.2
(Aunt Jemima/ Quaker)	1 cup (4 oz.)	404	88.8
Self-rising degermed:			
(USDA)	1 cup (5 oz.)	491	105.9
(Aunt Jemima)	1 cup (6 oz.)	582	126.0
Self-rising whole-ground (USDA)	1 cup (5 oz.)	489	101.4
Self-rising (Aunt Jemima)	1 cup (6 oz.)	594	122.4
Whole-ground, unbolted (USDA)	1 cup (4.3 oz.)	433	90.0
Cooked:			
(USDA)	1 cup (8.5 oz.)	120	25.7
Degermed (Albers)	1 cup	119	25.5
CORNMEAL MIX:			
Bolted (Aunt Jemima/ Quaker)	1 cup (4 oz.)	392	80.4
Degermed (Aunt Jemima/ Quaker)	1 cup (4 oz.)	392	84.0
CORN PUDDING, home recipe (USDA)	1 cup (8.6 oz.)	255	31.9
CORN SALAD, raw (USDA):			
Untrimmed	1 lb. (weighed untrimmed)	91	15.7
Trimmed	4 oz.	24	4.1
CORN SOUFFLÉ, frozen (Stouffer's)	12-oz. pkg.	492	57.0

(USDA): United States Department of Agriculture
(HEW/FAO): Health, Education and Welfare/Food and Agriculture Organization
* Prepared as Package Directs

Food and Description	Measure or Quantity	Calories	Carbohydrates (grams)
CORNSTARCH:			
(USDA)	1 cup (4.5 oz.)	463	112.1
(Argo)	1 T. (8 grams)	34	8.3
(Kingsford's)	1 T. (8 grams)	34	8.3
(Duryea's)	1 T. (8 grams)	34	8.3
CORN STICK (See **CORNBREAD**)			
CORN SYRUP, light & dark blend (USDA)	1 T. (.7 oz.)	61	15.8
CORN TOTAL, cereal	1¼ cup (1 oz.)	111	24.3
COTTAGE PUDDING, home recipe (USDA):			
Without sauce	2 oz.	195	30.8
With chocolate sauce	2 oz.	180	32.1
With strawberry sauce	2 oz.	166	27.4
COUGH DROP:			
(Beech-Nut)	1 drop (2 grams)	10	2.4
(Estee)	1 drop	12	3.0
(H-B)	1 drop	8	1.9
(Luden's):			
Honey lemon	1 drop	8	
Honey licorice	1 drop	8	
Menthol	1 drop	9	2.1
Wild cherry	1 drop	9	
(Pine Bros.)	1 drop (3 grams)	9	2.2
(Smith Brothers)	1 drop	7	2.1
COUNTRY-STYLE SAUSAGE, smoked links (USDA)	1 oz.	98	0.
COWPEA (USDA):			
Immature seeds:			
Raw, whole	1 lb. (weighed in pods)	317	54.4
Raw, shelled	½ cup (2.5 oz.)	91	15.7
Boiled, drained solids	½ cup (2.9 oz.)	88	14.8
Canned, solids and liq.	4 oz.	79	14.1
Frozen (See **BLACK-EYED PEAS,** frozen)			
Young pods with seeds:			
Raw, whole	1 lb. (weighed untrimmed)	182	39.2

Food and Description	Measure or Quantity	Calories	Carbo-hydrates (grams)
Boiled, drained solids	4 oz.	39	7.9
Mature seeds, dry:			
Raw	1 lb.	1556	279.9
Raw	½ cup (3 oz.)	288	51.8
Boiled	½ cup (4.4 oz.)	94	17.1
CRAB, all species:			
Fresh:			
Steamed, whole (USDA)	1 lb. (weighed in shell)	202	1.1
Steamed, meat only (USDA)	4 oz.	105	.6
Canned:			
Drained solids (USDA)	4 oz.	115	1.2
(Del Monte) Alaska King	7½-oz. can	202	3.6
Alaska King, drained solids (Icy Point)	7½-oz. can	215	2.3
Alaska King, drained solids (Pillar Rock)	7½-oz. can	215	2.3
Frozen:			
Alaska King, thawed & drained (Wakefield's)	4 oz.	96	.6
King Crab (Ship Ahoy)	8-oz. pkg.	211	.5
CRAB APPLE, fresh (USDA):			
Whole	1 lb. (weighed whole)	284	74.3
Flesh only	4 oz.	77	20.2
CRAB COCKTAIL, King crab (Sau-Sea)	4-oz. jar	80	18.4
CRAB, DEVILED:			
Home recipe (USDA)	1 cup (8.5 oz.)	451	31.9
Frozen (Mrs. Paul's)	3-oz. crab	173	17.1
CRAB IMPERIAL, home recipe (USDA)	1 cup (7.8 oz.)	323	8.6
CRAB NEWBURG, Alaska King, frozen (Stouffer's)	12-oz. pkg.	562	13.6

(USDA): United States Department of Agriculture
(HEW/FAO): Health, Education and Welfare/Food and Agriculture Organization
* Prepared as Package Directs

Food and Description	Measure or Quantity	Calories	Carbo- hydrates (grams)
CRAB SOUP (Crosse & Blackwell)	6½ oz. (½ can)	59	8.3
CRACKER, PUFFS and CHIPS:			
American Harvest (Nabisco)	1 piece (3 grams)	16	2.0
Arrowroot biscuit (Nabisco)	1 piece (5 grams)	22	3.5
Bacon flavored thins (Nabisco)	1 piece (2 grams)	11	1.2
Bacon Nips	1 oz.	147	15.6
Bacon rinds (Wonder)	1 oz.	146	0.
Bacon toast (Keebler)	1 piece (3 grams)	15	2.0
Bakon Tasters (Old London)	½-oz. bag	62	8.8
Bugles (General Mills)	15 pieces (½ oz.)	81	7.5
Butter (USDA)	1 oz.	130	19.1
Butter thins (Nabisco)	1 piece (3 grams)	15	2.4
Cheese flavored (See also individual brand names in this grouping):			
(USDA)	1 oz.	136	17.1
Cheese'n Bacon, sandwich (Nab)	6 pieces (1¼-oz. pkg.)	179	18.9
Cheese'n Cracker (Kraft)	4 crackers & ¾ oz. cheese	138	.7
Cheese *Nips* (Nab)	24 pieces (⅞-oz. pkg.)	114	16.5
Cheese *Nips* (Nabisco)	1 piece (1 gram)	5	.7
Cheese on Rye, sandwich (Nab)	6 pieces (1¼-oz. pkg.)	191	17.6
Cheese Pixies (Wise)	1-oz. bag	155	15.7
Chee•Tos, cheese-flavored puffs	1 oz.	156	14.4
Cheez Doodles (Old London)	1-oz. bag	155	15.7
Cheez-Its (Sunshine)	1 piece (1 gram)	6	.6
Cheez Waffles (Austin's)	1 piece	26	
Cheez Waffles (Old London)	1 piece (2 grams)	11	1.3
Che-zo (Keebler)	1 piece (<1 gram)	5	.6
Combo Cheez (Austin's)	1 piece	26	
Ritz (Nabisco)	1 piece (3 grams)	17	1.9
Sandwich (Nab)	6 pieces (1¼-oz. pkg.)	185	18.5

Food and Description	Measure or Quantity	Calories	Carbo-hydrates (grams)
Shapies, dip delights (Nabisco)	1 piece (2 grams)	9	.8
Shapies, shells (Nabisco)	1 piece (2 grams)	10	.9
Thins (Pepperidge Farm)	1 piece (3 grams)	12	1.8
Thins, dietetic (Estee)	1 piece (1 gram)	5	.7
Tid-Bit (Nab)	32 pieces (1⅛-oz. pkg.)	150	19.7
Tid-Bit (Nabisco)	1 piece (<1 gram)	4	.6
Toast (Keebler)	1 piece (3 grams)	16	1.9
Twists (Nalley)	1 oz.	155	14.2
Twists (Wonder)	1 oz.	154	14.7
Cheese & peanut butter sandwich:			
(USDA)	1 oz.	139	15.9
(Austin's)	1 ⅜-oz. pkg.	194	19.0
(Nab) *O-So-Gud*	4 pieces (1-oz. pkg.)	141	16.3
(Nab) squares	4 pieces (1-oz. pkg.)	139	14.7
(Nab) squares	6 pieces (1½-oz. pkg.)	208	22.1
(Nab) squares	6 pieces (1¾-oz. pkg.)	243	25.7
(Nab) variety pack	6 pieces (1½-oz. pkg.)	209	22.7
(Nab) variety pack	6 pieces (1¾-oz. pkg.)	244	26.5
Chicken in a Biskit (Nabisco)	1 piece (2 grams)	10	1.2
Chippers (Nabisco)	1 piece (3 grams)	14	1.8
Chipsters (Nabisco)	1 piece (<1 gram)	2	.3
Clam flavored crisps (Snow)	1 oz.	147	14.9
Club (Keebler)	1 piece (3 grams)	15	2.0
Corn Capers (Wonder)	1 oz.	158	15.4
Corn cheeze (Tom Houston)	10 pieces (5 grams)	29	1.9
Corn chips:			
Cornetts	1 oz.	153	16.3
Fritos	1 oz.	159	14.8
Korkers (Nabisco)	1 piece (2 grams)	8	.9

(USDA): United States Department of Agriculture
(HEW/FAO): Health, Education and Welfare/Food and Agriculture Organization
* Prepared as Package Directs

Food and Description	Measure or Quantity	Calories	Carbohydrates (grams)
(Old London)	1-oz. bag	162	15.6
(Wise) rippled	1-oz. bag	162	15.6
(Wonder)	1 oz.	162	14.8
Barbecue (Wise)	1 ¾-oz. bag	274	27.5
Corn Diggers (Nabisco)	1 piece (<1 gram)	4	.5
Crown Pilot (Nabisco)	1 piece (.6 oz.)	73	12.4
Dipsy Doodles (Old London)	1-oz. bag	162	15.6
Doo Dads (Nabisco)	1 piece (<1 gram)	2	.3
Escort (Nabisco)	1 piece (4 grams)	20	2.7
Flings, cheese flavored curls (Nabisco)	1 piece (2 grams)	11	.6
Flings, Swiss 'n ham (Nabisco)	1 piece (2 grams)	10	.8
Goldfish (Pepperidge Farm):			
Cheddar cheese	10 pieces (6 grams)	28	3.3
Lightly salted	10 pieces (6 grams)	28	3.6
Parmesan cheese	10 pieces (6 grams)	28	3.4
Pizza	10 pieces (6 grams)	29	3.6
Pretzel	10 pieces (7 grams)	29	5.0
Onion	10 pieces (6 grams)	28	3.6
Sesame garlic	10 pieces (6 grams)	29	3.5
Graham:			
(USDA)	2½" sq. (7 grams)	27	5.1
(Nabisco)	1 piece (7 grams)	30	5.4
Chocolate or coca-covered:			
(USDA)	1 oz.	135	19.2
(Keebler) Deluxe	1 piece (9 grams)	42	5.6
(Nabisco)	1 piece (.4 oz.)	55	7.0
(Nabisco) *Fancy*	1 piece (.5 oz.)	68	9.0
(Nabisco) *Pantry*	1 piece (.4 oz.)	62	8.5
Sweet-Tooth (Sunshine)	1 piece (.4 oz.)	45	6.4
Sugar-honey coated (USDA)	1 oz.	117	21.7
Sugar-honey coated (Nabisco) *Honey Maid*	1 piece (7 grams)	30	5.3
Hi-Ho (Sunshine)	1 piece (4 grams)	18	2.1
Hot Potatas (Old London)	⅝-oz. bag	82	12.0

Food and Description	Measure or Quantity	Calories	Carbo-hydrates (grams)
Matzo (See **MATZO**)			
Melba toast (See **MELBA**)			
Milk lunch (Nabisco)			
Royal Lunch	1 piece (.4 oz.)	55	7.9
Munchos	1 oz.	159	14.5
Onion flavored:			
Crisps (Snow)	1 oz.	157	15.9
French (Nabisco)	1 piece (2 grams)	12	1.6
Funyuns (Frito-Lay)	1 oz.	137	18.9
Meal Mates (Nabisco)	1 piece (4 grams)	19	3.4
Onyums (General Mills)	30 pieces (.5 oz.)	79	7.7
Rings (Old London)	½-oz. bag	68	10.4
Rings (Wise)	½-oz. bag	65	11.1
Rings (Wonder)	1 oz.	133	19.5
Thins (Pepperidge Farm)	1 piece (3 grams)	12	2.0
Toast (Keebler)	1 piece (3 grams)	18	2.1
OTC (Original Trenton Cracker)	1 cracker	23	4.4
Oyster:			
(USDA)	10 pieces (.4 oz.)	44	7.1
(USDA)	1 cup (1 oz.)	124	20.0
(Keebler)	1 piece (<1 gram)	2	.2
Dandy (Nabisco)	1 piece (<1 gram)	3	.5
Mini (Sunshine)	1 piece (<1 gram)	3	.6
Oysterettes (Nabisco)	1 piece (<1 gram)	3	.6
Peanut butter 'n cheez crackers (Kraft)	4 crackers & ¾ oz. peanut butter	191	13.4
Peanut butter sandwich:			
Adora (Nab)	6 pieces (1½-oz. pkg.)	201	26.8
Cheese crackers (Wise)	1 piece (6 grams)	30	3.4
Malted milk (Nab)	4 pieces (1-oz. pkg.)	137	16.0
Malted milk (Nab)	6 pieces (1⅜-oz. pkg.)	189	22.1
Toasted crackers (Wise)	1 piece (6 grams)	30	3.7
Pizza Spins (General Mills)	32 pieces (½ oz.)	72	8.0
Pizza Wheels (Wise)	¾-oz. bag	90	16.1
Potato crisps (General Mills)	16 pieces (½ oz.)	78	7.5

(USDA): United States Department of Agriculture
(HEW/FAO): Health, Education and Welfare/Food and Agriculture Organization
* Prepared as Package Directs

Food and Description	Measure or Quantity	Calories	Carbo-hydrates (grams)
Ritz, plain (Nabisco)	1 piece (3 grams)	16	2.1
Roman Meal Wafers	1 piece (4 grams)	15	2.4
Rye thins (Pepperidge Farm)	1 piece (3 grams)	10	2.0
Rye toast (Keebler)	1 piece (4 grams)	17	2.2
Rye wafers (Nabisco) *Meal Mates*	1 piece (4 grams)	19	3.4
Ry-Krisp:			
Seasoned	1 whole cracker (7 grams)	26	4.4
Traditional	1 whole cracker (6 grams)	24	4.9
Saltine:			
Flavor-Kist, any kind	1 piece	12	2.2
Krispy (Sunshine) salted tops	1 piece (3 grams)	11	2.0
Krispy (Sunshine) unsalted tops	1 piece (3 grams)	12	2.1
Premium (Nab)	8 pieces (¾-oz. pkg.)	91	15.3
Premium (Nabisco)	1 piece (3 grams)	12	2.0
Zesta (Keebler)	1 section (3 grams)	12	2.0
Sea toast (Keebler)	1 piece (.5 oz.)	62	11.1
Sesame:			
(Sunshine) *La Lanne*	1 piece (3 grams)	15	1.8
Buttery flavored (Nabisco)	1 piece (3 grams)	16	1.9
Wafer (Keebler)	1 piece (3 grams)	16	2.0
Wafer (Nabisco) *Meal Mates*	1 piece (5 grams)	21	3.2
Sesa Wheat (Austin's)	1 piece	34	3.7
Sip 'N Chips (Nabisco)	1 piece (2 grams)	9	1.0
Sociables (Nabisco)	1 piece (2 grams)	10	1.3
Soda:			
(USDA)	1 oz.	124	20.0
(USDA)	2½" sq. (6 grams)	24	3.9
(Nabisco) *Premium*, unsalted tops	1 piece (3 grams)	12	2.0
(Sunshine)	1 piece (4 grams)	20	3.3
Soya (Sunshine) *La Lanne*	1 piece (3 grams)	16	1.9
Star Lites (Wise)	1 cup (.5 oz.)	63	9.9
Swedish rye wafer (Keebler)	1 piece (5 grams)	5	3.8
Taco corn chips (Old London)	1¼-oz. bag	167	23.8
Taco tortilla chips (Wonder)	1 oz.	144	15.9
Taco tortilla chips (Frito-Lay) *Doritos*	1 oz.	150	17.8

Food and Description	Measure or Quantity	Calories	Carbo-hydrates (grams)
Tortilla chips (Frito-Lay) Doritos	1 oz.	137	18.3
Tortilla chips (Old London)	1½-oz. bag	207	27.8
Tortilla chips (Wonder)	1 oz.	148	17.2
Town House	1 piece (3 grams)	18	2.0
Triangle Thins (Nabisco)	1 piece (2 grams)	8	1.1
Triscuit (Nabisco)	1 piece (4 grams)	21	3.0
Twigs, sesame & cheese (Nabisco)	1 piece (3 grams)	14	1.6
Uneeda Biscuit (Nabisco) unsalted tops	1 piece (5 grams)	22	3.7
Wafer-ets (Hol-Grain):			
Rice, salted	1 piece (3 grams)	12	2.5
Rice, unsalted	1 piece (3 grams)	12	2.5
Wheat, salted	1 piece (2 grams)	7	1.4
Wheat, unsalted	1 piece (2 grams)	7	1.4
Waldorf, low salt (Keebler)	1 piece (3 grams)	14	2.4
Waverly wafer (Nabisco)	1 piece (4 grams)	18	2.6
Wheat chips (General Mills)	12 pieces (.5 oz.)	73	7.8
Wheat thins (Nabisco)	1 piece (2 grams)	9	1.2
Wheat toast (Keebler)	1 piece (3 grams)	16	2.0
Whistles (General Mills)	17 pieces (.5 oz.)	71	8.0
White thins (Pepperidge Farm)	1 piece (3 grams)	12	2.0
Whole-wheat (USDA)	1 oz.	114	19.3
Whole-wheat, natural (Froumine)	1 piece (.4 oz.)	46	7.5
CRACKER CRUMBS:			
Graham (USDA)	1 cup (3 oz.)	330	63.0
Graham (Keebler)	3 oz.	368	64.1
Graham (Nabisco)	9″ pie shell (1½ cups, 4.6 oz.)	563	100.3
CRACKER JACK (See POPCORN)			
CRACKER MEAL:			
(USDA)	1 T. (.4 oz.)	44	7.1
(Keebler): Fine, medium or coarse	3 oz.	316	68.5

(USDA): United States Department of Agriculture
(HEW/FAO): Health, Education and Welfare/Food and Agriculture Organization
* Prepared as Package Directs

Food and Description	Measure or Quantity	Calories	Carbohydrates (grams)
Zesty	3 oz.	363	61.5
(Nabisco) salted	1 cup (3 oz.)	309	65.7
(Nabisco) unsalted	1 cup (3 oz.)	319	67.9
(Sunshine)	3 oz.	340	71.2
CRACKER PIE CRUST MIX (See **PIECRUST MIX**)			
CRANAPPLE (Ocean Spray):			
Regular	½ cup (4.5 oz.)	94	22.9
Low calorie	½ cup (4.2 oz.)	19	4.7
CRANBERRY:			
Fresh:			
Untrimmed (USDA)	1 lb. (weighed with stems)	200	47.0
Stems removed (USDA)	1 cup (4 oz.)	52	12.2
(Ocean Spray)	1 oz.	15	2.7
Dehydrated (USDA)	1 oz.	104	23.9
CRANBERRY JUICE COCKTAIL (Ocean Spray):			
Regular	½ cup (4.4 oz.)	83	19.7
Frozen, drink	½ cup (4.4 oz.)	91	22.4
CRANBERRY-ORANGE RELISH:			
Uncooked (USDA)	4 oz.	202	51.5
(Ocean Spray)	4 oz.	209	51.8
CRANBERRY PIE			
(Tastykake)	4-oz. pie	376	57.7
CRANBERRY SAUCE:			
Home recipe, sweetened, unstrained (USDA)	4 oz.	202	51.6
Canned:			
Sweetened, strained (USDA)	½ cup (4.8 oz.)	199	51.0
Jellied (Ocean Spray)	4 oz.	184	42.9
Whole berry (Ocean Spray)	4 oz.	191	44.3
CRANBREAKER MIX			
(Bar-Tender's)	1 serving (⅝ oz.)	70	17.4
CRANPRUNE JUICE DRINK			
(Ocean Spray)	½ cup (4.4 oz.)	82	20.1

Food and Description	Measure or Quantity	Calories	Carbohydrates (grams)
CRAPPIE, white, raw, meat only (USDA)	4 oz.	90	0.
CRAYFISH, freshwater (USDA):			
Raw, in shell	1 lb. (weighed in shell)	39	.7
Raw, meat only	4 oz.	82	1.4
CREAM:			
Half and half:			
(Dean)	1 T. (.5 oz.)	22	.7
10.5% fat (Sealtest)	½ cup (4.2 oz.)	148	5.1
12.0% fat (Sealtest)	½ cup (4.2 oz.)	161	5.0
(Meadow Gold)	1 T.	30	.6
Light, table or coffee:			
(USDA)	1 T. (.5 oz.)	32	.6
16% fat (Sealtest)	1 T. (.5 oz.)	26	.6
18% fat (Sealtest)	1 T. (.5 oz.)	28	.6
25% fat (Sealtest)	1 T. (.5 oz.)	37	.5
Light whipping:			
(USDA)	1 cup (8.4 oz.)	717	8.6
(USDA)	1 T. (.5 oz.)	45	.5
30% fat (Sealtest)	1 T. (.5 oz.)	44	.5
Whipped topping, pressurized:			
(USDA)	1 cup (2.1 oz.)	155	.6
(USDA)	1 T. (3 grams)	10	.1
Heavy whipping:			
Unwhipped (USDA)	1 cup (8.4 oz.)	838	7.4
(Dean)	1 T. (.5 oz.)	51	.5
36% fat (Sealtest)	1 T. (.5 oz.)	52	.5
Sour:			
(USDA)	1 cup (8.1 oz.)	485	9.9
(Axelrod's)	8-oz. container	433	8.8
(Breakstone)	1 T. (.5 oz.)	29	.6
(Dean)	1 T. (.5 oz.)	28	.6
(Sealtest)	1 T. (.5 oz.)	28	.5
Imitation:			
(Borden) *Zest,* 13.5% vegetable fat	1 T.	24	.9

(USDA): United States Department of Agriculture
(HEW/FAO): Health, Education and Welfare/Food and Agriculture
Organization
* Prepared as Package Directs

Food and Description	Measure or Quantity	Calories	Carbo-hydrates (grams)
(Dean) Sour Slim	1 T. (1.1 oz.)	30	3.3
(Delite) Sour Treat	1 T. (.5 oz.)	25	.8
Sour cream, dried (Information supplied by General Mills Laboratory)	1 oz.	188	8.1
Sour dressing, cultured (Breakstone)	1 T.	27	.7
CREAMIES (Tastykake):			
Banana cake	1 pkg. (1⅞ oz.)	238	34.5
Chocolate	1 pkg. (1⅞ oz.)	290	29.3
Koffee Kake	1 pkg. (1⅞ oz.)	303	47.2
Vanilla	1 pkg. (1⅞ oz.)	292	32.3
***CREAM OF RICE**, cereal	4 oz.	82	17.9
CREAMSICLE (Popsicle Industries)	2½ fl. oz. (1.9 oz.)	78	12.8
CREAM or CREME SOFT DRINK:			
Sweetened:			
(Canada Dry) vanilla	6 fl. oz.	97	24.0
(Dr. Brown's)	6 fl. oz.	84	20.9
(Fanta)	6 fl. oz.	94	24.2
(Hoffman)	6 fl. oz.	85	21.3
(Key Food)	6 fl. oz.	84	20.9
(Kirsch)	6 fl. oz.	77	19.6
(Shasta)	6 fl. oz.	84	21.3
(Waldbaum)	6 fl. oz.	84	20.9
(Yukon Club)	6 fl. oz.	85	21.3
Low calorie:			
(Canada Dry)	6 fl. oz.	5	.2
(Hoffman)	6 fl. oz.	1	.2
(No-Cal)	6 fl. oz.	2	<.1
(Shasta)	6 fl. oz.	<1	<.1
CREAM SUBSTITUTE (See individual brand names)			
CREAM OF WHEAT, cereal:			
Instant or quick, dry	1 oz. (¾ cup cooked)	99	21.2
Mix'n Eat, regular, dry	3½ T. (1 oz.)	99	20.8
Regular, dry	1 oz. (¾ cup cooked)	102	21.7

Food and Description	Measure or Quantity	Calories	Carbo-hydrates (grams)
CREME D'AMANDE			
LIQUEUR (Garnier) 60 proof	1 fl. oz.	111	15.6
CREME D'APRICOT			
LIQUEUR (Old Mr. Boston)			
42 proof	1 fl. oz.	66	6.0
CREME DE BANANE			
LIQUEUR:			
(Garnier) 60 proof	1 fl. oz.	80	8.0
(Old Mr. Boston) 42 proof	1 fl. oz.	66	6.0
CREME DE BLACKBERRY			
LIQUEUR (Old Mr. Boston)			
42 proof	1 fl. oz.	66	6.0
CREME DE CACAO			
LIQUEUR, brown or white:			
(Bols) 54 proof	1 fl. oz.	101	11.8
(Garnier) 54 proof	1 fl. oz.	97	13.1
(Hiram Walker) 54 proof	1 fl. oz.	104	15.0
(Leroux) brown, 54 proof	1 fl. oz.	101	14.3
(Leroux) white, 54 proof	1 fl. oz.	98	13.3
(Old Mr. Boston) 42 proof	1 fl. oz.	84	7.0
(Old Mr. Boston) 54 proof	1 fl. oz.	95	7.0
CREME DE CAFE LIQUEUR			
(Leroux) 60 proof	1 fl. oz.	104	13.6
CREME DE CASSIS			
LIQUEUR:			
(Garnier) 36 proof	1 fl. oz.	83	13.5
(Leroux) 35 proof	1 fl. oz.	88	14.9
CREME DE CHERRY			
LIQUEUR, black cherry (Old			
Mr. Boston) 42 proof	1 fl. oz.	66	6.0
CREME DE COFFEE			
LIQUEUR (Old Mr. Boston)			
42 proof	1 fl. oz.	66	6.0

(USDA): United States Department of Agriculture
(HEW/FAO): Health, Education and Welfare/Food and Agriculture
          Organization
* Prepared as Package Directs

Food and Description	Measure or Quantity	Calories	Carbo-hydrates (grams)
CREME DE MENTHE			
LIQUEUR, green or white:			
(Bols) 60 proof	1 fl. oz.	122	13.0
(Garnier) 60 proof	1 fl. oz.	110	15.3
(Hiram Walker) 60 proof	1 fl. oz.	94	11.2
(Leroux) green, 60 proof	1 fl. oz.	110	15.2
(Leroux) white, 60 proof	1 fl. oz.	101	12.8
(Old Mr. Boston) 42 proof	1 fl. oz.	66	6.0
(Old Mr. Boston) 60 proof	1 fl. oz.	94	8.5
CREME DE NOYAUX			
LIQUEUR:			
(Bols) 60 proof	1 fl. oz.	115	13.7
(Leroux) 60 proof	1 fl. oz.	108	14.6
CREME DE PEACH			
LIQUEUR (Old Mr. Boston)			
42 proof	1 fl. oz.	66	6.0
CREME SOFT DRINK (See **CREAM SOFT DRINK**)			
CREMORA, non-dairy			
(Borden)	1 tsp. (2 grams)	11	1.1
CRESS, GARDEN (USDA):			
Raw, whole	1 lb. (weighed untrimmed)	103	17.7
Boiled in small amount of water, short time, drained	1 cup (6.3 oz.)	41	6.8
Boiled in large amount of water, long time, drained	1 cup (6.3 oz.)	40	6.5
CRISP RICE (Van Brode)	1 oz.	106	24.7
CRISPY CRITTERS, cereal	1 cup (1 oz.)	113	23.0
CRISPY RICE, cereal (Ralston Purina)	1 cup (1 oz.)	109	24.1
CROAKER (USDA):			
Atlantic:			
Raw, whole	1 lb. (weighed whole)	148	0.
Raw, meat only	4 oz.	109	0.
Baked	4 oz.	151	0.
White, raw, meat only	4 oz.	95	0.
Yellowfin, raw, meat only	4 oz.	101	0.

Food and Description	Measure or Quantity	Calories*	Carbo-hydrates (grams)

CRULLER (See **DOUGHNUT**)

CUCUMBER, fresh (USDA):

Eaten with skin	½ lb. (weighed whole)	32	7.4
Eaten without skin	½ lb. (weighed with skin)	23	5.3
Unpared, 10-oz. cucumber	7½″ x 2″ pared cucumber (7.3 oz.)	29	6.6
Pared	6 slices (2″ x ⅛″)	7	1.6
Pared & diced	½ cup (2.5 oz.)	10	2.3

CUPCAKE:
Home recipe (USDA):

Without icing	1.4-oz. cupcake (2¾″)	146	22.4
With chocolate icing	1.8-oz. cupcake (2¾″)	184	29.7
With boiled white icing	1.8-oz. cupcake (2¾″)	176	30.9
With uncooked white icing	1.8-oz. cupcake (2¾″)	184	31.6

Commercial:

Chocolate (Tastykake)	1 cupcake (1 oz.)	192	33.0
Chocolate, chocolate creme filled (Tastykake)	1 cupcake (1¼ oz.)	128	23.2
Chocolate, creme filled (Drake's)	1 cupcake (1½ oz.)	187	25.6
Coconut (Tastykake)	1 cupcake (¾ oz.)	92	16.7
Creme filled, chocolate butter cream (Tastykake)	1 cupcake (1⅛ oz.)	161	23.1
Devil's Food Cake (Hostess)	1 cupcake (1½ oz.)	162	25.9

(USDA): United States Department of Agriculture
(HEW/FAO): Health, Education and Welfare/Food and Agriculture Organization
* Prepared as Package Directs

Food and Description	Measure or Quantity	Calories	Carbo-hydrates (grams)
Lemon creme filled (Tastykake)	1 cupcake (⅞ oz.)	124	17.1
Orange (Hostess)	1 cupcake (⅞ oz.)	133	17.1
Orange creme filled (Tastykake)	1 cupcake (⅞ oz.)	133	17.1
Raisin Snack (Drake's):			
Junior	1 cupcake (1.1 oz.)	112	19.2
Small	1 cupcake (2¼ oz.)	233	41.8
Vanilla creme filled (Tastykake)	1 cupcake (⅞ oz.)	123	16.4
Vanilla *Triplets* (Tastykake)	1 cupcake (.8 oz.)	101	16.1
CUPCAKE MIX:			
*(Flako)	1 cupcake (1⁄12 of pkg.)	140	21.9
*(Pillsbury):			
Devil's Food Cake, frosted	1 cupcake	170	30.0
Fudge, frosted	1 cupcake	180	32.0
Yellow, frosted	1 cupcake	170	31.0
CURACAO LIQUEUR:			
Blue (Bols) 64 proof	1 fl. oz.	105	10.3
Orange (Bols) 64 proof	1 fl. oz.	100	8.8
(Garnier) 60 proof	1 fl. oz.	100	12.7
(Hiram Walker) 60 proof	1 fl. oz.	96	11.8
(Leroux) 60 proof	1 fl. oz.	84	9.5
CURRANT:			
Fresh (USDA):			
Black European:			
Whole	1 lb. (weighed with stems)	240	58.2
Stems removed	4 oz.	61	14.9
Red & white:			
Whole	1 lb. (weighed with stems)	220	53.2
Stems removed	1 cup (3.9 oz.)	55	13.3
Dried, Zante (Del Monte)	½ cup (2.5 oz.)	205	54.2

Food and Description	Measure or Quantity	Calories	Carbo-hydrates (grams)
CURRANT JELLY (Smucker's)	1 T. (.7 oz.)	50	12.9
CURRY POWDER (Crosse & Blackwell)	1 T. (6 grams)	21	3.9
CUSK (USDA):			
Raw, drawn	1 lb. (weighed drawn, head & tail on)	197	0.
Raw, meat only	4 oz.	85	0.
Steamed	4 oz.	120	0.
CUSTARD:			
Home recipe, baked (USDA)	½ cup (4.7 oz.)	152	14.7
Chilled (Sealtest)	4 oz.	149	24.3
CUSTARD APPLE, bullock's-heart, raw (USDA):			
Whole	1 lb. (weighed with skin & seeds)	266	66.3
Flesh only	4 oz.	115	28.6
CUSTARD PIE:			
Home recipe (USDA)	⅙ of 9" pie (5.4 oz.)	331	35.6
Frozen (Banquet)	5 oz.	274	41.2
Frozen (Mrs. Smith's)	⅛ of 8" pie (4 oz.)	296	43.3
CUSTARD PUDDING MIX:			
Dry, with vegetable gum base (USDA)	1 oz.	109	28.0
*Prepared with whole milk (USDA)	4 oz.	149	25.6
*(Jell-O) no egg yolk	½ cup (5 oz.)	165	22.9
Real egg (Lynden Farms)	4-oz. pkg.	441	69.2
*Regular (Royal)	½ cup (5.1 oz.)	132	18.5

(USDA): United States Department of Agriculture
(HEW/FAO): Health, Education and Welfare/Food and Agriculture Organization
* Prepared as Package Directs

Food and Description	Measure or Quantity	Calories	Carbohydrates (grams)

D

DAIQUIRI COCKTAIL:
(Hiram Walker) 52.5 proof	3 fl. oz.	177	12.0
(National Distillers) *Duet*, 12% alcohol	8-fl.-oz. can	280	24.0
Canned (Party Tyme) 12.5% alcohol	2 fl. oz.	65	5.4
Canned, banana (Party Tyme) 12.5% alcohol	2 fl. oz.	66	5.7
Dry mix (Bar-Tender's)	1 serving (⅝ oz.)	70	17.2

DAMSON PLUM (See PLUM)

DANDELION GREENS, raw (USDA):
Trimmed	1 lb.	204	41.7
Boiled, drained	½ cup (3.2 oz.)	30	5.8

DANISH PASTRY (See COFFEE CAKE)

DANISH-STYLE VEGETABLES, frozen (Birds Eye)
	⅓ of 10-oz. pkg.	92	7.6

DATE, dry:
Domestic:
With pits (USDA)	1 lb. (weighed with pits)	1081	287.7
Without pits (USDA)	4 oz.	311	82.7
Without pits, chopped (USDA)	1 cup (6.1 oz.)	477	126.8
Whole (Cal-Date)	1 date (.8 oz.)	62	16.4
Diced (Cal-Date)	2 oz.	161	42.8
Chopped (Dromedary)	1 cup (5 oz.)	493	114.2
Pitted (Dromedary)	1 cup (5 oz.)	470	112.3
Imported (Bordo):			
Iraq, diced	¼ cup (2 oz.)	159	39.8
Iraq, whole	4 average dates (.9 oz.)	73	18.2

Food and Description	Measure or Quantity	Calories	Carbohydrates (grams)
DELAWARE WINE:			
(Gold Seal) 12% alcohol	3 fl. oz.	87	2.6
(Great Western) 12% alcohol	3 fl. oz.	75	3.0
DEVIL DOGS (Drake's)	1 cake (1.6 oz.)	178	24.9
DEVIL'S FOOD CAKE:			
Home recipe (USDA):			
Without icing	3″ x 2″ x 1½″ (1.9 oz.)	201	28.6
With chocolate icing	⅟₁₆ of 10″ layer cake (4.2 oz.)	443	67.0
With uncooked white icing	⅟₁₆ of 10″ layer cake (4.2 oz.)	443	71.0
Commercial, frozen:			
With chocolate icing (USDA)	2 oz.	215	31.5
With whipped cream filling & chocolate icing (USDA)	2 oz.	210	24.8
(Pepperidge Farm)	⅙ of cake (3.1 oz.)	326	47.0
DEVIL'S FOOD CAKE MIX:			
Dry (USDA)	1 oz.	115	21.8
*With chocolate icing (USDA)	⅟₁₆ of 9″ cake	234	40.2
*(Betty Crocker)	⅟₁₂ of cake	199	35.8
*Butter recipe (Betty Crocker)	⅟₁₂ of cake	269	37.0
*(Duncan Hines)	⅟₁₂ of cake (2.7 oz.)	205	35.0
*Red Devil (Pillsbury)	⅟₁₂ of cake	210	33.0
*(Swans Down)	⅟₁₂ of cake (2.4 oz.)	184	35.3
DEWBERRY, fresh (See **BLACKBERRY,** fresh)			

(USDA): United States Department of Agriculture
(HEW/FAO): Health, Education and Welfare/Food and Agriculture Organization
* Prepared as Package Directs

Food and Description	Measure or Quantity	Calories	Carbo-hydrates (grams)
DIAMOND WINE (Great Western) 12% alcohol	3 fl. oz.	76	1.7
DING DONG (Hostess)	1 cake (1.3 oz.)	185	21.5
DINNER, frozen (See individual listings such as **BEEF DINNER, CHICKEN DINNER, CHINESE DINNER, ENCHILADA DINNER,** etc.)			
DIP:			
Bacon & horseradish:			
(Borden)	1 oz.	58	1.7
(Breakstone)	1 T. (.6 oz.)	31	.7
Bacon & smoke (Sealtest) *Dip'n Dressing*	1 oz.	47	1.7
Blue cheese, neufchâtel cheese (Kraft) *Ready Dip*	1 oz.	69	1.6
Blue cheese (Kraft) *Teez*	1 oz.	51	1.3
Clam, neufchâtel cheese (Kraft) *Ready Dip*	1 oz.	67	1.8
Clam (Kraft) *Teez*	1 oz.	45	1.5
Dill pickle & neufchâtel cheese (Kraft) *Ready Dip*	1 oz.	67	2.4
Garlic (Kraft) *Teez*	1 oz.	47	1.5
Green Goddess (Kraft) *Teez*	1 oz.	46	1.5
Onion:			
(Borden) French	1 oz.	58	1.7
Neufchâtel cheese (Kraft) *Ready Dip*	1 oz.	68	2.0
French onion (Kraft) *Teez*	1 oz.	43	1.5
French onion (Sealtest) *Dip'n Dressing*	1 oz.	46	2.2
Tasty Tartar (Borden)	1 oz.	48	1.8
Western Bar B-Q (Borden)	1 oz.	48	1.8
DIP MIX:			
Bacon onion (Fritos)	1 pkg. (.6 oz.)	47	7.2
Bleu cheese (Fritos)	1 pkg. (.6 oz.)	48	8.1
Chili con queso (Fritos)	1 pkg. (.6 oz.)	72	7.5
Green onion (Lawry's)	1 pkg. (.6 oz.)	50	10.6
Guacamole	1 pkg. (.6 oz.)	50	5.5

Food and Description	Measure or Quantity	Calories	Carbo-hydrates (grams)
Taco (Fritos)	1 pkg. (.6 oz.)	43	10.0
Toasted onion (Lawry's)	1 pkg. (.6 oz.)	48	9.8

DISTILLED LIQUOR. The values below apply to un-flavored bourbon whiskey, brandy, Canadian whisky, gin, Irish whiskey, rum, rye whiskey, Scotch whisky, te-quila, and vodka. The caloric content of distilled liquors depends on the percentage of alcohol. The proof is twice the alcohol percent and the following values apply to all brands. (USDA):

80 proof	1 fl. oz.	65	Tr.
86 proof	1 fl. oz.	70	Tr.
90 proof	1 fl. oz.	74	Tr.
94 proof	1 fl. oz.	77	Tr.
100 proof	1 fl. oz.	83	Tr.

DOCK, including **SHEEP SORREL:**

Raw, whole (USDA)	1 lb. (weighed untrimmed)	89	17.8
Boiled, drained (USDA)	4 oz.	22	4.4

DOGFISH, spiny, raw, meat only (USDA) 4 oz. 177 0.

DOLLY VARDEN, raw, meat & skin (USDA) 4 oz. 163 0.

DOUGHNUT:

Cake type (USDA)	1 piece (1.1 oz.)	125	16.4
Chocolate: (Hostess) 10 to pkg.	1 piece (1.2 oz.)	139	18.2
Coated gem (Hostess)	1 piece (.6 oz.)	110	
Long John (Van de Kamp's)	1 piece (2.1 oz.)	179	

(USDA): United States Department of Agriculture
(HEW/FAO): Health, Education and Welfare/Food and Agriculture Organization
* Prepared as Package Directs

Food and Description	Measure or Quantity	Calories	Carbohydrates (grams)
Cruller (Van de Kamp's)	1 piece (1½ oz.)	161	
Cruller, old-fashioned (Hostess)	1 piece	100	
Powdered, frozen (Morton)	1 piece (.6 oz.)	82	9.2
Sugared (Hostess):			
Regular	1 piece (1.8 oz.)	233	
Gem, mini	1 piece (½ oz.)	95	
Gem, chocolate inside	1 piece (½ oz.)	100	
Sugar & spice, frozen (Morton)	1 piece (.6 oz.)	82	8.6
Yeast-leavened (USDA)	4 oz.	469	42.8
DRAMBUIE LIQUEUR, 80 proof (Hiram Walker)	1 fl. oz.	110	11.0
DR. BROWN'S CEL-RAY TONIC, soft drink	6 fl. oz.	66	16.5
DREAMSICLE (Popsicle Industries)	3 fl. oz.	87	
DR. PEPPER, soft drink:			
Regular	6 fl. oz.	71	17.4
Sugar free	6 fl. oz.	2	.4
DRUM, raw (USDA):			
Freshwater:			
Whole	1 lb. (weighed whole)	143	0.
Meat only	4 oz.	137	0.
Red:			
Whole	1 lb. (weighed whole)	149	0.
Meat only	4 oz.	91	0.
DUCK, raw (USDA):			
Domesticated:			
Ready-to-cook	1 lb. (weighed with bones)	1213	0.
Meat only	4 oz.	187	0.
Wild:			
Dressed	1 lb. (weighed dressed)	613	0.
Meat only	4 oz.	156	0.

Food and Description	Measure or Quantity	Calories	Carbo-hydrates (grams)

E

ECLAIR, home recipe, with custard filling & chocolate icing (USDA) | 4 oz. | 271 | 26.3

EEL (USDA):
| Raw, meat only | 4 oz. | 264 | 0. |
| Smoked, meat only | 4 oz. | 374 | 0. |

EGG: CHICKEN (USDA):
Raw:

White only	1 large egg (1.2 oz.)	17	.3
White only	1 cup (9 oz.)	130	2.0
Yolk only	1 large egg (.6 oz.)	59	.1
Yolk only	1 cup (8.5 oz.)	835	1.4
Whole, small	1 egg (1.3 oz.)	60	.3
Whole, medium	1 egg (1.5 oz.)	71	.4
Whole, large	1 egg (1.8 oz.)	81	.4
Whole	1 cup (8.8 oz.)	409	2.3
Whole, extra large	1 egg (2 oz.)	94	.5
Whole, jumbo	1 egg (2.3 oz.)	105	.6

Cooked:
Boiled	1 large egg (1.8 oz.)	81	.4
Fried in butter	1 large egg	99	.1
Omelet, mixed with milk & cooked in fat	1 large egg	107	1.5
Poached	1 large egg	78	.4
Scrambled, mixed with milk & cooked in fat	1 large egg	111	1.5
Scrambled, mixed with milk & cooked in fat	1 cup (7.8 oz.)	381	5.3

(USDA): United States Department of Agriculture
(HEW/FAO): Health, Education and Welfare/Food and Agriculture Organization
* Prepared as Package Directs

Food and Description	Measure or Quantity	Calories	Carbo-hydrates (grams)
Dried:			
Whole	1 cup (3.8 oz.)	639	4.4
White, powder	1 oz.	105	1.6
Yolk	1 cup (3.4 oz.)	637	2.4
EGG, DUCK, raw (USDA)	1 egg (2.8 oz.)	153	.6
EGG, GOOSE, raw (USDA)	1 egg (5.8 oz.)	303	2.1
EGG, TURKEY, raw (USDA)	1 egg (3.1 oz.)	150	1.5
EGG FOO YOUNG, frozen (Chun King)	6 oz. (½ pkg.)	120	10.9
EGG McMUFFIN (McDonald's)	1 piece (4.5 oz.)	313	35.3
EGG NOG:			
Dairy:			
(Borden) 4.69% fat	½ cup (4.2 oz.)	132	16.3
(Borden) 6.0% fat	½ cup (4.4 oz.)	154	16.6
(Borden) 8.0% fat	½ cup (4.4 oz.)	175	16.0
(Sealtest) 6% fat	½ cup (4.6 oz.)	174	18.0
(Sealtest) 8% fat	½ cup (4.6 oz.)	192	17.3
With alcohol (Old Mr. Boston) 30 proof	1 fl. oz.	83	4.5
EGGPLANT:			
Raw, whole (USDA)	1 lb. (weighed untrimmed)	92	20.6
Boiled, drained, diced (USDA)	1 cup (7.1 oz.)	38	8.2
Frozen, parmagiana (Buitoni)	4 oz.	189	16.2
Frozen, sticks (Mrs. Paul's)	7-oz. pkg.	517	57.3
EGG ROLL, frozen:			
Lobster & meat (Chun King)	½-oz. roll	26	3.7
Shrimp (Chun King)	½-oz. roll	24	3.8
Shrimp (Hung's)	1 piece	131	15.7
Vegetable (Mow Sang)	1 roll	66	7.0
***EGGSTRA** (Tillie Lewis)	½ of 7-oz. dry pkg. (1 large egg)	42	2.2

Food and Description	Measure or Quantity	Calories	Carbo-hydrates (grams)
ELDERBERRY, fresh (USDA):			
Whole	1 lb. (weighed with stems)	307	69.9
Stems removed	4 oz.	82	18.6
ENCHILADA, frozen:			
Beef:			
With cheese (Banquet)	8 pieces (2 lbs.)	1297	136.0
With chili gravy (Patio)	4-oz. piece (2 in pkg.)	371	23.7
Cheese:			
(Patio)	4-oz. piece (2 in pkg.)	130	18.9
(Van de Kamp's)	1 pkg.	387	
ENCHILADA DINNER, frozen:			
Beef:			
(Banquet)	12-oz. dinner	479	63.6
(Morton)	12-oz. dinner	524	57.8
(Patio) 5-compartment	13-oz. dinner	610	93.0
(Rosarita)	12-oz. dinner	511	
(Swanson)	15-oz. dinner	561	59.5
Cheese:			
(Banquet)	12-oz. dinner	282	38.8
(Patio) 5-compartment	12-oz. dinner	380	55.0
(Rosarita)	12-oz. dinner	436	
ENDIVE, BELGIAN or **FRENCH** (See **CHICORY, WITLOOF**)			
ENDIVE, CURLY, raw (USDA):			
Untrimmed	1 lb. (weighed untrimmed)	80	16.4
Trimmed	½ lb.	45	9.3
Cut up or shredded	1 cup (2.5 oz.)	14	2.9

(USDA): United States Department of Agriculture
(HEW/FAO): Health, Education and Welfare/Food and Agriculture Organization
* Prepared as Package Directs

Food and Description	Measure or Quantity	Calories	Carbo-hydrates (grams)
ESCAROLE, raw (USDA):			
Untrimmed	1 lb. (weighed untrimmed)	80	16.4
Trimmed	½ lb.	46	9.2
Cut up or shredded	1 cup (2.5 oz.)	14	2.9
EULACHON or **SMELT,** raw, meat only (USDA)	4 oz.	134	0.
EXTRACT (See individual listings)			

F

Food and Description	Measure or Quantity	Calories	Carbo-hydrates (grams)
FARINA (See also *CREAM OF WHEAT*):			
Regular:			
Dry:			
(USDA)	1 cup (6 oz.)	627	130.1
Cream, enriched (H-O)	1 cup (6.1 oz.)	646	134.3
Cream, enriched (H-O)	1 T.	40	8.5
(Pearls of Wheat)	1 cup	608	128.6
Cooked:			
*(USDA)	1 cup (8.4 oz.)	100	20.7
*(USDA)	4 oz.	48	9.9
*(Quaker)	1 cup (1 oz. dry)	100	22.1
Quick-cooking (USDA):			
Dry	1 oz.	103	21.2
Cooked	1 cup (8.6 oz.)	105	21.8
Instant-cooking (USDA):			
Dry	1 oz.	103	21.2
Cooked	4 oz.	62	12.9
FAT, COOKING, vegetable:			
(USDA)	1 cup (7.1 oz.)	1768	0.
(USDA)	1 T. (.4 oz.)	106	0.
Snowdrift	1 T.	110	0.
Light Spry	¼ lb.	1002	0.
Light Spry	1 T. (.4 oz.)	93	0.

FIG   [169]

Food and Description	Measure or Quantity	Calories	Carbo-hydrates (grams)
FENNEL LEAVES, raw (USDA):			
Untrimmed	1 lb. (weighed untrimmed)	118	21.5
Trimmed	4 oz.	32	5.8
FESTIVAL MAIN MEAL *MEAT, canned (Wilson Sinclair):			
Beef roast	3 oz.	100	0.
Corned beef brisket	3 oz.	135	0.
Ham	3 oz.	129	.8
Picnic	3 oz.	137	.8
Pork loin, smoked	3 oz.	114	.8
Pork roast	3 oz.	133	0.
Turkey & dressing	3 oz.	159	8.5
Turkey roast	3 oz.	87	0.
FIG:			
Fresh:			
(USDA)	1 lb.	363	92.1
Small (USDA)	1.3-oz. fig (1½″ dia.)	30	7.7
Candied (Bama)	1 T. (.7 oz.)	37	9.6
Canned, regular pack (USDA):			
Light syrup, solids & liq.	4 oz.	74	19.1
Heavy syrup, solids & liq.	3 figs & 2 T. syrup (4 oz.)	96	24.9
Heavy syrup, solids & liq.	½ cup (4.4 oz.)	106	27.5
Extra heavy syrup, solids & liq.	4 oz.	117	30.3
Canned, unsweetened or dietetic pack:			
Water pack, solids & liq. (USDA)	4 oz.	54	14.1
Kadota, solids & liq. (Diet Delight)	½ cup (4.4 oz.)	76	18.2
Whole, unsweetened (S and W) *Nutradiet*	6 figs (3.5 oz.)	52	12.7

(USDA): United States Department of Agriculture
(HEW/FAO): Health, Education and Welfare/Food and Agriculture Organization
* Prepared as Package Directs

Food and Description	Measure or Quantity	Calories	Carbo-hydrates (grams)
Solids & liq. (Tillie Lewis)	½ cup (4.5 oz.)	64	14.9
Dried:			
Chopped (USDA)	1 cup (6 oz.)	469	118.2
(USDA)	.7-oz. fig (2″ x 1″)	58	14.5
Calimyrna (Del Monte)	1 cup (5.4 oz.)	386	96.4
FIG JUICE, *Real Fig*	½ cup (4.5 oz.)	61	15.8
FILBERT or **HAZELNUT** (USDA):			
Whole	4 oz. (weighed in shell)	331	8.7
Shelled	1 oz.	180	4.7
FINNAN HADDIE, meat only (USDA)	4 oz.	117	0.
FISH (See individual listings)			
FISH CAKE:			
Home recipe, fried (USDA)	2 oz.	98	5.3
Frozen:			
(Commodore)	2 oz.	102	9.8
Breaded & fried (Mrs. Paul's)	2-oz. cake	105	10.4
FISH CHOWDER, New England (Snow)	8 oz.	144	11.9
FISH & CHIPS, frozen:			
(Gorton)	½ of 1-lb. pkg.	395	39.0
(Mrs. Paul's)	14-oz. pkg.	706	93.5
(Swanson)	5-oz. pkg.	263	28.4
FISH FILLET:			
Sandwich (McDonald's)	1 sandwich (4.8 oz.)	407	37.6
Frozen, breaded (Mrs. Paul's)	2-oz. piece	104	11.5
FISH FLAKES, canned (USDA)	4 oz.	126	0.
FISH LOAF, home recipe (USDA)	4 oz.	141	8.3

Food and Description	Measure or Quantity	Calories	Carbo-hydrates (grams)
FISH MEAL, frozen:			
(Morton)	8¾-oz. dinner	374	42.2
With French fries (Swanson)	9¾-oz. dinner	429	41.4
With green beans & peach (Weight Watchers)	18-oz. dinner	266	21.9
With pineapple chunks (Weight Watchers)	9½-oz. luncheon	175	17.2
FISH STICK, frozen:			
Cooked, commercial, 3¾″ x 1″ x ½″ sticks (USDA)	10 sticks (8-oz. pkg.)	400	14.8
(Commodore)	4 oz.	200	7.6
(Mrs. Paul's)	14-oz. pkg.	756	72.6
FLIP, soft drink	6 fl. oz. (6.5 oz.)	75	18.4
FLOUNDER:			
Raw:			
Whole (USDA)	1 lb. (weighed whole)	118	0.
Meat only (USDA)	4 oz.	90	0.
Baked (USDA)	4 oz.	229	0.
Frozen (Gorton)	1-lb. pkg.	360	0.
Frozen (Ship Ahoy)	1-lb. pkg.	316	0.
Frozen, dinner (Weight Watchers)	16-oz. dinner	296	28.8
Frozen, dinner (Weight Watchers)	18-oz. dinner	269	18.9
Frozen, & broccoli (Weight Watchers)	9½-oz. luncheon	170	8.8
FLOUR:			
Buckwheat, dark, sifted (USDA)	1 cup (3.5 oz.)	326	70.6
Buckwheat, light, sifted (USDA)	1 cup (3.5 oz.)	340	77.9
Carob or St. John's-bread (USDA)	1 oz.	51	22.9
Chestnut (USDA)	1 oz.	103	21.6

(USDA): United States Department of Agriculture
(HEW/FAO): Health, Education and Welfare/Food and Agriculture Organization
* Prepared as Package Directs

Food and Description	Measure or Quantity	Calories	Carbo-hydrates (grams)
Corn (USDA)	1 cup (3.9 oz.)	405	84.5
Cottonseed (USDA)	1 oz.	101	9.4
Fish, from whole fish (USDA)	1 oz.	95	0.
Lima bean (USDA)	1 oz.	97	17.9
Potato (USDA)	1 oz.	100	22.7
Rice, stirred, spooned (USDA)	1 cup (5.6 oz.)	574	125.6
Rye:			
Light:			
Unsifted, spooned (USDA)	1 cup (3.6 oz.)	361	78.7
Sifted, spooned (USDA)	1 cup (3.1 oz.)	314	68.6
Medium (USDA)	1 oz.	99	21.2
Dark:			
(USDA)	1 oz.	93	19.3
Unstirred (USDA)	1 cup (4.5 oz.)	419	87.2
Stirred (USDA)	1 cup (4.5 oz.)	415	86.5
Soybean, defatted, stirred (USDA)	1 cup (3.6 oz.)	329	38.5
Soybean, high fat (USDA)	1 oz.	108	9.4
Sunflower seed, partially defatted (USDA)	1 oz.	96	10.7
Wheat:			
All-purpose:			
(USDA)	1 oz.	103	21.6
Unsifted, dipped (USDA)	1 cup (5 oz.)	521	108.8
Unsifted, spooned (USDA)	1 cup (4.4 oz.)	459	95.9
Sifted, spooned (USDA)	1 cup (4.1 oz.)	422	88.3
Bread:			
(USDA)	1 oz.	103	21.2
Unsifted, dipped (USDA)	1 cup (4.8 oz.)	496	101.6
Unsifted, spooned (USDA)	1 cup (4.3 oz.)	449	91.9
Sifted, spooned (USDA)	1 cup (4.1 oz.)	427	87.4
Cake:			
(USDA)	1 oz.	103	22.5
Unsifted, dipped (USDA)	1 cup (4.2 oz.)	433	94.5
Unsifted, spooned (USDA)	1 cup (3.9 oz.)	404	88.1
Sifted, spooned (USDA)	1 cup (3.5 oz.)	360	78.6

Food and Description	Measure or Quantity	Calories	Carbo-hydrates (grams)
Gluten:			
(USDA)	1 oz.	107	13.4
Unsifted, dipped			
(USDA)	1 cup (5 oz.)	537	67.0
Unsifted, spooned			
(USDA)	1 cup (4.8 oz.)	510	63.7
Sifted, spooned (USDA)	1 cup (4.8 oz.)	514	64.2
Self-rising:			
(USDA)	1 oz.	100	21.0
Unsifted, dipped			
(USDA)	1 cup (4.6 oz.)	458	96.5
Unsifted, spooned			
(USDA)	1 cup (4.5 oz.)	447	94.2
Sifted, spooned (USDA)	1 cup (3.7 oz.)	373	78.7
Whole wheat (USDA)	1 oz.	94	20.1
Aunt Jemima, self-rising			
(Quaker Oats)	1 cup (4 oz.)	384	83.2
Gold Medal, regular			
(Betty Crocker)	1 cup	483	100.7
Gold Medal, self-rising			
(Betty Crocker)	1 cup	476	100.5
Presto, self-rising	1 cup (3.9 oz.)	392	84.5
(Quaker)	1 cup (4 oz.)	400	87.2
Robin Hood, all purpose	1 cup (4 oz.)	401	86.0
Robin Hood, self-rising	1 cup (4 oz.)	381	82.0
Softasilk (Betty Crocker)	1 cup	412	88.4
FOLLE BLANCHE WINE			
(Louis M. Martini) 12.5% alcohol	3 fl. oz.	90	.2
FOURNIER NATURE (Gold Seal) 12% alcohol	3 fl. oz.	82	.4
FRANKFURTER:			
Raw:			
All kinds (USDA)	1 frankfurter (10 per lb.)	140	.8
All meat (USDA)	1 frankfurter (10 per lb.)	134	1.1

(USDA): United States Department of Agriculture
(HEW/FAO): Health, Education and Welfare/Food and Agriculture
  Organization
♦ Prepared as Package Directs

Food and Description	Measure or Quantity	Calories	Carbo-hydrates (grams)
With cereal (USDA)	1 frankfurter (10 per lb.)	112	<.1
All meat (Armour Star)	1 frankfurter (10 per lb.)	155	0.
All beef (Eckrich)	1 frankfurter (1.6 oz.)	152	2.0
All beef (Hormel)	1 frankfurter (1.6 oz.)	140	.6
Pure beef (Oscar Mayer)	1 frankfurter (1.6 oz.)	143	1.4
(Vienna)	1 frankfurter	121	1.0
All beef (Wilson)	1 frankfurter (1.6 oz.)	136	.8
Skinless (Wilson)	1 frankfurter (1.6 oz.)	140	.8
Cooked, all kinds (USDA)	1 frankfurter (10 per lb., raw)	136	.7
Canned (USDA)	2 oz.	125	.1
Canned (Hormel)	12-oz. can	966	2.4
FRANKS & BEANS (See **BEANS & FRANKS**)			
FRANKS-N-BLANKETS, frozen (Durkee)	1 piece (.4 oz.)	45	1.0
FRENCH TOAST, frozen:			
(Aunt Jemima)	1 slice (1.5 oz.)	88	13.6
(Swanson)	4½-oz. breakfast	290	20.9
FRESCA, soft drink	6 fl. oz.	<1	<.1
FROG LEGS, raw (USDA):			
Bone in	1 lb. (weighed with bone)	215	0.
Meat only	4 oz.	83	0.
FROOT LOOPS, cereal (Kellogg's)	1 cup (1 oz.)	115	25.3
FROSTED SHAKE, any flavor (Borden)	9¼-oz. can	320	43.0
FROSTED TREAT (Weight Watchers)	1 serving (4.8 oz.)	140	23.5
FROSTING (See **CAKE ICING**)			

Food and Description	Measure or Quantity	Calories	Carbohydrates (grams)
FROSTY O's, cereal	1 cup (1 oz.)	112	24.0
FROZEN CUSTARD (See ICE CREAM)			
FROZEN DESSERT (Sugar Lo):			
Chocolate, ice milk	⅓ pt. (3.5 oz.)	140	20.3
Vanilla, ice cream	⅓ pt. (3.5 oz.)	187	19.3
FRUIT CAKE (USDA):			
Dark, home recipe	1.1-oz. piece (2" x 2" x ½")	114	17.9
Light, home recipe	1.1-oz. piece (2" x 2" x ½")	117	17.2
FRUIT COCKTAIL:			
Canned, regular pack, solids & liq.:			
Light syrup (USDA)	4 oz.	68	17.8
Heavy syrup:			
(USDA)	½ cup (4.5 oz.)	97	25.2
(Del Monte)	½ cup (4.3 oz.)	87	23.5
(Dole)	½ cup (with 3 T. liq., 4.4 oz.)	94	24.4
(Hunt's)	½ cup (4.5 oz.)	89	23.9
Extra heavy syrup (USDA)	4 oz.	104	26.9
Canned, unsweetened or dietetic pack, solids & liq.:			
Water pack (USDA)	4 oz.	42	11.0
Solids & liq. (Diet Delight)	½ cup (4.4 oz.)	67	16.0
(Libby's)	4 oz.	36	11.0
(S and W) *Nutradiet*, low calorie	4 oz.	41	9.7
(Tillie Lewis)	½ of 8-oz. can	44	11.6
FRUIT CUP (Del Monte) fruit cocktail	5¼-oz. cont.	106	28.5

(USDA): United States Department of Agriculture
(HEW/FAO): Health, Education and Welfare/Food and Agriculture Organization
* Prepared as Package Directs

Food and Description	Measure or Quantity	Calories	Carbo-hydrates (grams)
FRUITFORT, cereal	1 oz.	111	
FRUIT ICE MILK (See individual sherbet flavors)			
FRUIT, MIXED, frozen, quick thaw (Birds Eye)	½ cup (5 oz.)	111	28.4
FRUIT PUNCH:			
Canned (Del Monte)	6 fl. oz.	82	15.0
*Mix (Wyler's)	6 fl. oz.	64	15.8
FRUIT SALAD:			
Bottled, chilled (Kraft)	4 oz.	57	13.3
Canned, regular pack, solids & liq.:			
Light syrup (USDA)	4 oz.	67	17.6
Heavy syrup (USDA)	½ cup (4.3 oz.)	85	22.0
Extra heavy syrup (USDA)	4 oz.	102	26.5
Tropical (Del Monte)	½ cup (4.4 oz.)	110	29.2
Canned, unsweetened or dietetic pack:			
Water pack, solids & liq. (USDA)	4 oz.	40	10.3
Solids & liq. (Diet Delight)	½ cup (4.4 oz.)	67	16.1
(S and W) *Nutradiet*, unsweetened	4 oz.	43	10.3
FRUIT-SICLE (Popsicle Industries)	2½ fl. oz.	59	
FUDGE CAKE MIX:			
*Butter recipe (Duncan Hines)	1/12 of cake (3.3 oz.)	283	35.2
*Cherry (Betty Crocker)	1/12 of cake	199	35.8
*Chocolate (Pillsbury)	1/12 of cake	210	34.0
*Dark chocolate (Betty Crocker)	1/12 of cake	198	35.2
*Macaroon (Pillsbury)	1/12 of cake	220	33.0
*Marble (Duncan Hines)	1/12 of cake (2.7 oz.)	202	35.0
*Sour cream, chocolate flavor (Betty Crocker)	1/12 of cake	195	35.4
*Sour cream flavor (Pillsbury)	1/12 of cake	210	33.0

Food and Description	Measure or Quantity	Calories	Carbohydrates (grams)
FUDGE PUDDING (Thank You)	½ cup (4.5 oz.)	202	34.3
FUDGSICLE, chocolate (Popsicle Industries)	2½ fl. oz.	102	23.7
FUNNY BONES (Drake's)	1¼-oz. cake	153	20.0
FUNNY FACE (Pillsbury) Orange	8 fl. oz.	90	22.0

G

Food and Description	Measure or Quantity	Calories	Carbohydrates (grams)
GARBANZO, dry (See **CHICK-PEA**, dry)			
GARBANZO SOUP, canned (Hormel)	15-oz. can	459	30.6
GARLIC, raw (USDA): Whole	2 oz. (weighed with skin)	68	15.4
Peeled	1 oz.	39	8.7
GARLIC SPREAD (Lawry's)	1 T. (.5 oz.)	79	1.2
GATORADE, soft drink	6 fl. oz. (6.3 oz.)	53	16.0
GAZPACHO SOUP, canned (Crosse & Blackwell)	½ can (6½ oz.)	61	6.8
GEFILTE FISH, canned: (Manischewitz) 4-portion can	1 piece (3.7 oz.)	100	3.9
(Manischewitz) 2-lb. jar	1 piece (2.4 oz.)	64	2.5
Fish balls (Manischewitz)	1 piece (1.5 oz.)	40	1.6
Fishlet (Manischewitz)	1 piece (7 grams)	70	.3

(USDA): United States Department of Agriculture
(HEW/FAO): Health, Education and Welfare/Food and Agriculture Organization
* Prepared as Package Directs

Food and Description	Measure or Quantity	Calories	Carbohydrates (grams)
Whitefish & pike (Manischewitz):			
4-portion can	1 piece (3.8 oz.)	87	3.3
2-lb. jar	1 piece (1.7 oz.)	40	1.5
GELATIN, unflavored, dry:			
(USDA)	1 envelope (7 grams)	23	0.
(Knox)	1 envelope (7 grams)	28	0.
GELATIN DESSERT POWDER:			
Regular:			
(USDA)	3-oz. pkg.	315	74.8
*Prepared (USDA)	½ cup (4.2 oz.)	71	16.9
*Prepared with fruit added (USDA)	½ cup (4.2 oz.)	81	19.8
*All fruit flavors (Jell-O)	½ cup (4.9 oz.)	81	18.2
*All flavors (Jells Best)	½ cup	80	18.7
*All flavors (Royal)	½ cup (4.2 oz.)	82	18.9
*Wild flavors (Jell-O)	½ cup (4.9 oz.)	81	17.8
Dietetic or low calorie:			
*All flavors (D-Zerta)	½ cup (4.3 oz.)	8	Tr.
All flavors (Dia-Mel)			
Gela-thin	1 envelope (7 grams)	19	0.
*All flavors (Louis Sherry) *Shimmer*	½ cup (4.4 oz.)	10	.6
GELATIN DRINK (Knox):			
Grapefruit or orange	1 envelope (8 grams)	30	1.0
Plain	1 envelope (7 grams)	25	9.
GERMAN DINNER, frozen (Swanson)	11-oz. dinner	405	42.2
GEVREY-CHAMBERTIN, French red Burgundy (Cruse) 12% alcohol	3 fl. oz.	72	
GEWURZTRAMINER WINE:			
(Louis M. Martini) 12.5% alcohol	3 fl. oz.	90	.2

Food and Description	Measure or Quantity	Calories	Carbohydrates (grams)
(Willm) Alsatian, 11–14% alcohol	3 fl. oz.	66	3.6
(Willm) *Clos Gaensbronnel*, 11–14% alcohol	3 fl. oz.	66	3.6
GIN, unflavored (See **DISTILLED LIQUOR**)			
GIN, FLAVORED:			
Lemon (Old Mr. Boston) 70 proof	1 fl. oz.	76	1.4
Mint (Old Mr. Boston) 70 proof	1 fl. oz.	100	8.0
Orange (Old Mr. Boston) 70 proof	1 fl. oz.	76	1.4
GIN, SLOE:			
(Bols) 66 proof	1 fl. oz.	85	4.7
(DeKuyper) 60 proof	1 fl. oz.	70	5.2
(Garnier) 60 proof	1 fl. oz.	82	8.5
(Hiram Walker) 60 proof	1 fl. oz.	68	4.8
(Old Mr. Boston) 42 proof	1 fl. oz.	50	2.0
(Old Mr. Boston) 70 proof	1 fl. oz.	76	1.4
GIN & TONIC, canned (Party Tyme) 10% alcohol	2 fl. oz.	55	5.1
GINGER ALE, soft drink:			
Sweetened:			
(Canada Dry)	6 fl. oz.	65	16.2
(Canada Dry) golden	6 fl. oz.	72	18.0
(Clicquot Club)	6 fl. oz.	62	15.0
(Cott)	6 fl. oz.	62	15.0
(Dr. Brown's)	6 fl. oz.	60	15.0
(Fanta)	6 fl. oz.	62	15.9
(Hoffman)	6 fl. oz.	58	14.6
(Key Food)	6 fl. oz.	60	15.0
(Kirsch)	6 fl. oz.	59	14.8
(Mission)	6 fl. oz.	62	15.0
(Salute)	6 fl. oz.	65	16.4
(Schweppes)	6 fl. oz.	66	16.3

(USDA): United States Department of Agriculture
(HEW/FAO): Health, Education and Welfare/Food and Agriculture Organization
* Prepared as Package Directs

Food and Description	Measure or Quantity	Calories	Carbohydrates (grams)
(Shasta)	6 fl. oz.	65	16.5
(Waldbaum)	6 fl. oz.	60	15.0
(Yukon Club) golden	6 fl. oz.	64	16.1
Low calorie:			
(Canada Dry)	6 fl. oz.	18	0.
(Dr. Brown's)	6 fl. oz.	1	.2
(Hoffman)	6 fl. oz.	1	.2
(No-Cal)	6 fl. oz.	2	<.1
(Shasta)	6 fl. oz.	<1	<.1
GINGER BEER, soft drink			
(Schweppes)	6 fl. oz.	72	17.6
GINGERBREAD, home recipe (USDA)	1.9-oz. piece (2" x 2" x 2")	174	28.6
GINGERBREAD MIX:			
Dry (USDA)	4 oz.	482	88.7
*Prepared (USDA)	⅑ of 8" sq. (2.2 oz.)	174	32.2
*(Betty Crocker)	⅑ of cake	171	36.1
*(Dromedary)	1.2-oz. piece (2" x 2")	100	18.8
*(Pillsbury)	3" sq.	190	36.0
GINGER, CANDIED			
(USDA)	1 oz.	96	24.7
GINGER ROOT, fresh (USDA):			
With skin	1 oz.	13	2.5
Without skin	1 oz.	14	2.7
GIN SOUR COCKTAIL			
(Calvert) 60 proof	3 fl. oz.	195	10.4
GOLD-O-MINT LIQUEUR			
(Leroux) 25 proof	1 fl. oz.	110	15.2
GOOD HUMOR:			
Bar, ice cream:			
Chocolate chip	1 piece (3 fl. oz.)	239	
Chocolate chip candy, *Super Humor*	1 piece	383	
Chocolate eclair	1 piece (2.4 oz.)	224	23.9

Food and Description	Measure or Quantity	Calories	Carbo-hydrates (grams)
Chocolate fudge cake, *Super Humor*	1 piece	345	
Chocolate malt	1 piece	205	13.6
Strawberry shortcake	1 piece (2.2 oz.)	179	21.4
Toasted almond	1 piece (2.4 oz.)	229	23.8
Vanilla	1 piece (2.1 oz.)	197	15.8
Cone:			
Ice cream, chocolate burst	1 piece	165	
Ice milk, chocolate	1 piece	88	
Ice milk, vanilla	1 piece	85	
Cup:			
Ice:			
Bon Joy Swirl	1 piece	138	
Italian	1 piece	232	
Venetian	1 piece	115	
Ice cream:			
Chocolate	3 oz.	113	
Chocolate	5 oz.	189	
Vanilla	3 oz.	110	11.6
Vanilla	5 oz.	183	
Frostee Humor bar	1 piece	150	
Frostee shake	1 piece	287	
Humorette	1 piece	103	
Ice Stix:			
Chocolate	1 piece	119	
Chocolate, double	1 piece	151	
Fruit	1 piece	89	
Fruit, double	1 piece	138	
Lollie Jets	1 piece	109	
Wahoos	1 piece	52	
X-5 Jetstars	1 piece	57	
Pint, deluxe French	1 oz.	50	
Sandwich, without crackers:			
Ice cream, grocery pack:			
Chocolate	1 piece	53	
Vanilla	1 piece	51	
Ice milk	1 piece	88	
Sundae:			
Bittersweet	1 piece	282	

(USDA): United States Department of Agriculture
(HEW/FAO): Health, Education and Welfare/Food and Agriculture Organization
* Prepared as Package Directs

Food and Description	Measure or Quantity	Calories	Carbohydrates (grams)
Chocolate nut fudge supreme	1 piece	448	
Strawberry	1 piece	221	
Whammy:			
Assorted stick	1 piece (1.4 oz.)	136	11.4
Vanilla	1 piece (1.4 oz.)	137	11.2
Ice milk	1 piece (1¾ fl. oz.)	128	
GOOSE, domesticated (USDA):			
Raw	1 lb. (weighed ready-to-cook)	1172	0.
Roasted, meat & skin	4 oz.	500	0.
Roasted, meat only	4 oz.	264	0.
GOOSEBERRY (USDA):			
Fresh	1 lb.	177	44.0
Fresh	1 cup (5.3 oz.)	58	14.6
Canned, water pack, solids & liq.	4 oz.	29	7.5
GOOSE, GIZZARD, raw (USDA)	4 oz.	158	0.
GOULASH DINNER (Chef Boy-Ar-Dee)	7⅓-oz. pkg.	262	32.4
GRAACHER HIMMELREICH, German Moselle (Julius Kayser) 10% alcohol	3 fl. oz.	60	2.5
GRAHAM CRACKER (See **CRACKER**)			
GRANOLA:			
(Pillsbury)	¼ cup	120	19.0
Sun Country, raisin	¼ cup	126	19.0
GRAPE:			
Fresh:			
American type (slip skin), Concord, Delaware, Niagara, Catawba & Scuppernong:			
(USDA)	½ lb. (weighed with stem, skin & seeds)	98	22.4

Food and Description	Measure or Quantity	Calories	Carbohydrates (grams)
(USDA)	½ cup (2.7 oz.)	52	11.9
(USDA)	3½″ x 3″ bunch (3.5 oz.)	43	9.9
European type (adherent skin), Malaga, Muscat, Thompson seedless, Emperor & Flame Tokay:			
(USDA)	½ lb. (weighed with stem & seeds)	135	34.9
Whole (USDA)	20 grapes (¾″ dia.)	54	13.8
Whole (USDA)	½ cup (.3 oz.)	58	15.1
Halves (USDA)	½ cup (.3 oz.)	58	14.9
Canned, solids & liq. (USDA):			
Thompson seedless, heavy syrup	4 oz.	87	22.7
Thompson seedless, water pack	4 oz.	58	15.4
GRAPEADE, chilled (Sealtest)	6 fl. oz. (6.5 oz.)	96	24.2
GRAPE DRINK:			
(Del Monte)	6 fl. oz. (6.5 oz.)	90	24.6
(Hi-C)	6 fl. oz. (6.3 oz.)	98	22.0
(Salada)	6 fl. oz.	80	19.4
(Wagner's)	6 fl. oz.	97	24.3
(Wyler's)	6 fl. oz.	64	15.8
GRAPE JELLY, dietetic or low calorie:			
(Dia-Mel)	1 T. (.5 oz.)	6	1.4
Concord (Diet Delight)	1 T. (.6 oz.)	21	5.3
(Kraft)	1 oz.	34	8.4
(Louis Sherry)	1 T. (.4 oz.)	6	1.5
(Slenderella)	1 T. (.7 oz.)	26	6.4
(Tillie Lewis)	1 T. (.8 oz.)	11	3.0

(USDA): United States Department of Agriculture
(HEW/FAO): Health, Education and Welfare/Food and Agriculture Organization
* Prepared as Package Directs

Food and Description	Measure or Quantity	Calories	Carbo-hydrates (grams)
GRAPE JUICE:			
Canned:			
(Heinz)	5½-fl.-oz. can	130	31.3
Unsweetened (S and W) Nutradiet	4 oz. (by wt.)	68	17.5
Sweetened (Seneca)	½ cup (4.4 oz.)	115	29.0
Unsweetened (Seneca)	½ cup (4.4 oz.)	84	20.9
Frozen, concentrate, sweetened:			
(USDA)	6-fl.-oz. can	395	100.0
*Diluted (USDA)	½ cup (4.4 oz.)	66	16.6
*(Minute Maid)	½ cup (4.2 oz.)	66	15.8
*(Seneca)	½ cup (4.4 oz.)	66	17.2
*(Snow Crop)	½ cup (4.2 oz.)	66	15.8
GRAPE JUICE DRINK, canned, approx. 30% grape juice (USDA)	1 cup (8.8 oz.)	135	34.5
GRAPE-NUTS, cereal	¼ cup (1 oz.)	104	23.0
GRAPE-NUTS FLAKES, cereal	⅔ cup (1 oz.)	101	22.0
GRAPE PIE (Tastykake)	4-oz. pie	369	51.8
GRAPE SOFT DRINK:			
Sweetened:			
(Canada Dry)	6 fl. oz. (6.4 oz.)	96	24.0
(Dr. Brown's)	6 fl. oz.	87	21.9
(Fanta)	6 fl. oz.	92	23.9
Grapette	6 fl. oz.	91	23.4
(Hoffman)	6 fl. oz.	93	23.2
(Key Food)	6 fl. oz.	87	21.9
(Kirsch)	6 fl. oz.	88	21.8
(Mission)	6 fl. oz.	105	25.1
(Nedick's)	6 fl. oz.	93	23.2
(Nehi)	6 fl. oz. (6.6 oz.)	93	23.2
(Patio)	6 fl. oz.	96	24.0
(Salute)	6 fl. oz.	101	25.5
(Shasta)	6 fl. oz.	88	22.2
(Waldbaum)	6 fl. oz.	87	21.9
(Yoo-Hoo) high-protein	6 fl. oz. (6.4 oz.)	100	18.9
(Yukon Club)	6 fl. oz.	93	23.2
Low calorie:			
(Canada Dry)	6 fl. oz.	1	0.

Food and Description	Measure or Quantity	Calories	Carbo- hydrates (grams)
(Dr. Brown's)	6 fl. oz.	2	.4
(Hoffman)	6 fl. oz.	2	.4
(Key Food)	6 fl. oz.	2	.4
(No-Cal)	6 fl. oz.	2	0.
(Shasta)	6 fl. oz.	<1	.1

GRAPE SYRUP, dietetic
(No-Cal)	1 tsp. (5 grams)	<1	0.

GRAPEFRUIT:
Fresh:
White:

Seeded type (USDA)	1 lb. (weighed with seeds & skin)	84	22.0
Seedless type (USDA)	1 lb. (weighed with skin)	87	22.4
Seeded type (USDA)	½ med. grapefruit (3¾" dia., 8.5 oz.)	44	11.7
(Sunkist)	½ grapefruit (8.5 oz.)	44	11.0
Sections, seedless (USDA)	1 cup (7 oz.)	78	20.2

Pink and red:

Seeded type (USDA)	1 lb. (weighed with seeds & skin)	87	22.6
Seedless type (USDA)	1 lb. (weighed with skin)	93	24.1
Seeded type (USDA)	½ med. grapefruit (3¾" dia., 8.5 oz.)	46	12.0
Bottled, chilled sections, sweetened (Kraft)	4 oz.	53	12.5
Canned, syrup pack, solids & liq. (Del Monte)	½ cup (4.5 oz.)	69	18.6

Canned, unsweetened or dietetic pack, solids & liq.:

Water pack (USDA)	½ cup (4.2 oz.)	36	9.1
Solids & liq. (Diet Delight)	½ cup (4.3 oz.)	41	9.4
(Tillie Lewis)	½ cup (4.4 oz.)	45	10.4

(USDA): United States Department of Agriculture
(HEW/FAO): Health, Education and Welfare/Food and Agriculture
    Organization
* Prepared as Package Directs

Food and Description	Measure or Quantity	Calories	Carbo-hydrates (grams)
GRAPEFRUIT DRINK, sweetened (Wagner)	6 fl. oz.	86	21.6
GRAPEFRUIT JUICE:			
Fresh, pink, red or white, all varieties (USDA)	½ cup (4.3 oz.)	48	11.3
Bottled, chilled, unsweetened (Kraft)	½ cup (4.3 oz.)	48	11.1
Bottled, chilled, sweetened (Kraft)	½ cup (4.3 oz.)	60	14.0
Canned:			
Sweetened:			
(USDA)	½ cup (4.4 oz.)	66	16.0
(Del Monte)	½ cup (4.3 oz.)	48	12.7
(Heinz)	5½-fl.-oz. can	73	16.1
(Libby's)	½ cup (4.3 oz.)	59	14.5
(Stokely-Van Camp)	½ cup (4.4 oz.)	67	16.2
Unsweetened:			
(USDA)	½ cup (4.4 oz.)	51	12.2
(Del Monte)	½ cup (4.3 oz.)	46	11.8
(Diet Delight)	½ cup (4 oz.)	39	9.5
(Heinz)	5½-fl.-oz. can	56	11.8
(Libby's)	½ cup (4.3 oz.)	48	11.4
(Stokely-Van Camp)	½ cup (4.5 oz.)	52	12.4
Frozen, concentrate:			
Sweetened:			
(USDA)	6-fl.-oz. can	348	84.8
*Diluted with 3 parts water (USDA)	½ cup (4.4 oz.)	58	14.1
Unsweetened:			
(USDA)	6-fl.-oz. can	300	71.6
*Diluted with 3 parts water (USDA)	½ cup (4.4 oz.)	51	12.2
*(Florida Diet)	½ cup (4.3 oz.)	50	10.7
*(Minute Maid)	½ cup (4.2 oz.)	50	11.6
*(7L)	½ cup	50	12.0
*(Snow Crop)	½ cup (4.2 oz.)	50	11.6
Dehydrated, crystals:			
(USDA)	4-oz. can	429	102.4
*Reconstituted (USDA)	½ cup (4.4 oz.)	50	11.9
GRAPEFRUIT-ORANGE JUICE (See ORANGE-GRAPEFRUIT JUICE)			
GRAPEFRUIT PEEL, CANDIED (Liberty)	1 oz.	93	22.6

Food and Description	Measure or Quantity	Calories	Carbo-hydrates (grams)
GRAPEFRUIT SOFT DRINK:			
Sweetened:			
(Clicquot Club)	6 fl. oz.	83	20.0
(Fanta)	6 fl. oz.	84	21.5
(Salute)	6 fl. oz.	80	20.3
(Shasta)	6 fl. oz.	81	20.5
Low calorie, pink:			
(Canada Dry)	6 fl. oz.	1	.2
(Hoffman)	6 fl. oz.	2	.4
(No-Cal)	6 fl. oz.	2	0.
(Shasta)	6 fl. oz.	<1	.1
GRAVES WINE (See also individual regional, vineyard or brand names):			
(Barton & Guestier) 12.5% alcohol	3 fl. oz.	65	.6
(Cruse) 11.5% alcohol	3 fl. oz.	69	
GRAVY, canned:			
Beef (Franco-American)	¼ cup	44	3.6
Chicken (Franco-American)	¼ cup	51	3.2
Chicken giblet (Franco-American)	¼ cup	28	2.8
Giblet (Lynden)	7¾-oz. can	264	16.0
Mushroom (Franco-American)	¼ cup	27	2.8
Ready Gravy	¼ cup (2.2 oz.)	44	7.4
GRAVY MASTER	1 fl. oz. (1.3 oz.)	66	13.9
GRAVY with **MEAT** or **TURKEY,** canned or frozen:			
Sliced beef (Morton House)	½ of 12½-oz. can	189	7.7
Sliced liver (Bunker Hill)	½ of 15-oz. can	199	15.0
Sliced pork (Morton House)	½ of 12½-oz. can	193	9.4
Sliced beef, buffet, frozen (Banquet)	2 lb.	956	21.2
Sliced beef, frozen (Banquet)	5-oz. bag	158	4.2

(USDA): United States Department of Agriculture
(HEW/FAO): Health, Education and Welfare/Food and Agriculture Organization
* Prepared as Package Directs

Food and Description	Measure or Quantity	Calories	Carbo-hydrates (grams)
Sliced turkey, frozen (Banquet)	2 lb.	677	22.0
Sliced turkey, frozen (Banquet)	5-oz. bag	129	4.2
Sliced turkey (Morton House)	½ of 12½-oz. can	140	7.2
GRAVY MIX:			
Au jus (Durkee)	1-oz. pkg.	67	12.8
Au jus (French's)	¾-oz. pkg.	44	8.7
Beef:			
(Swiss)	1¼-oz. pkg.	107	22.6
*(Wyler's)	2-oz. serving	25	3.9
Brown:			
*(Durkee)	1 cup (.8-oz. pkg.)	56	11.2
(French's)	¾-oz. pkg.	72	11.7
*(Kraft)	1 oz.	10	1.4
(Lawry's)	1¼-oz. pkg.	136	16.3
(McCormick)	⅞-oz. pkg.	100	10.0
Chicken:			
*(Durkee)	1 cup (1-oz. pkg.)	96	12.8
(French's)	1¼-oz. pkg.	130	14.7
(Lawry's)	1-oz. pkg.	110	13.6
*(McCormick)	2-oz. serving	20	3.0
*(Pillsbury)	1 cup	120	16.0
(Swiss)	1¼-oz. pkg.	107	22.7
*(Wyler's)	2-oz. serving	25	3.7
*Herb (McCormick)	2-oz. serving	22	2.5
Mushroom:			
*(Durkee)	1 cup (.8-oz. pkg.)	72	13.6
(French's)	¾-oz. pkg.	62	7.0
(Lawry's)	1.3-oz. pkg.	145	15.6
*(McCormick)	2-oz. serving	17	2.5
*(Wyler's)	2-oz. serving	15	1.8
Onion:			
*(Durkee)	1 cup (1-oz. pkg.)	88	16.8
(French's)	1-oz. pkg.	72	12.3
*(Kraft)	2-oz. serving	22	3.7
*(McCormick)	2-oz. serving	29	3.5
*(Wyler's)	2-oz. serving	17	2.7
GREEN PEA (See **PEA**)			
GERENADINE SYRUP:			
(Garnier) nonalcoholic	1 fl. oz.	103	26.0

Food and Description	Measure or Quantity	Calories	Carbo-hydrates (grams)
(Giroux) nonalcoholic	1 fl. oz.	100	25.0
(Leroux) 25 proof	1 fl. oz.	81	15.2
GRITS (See **HOMINY GRITS**)			
GROUND-CHERRY, Poha or Cape Gooseberry:			
Whole (USDA)	1 lb. (weighed with husks & stems)	221	46.7
Flesh only (USDA	4 oz.	60	12.7
GROUPER, raw (USDA):			
Whole	1 lb. (weighed whole)	170	0.
Meat only	4 oz.	99	0.
GUAVA, COMMON, fresh:			
Whole (USDA)	1 lb. (weighed untrimmed)	273	66.0
Whole (USDA)	1 guava (2.8 oz.)	48	11.7
Fresh only (USDA)	4 oz.	70	17.0
GUAVA, STRAWBERRY, fresh:			
Whole (USDA)	1 lb. (weighed untrimmed)	289	70.2
Flesh only (USDA)	4 oz.	74	17.9
GUINEA HEN, raw (USDA):			
Ready-to-cook	1 lb. (weighed ready-to-cook)	594	0.
Meat & skin	4 oz.	179	0.

(USDA): United States Department of Agriculture
(HEW/FAO): Health, Education and Welfare/Food and Agriculture Organization
* Prepared as Package Directs

Food and Description	Measure or Quantity	Calories	Carbohydrates (grams)

H

HADDOCK:
  Raw:

Whole (USDA)	1 lb. (weighed whole)	172	0.
Meat only (USDA)	4 oz.	90	0.
Fried, breaded (USDA)	4″ x 3″ x ½″ fillet (3.5 oz.)	165	5.8
Frozen (Gorton)	⅓ of 1-lb. pkg.	120	0.
Smoked, canned or not (USDA)	4 oz.	117	0.

HADDOCK MEALS, frozen:

(Banquet)	8¾-oz. dinner	419	45.4
(Swanson)	12¼-oz. dinner	397	36.5
(Weight Watchers)	18-oz. dinner	256	17.3
& spinach (Weight Watchers)	8-oz. luncheon	150	7.4

HAKE, raw (USDA):

Whole	1 lb. (weighed whole)	144	0.
Meat only	4 oz.	84	0.

HALF & HALF (milk & cream)
  (See **CREAM**)

HALF & HALF SOFT DRINK:
  Sweetened:

(Canada Dry)	6 fl. oz. (6.4 oz.)	79	19.8
(Dr. Brown's)	6 fl. oz.	77	19.4
(Hoffman)	6 fl. oz.	77	19.4
(Key Food)	6 fl. oz.	77	19.4
(Kirsch)	6 fl. oz.	81	20.3
(Yukon Club)	6 fl. oz.	89	22.1
Low calorie (Hoffman)	6 fl. oz.	3	.8

HALF & HALF WINE:

(Gallo) 20% alcohol	3 fl. oz.	100	5.7
(Lejon) 18.5% alcohol	3 fl. oz.	116	6.7

Food and Description	Measure or Quantity	Calories	Carbo-hydrates (grams)
HALIBUT:			
Atlantic & Pacific:			
Raw:			
Whole (USDA)	1 lb. (weighed whole)	268	0.
Meat only (USDA)	4 oz.	113	0.
Broiled (USDA)	4 oz.	194	0.
Broiled (USDA)	4" x 3" x ½" steak (4.4 oz.)	214	0.
Smoked (USDA)	4 oz.	254	0.
California, raw meat only (USDA)	4 oz.	110	0.
Greenland (See **TURBOT**)			
HAM (See also **PORK**):			
Cooked:			
(Hormel)	1 oz.	35	0.
Chopped, sliced (Hormel)	1 oz.	70	<1.0
Minced (Oscar Mayer)	1 slice (.9 oz.)	56	.3
Smoked (Oscar Mayer)	.7-oz. slice	29	0.
Canned:			
(Armour Golden Star)	1 oz.	36	0.
(Armour Star)	1 oz.	53	0.
(Oscar Mayer):			
Jubilee, bone in	1 lb.	835	1.8
Jubilee, boneless	1 lb.	826	4.5
Jubilee, special trim, as purchased	1 oz.	41	0.
Jubilee, special trim, cooked	1 oz.	37	0.
Steak	1 slice (2 oz.)	74	0.
(Swift)	5" x 2¼" x ¼" slice (1¾ oz.)	111	.4
(Wilson)	1 oz.	48	.3
(Wilson) *Tender Made*	1 oz.	44	.3
Chopped or minced, canned:			
(Armour Star)	1 oz.	84	.4
(Hormel)	1 oz. (8-lb. can)	90	<1.0
Deviled, canned:			
(USDA)	1 T. (.5 oz.)	46	0.
(Armour Star)	1 oz.	79	0.

(USDA): United States Department of Agriculture
(HEW/FAO): Health, Education and Welfare/Food and Agriculture Organization
* Prepared as Package Directs

Food and Description	Measure or Quantity	Calories	Carbo-hydrates (grams)
(Libby's)	1 oz.	83	.2
(Underwood)	1 T. (.5 oz.)	46	Tr.
Spiced or unspiced, canned			
(Hormel)	1 oz. (5-lb. can)	78	.4
HAM & CHEESE:			
Loaf (Oscar Mayer)	1-oz. slice	69	.3
Roll (Oscar Mayer)	1 oz.	64	.3
Spread (Oscar Mayer)	1 oz.	75	.5
HAM DINNER:			
*Mix, au gratin (Jeno's)	35-oz. pkg.	1627	143.9
Frozen: (Banquet)	10-oz. dinner	369	47.7
(Morton)	10½-oz. dinner	447	50.7
(Swanson)	10¼-oz. dinner	366	42.1
HAMBURGER (Also see **BEEF,** Ground), (McDonald's): *Big Mac* (See **BIG MAC**)			
Regular	1 hamburger (3.4 oz.)	251	28.3
Regular, cheese	1 hamburger (3.9 oz.)	310	30.3
¼ pound	1 hamburger (5.5 oz.)	416	34.0
¼ pound, cheese	1 hamburger (6.6 oz.)	523	36.9
HAWAIIAN PUNCH, orange	6 fl. oz.	90	24.0
HAWS, SCARLET, raw (USDA):			
Whole	1 lb. (weighed with core)	316	75.5
Flesh & skin	4 oz.	99	23.6
HAZELNUT (See **FILBERT**)			
HEADCHEESE (Sugardale)	1-oz. slice	77	Tr.
HEART (USDA)			
Beef:			
Lean, braised	4 oz.	213	.8
Lean with visible fat, braised	4 oz.	422	.1
Calf, braised	4 oz.	236	2.0

Food and Description	Measure or Quantity	Calories	Carbo-hydrates (grams)
Chicken, raw	1 lb.	608	.5
Chicken, simmered	1 heart (5 grams)	9	<.1
Hog, braised	4 oz.	221	.3
Lamb, braised	4 oz.	295	1.1
Turkey, simmered	4 oz.	245	.2
HERRING (USDA):			
Raw:			
Atlantic, whole	1 lb. (weighed whole)	407	0.
Atlantic, meat only	4 oz.	200	0.
Pacific, meat only	4 oz.	111	0.
Canned:			
Plain, solids & liq.	4 oz.	236	0.
Bismarck, drained (Vita)	5-oz. jar	273	6.9
Cocktail, drained (Vita)	8-oz. jar	342	24.8
In cream sauce (Vita)	8-oz. jar	397	18.1
In tomato sauce, solids & liq.	4 oz.	200	4.2
In wine sauce, drained (Vita)	8-oz. jar	401	16.6
Lunch, drained (Vita)	8-oz. jar	483	13.1
Matjes, drained (Vita)	8-oz. jar	304	26.2
Party Snacks, drained (Vita)	8-oz. jar	401	16.6
Tastee Bits, drained (Vita)	8-oz. jar	361	24.7
Pickled, Bismarck type	4 oz.	253	0.
Salted or brined	4 oz.	247	0.
Smoked:			
Bloaters	4 oz.	222	0.
Hard	4 oz.	340	0.
Kippered	4 oz.	239	0.
HICKORY NUT (USDA):			
Whole	1 lb. (weighed in shell)	1068	20.3
Shelled	4 oz.	763	14.5
HI-SPOT (Canada Dry)	6 fl. oz. (6.4 oz.)	74	18.6

(USDA): United States Department of Agriculture
(HEW/FAO): Health, Education and Welfare/Food and Agriculture Organization
* Prepared as Package Directs

Food and Description	Measure or Quantity	Calories	Carbohydrates (grams)
HO-HO (Hostess)	1 cake (1 oz.)	133	17.3
HOMINY GRITS:			
Dry:			
Degermed (USDA)	1 oz.	103	22.1
Degermed (USDA)	½ cup (2.8 oz.)	282	60.9
Instant (Quaker)	.8-oz. packet	78	17.5
Cooked:			
Degermed (USDA)	⅔ cup (5.6 oz.)	84	18.0
Enriched (Albers)	⅔ cup	82	17.7
(Aunt Jemima/Quaker)	⅔ cup	100	22.0
HONEY, strained:			
(USDA)	½ cup (5.7 oz.)	496	134.1
(USDA)	1 T. (.7 oz.)	61	16.5
HONEY CAKE (Holland Honey Cake)	½" slice	63	
HONEYCOMB, cereal (Post)	1 cup	108	25.0
HONEYDEW, fresh (USDA):			
Whole	1 lb. (weighed whole)	94	22.0
Wedge	2" x 7" wedge (5.3 oz.)	31	7.2
Flesh only	4 oz.	37	8.7
Flesh only, diced	1 cup (5.9 oz.)	55	12.9
HORSERADISH:			
Raw (USDA):			
Whole	1 lb. (weighed unpared)	288	65.2
Pared	1 oz.	25	5.6
Dehydrated (Heinz)	1 T.	25	5.0
Prepared:			
(USDA)	1 oz.	11	2.7
(Gold's)	1 tsp.	3	
(Kraft)	1 oz.	3	.4
Cream style (Kraft)	1 oz.	9	.7
Oil style (Kraft)	1 oz.	20	.5
*HOT DOG BEAN SOUP (Campbell)	1 cup	154	21.0
HUSH PUPPIES, refrigerated (Borden)	1 piece (.8 oz.)	58	10.7

Food and Description	Measure or Quantity	Calories	Carbo- hydrates (grams)
HYACINTH BEAN (USDA):			
Young pod, raw:			
Whole	1 lb. (weighed untrimmed)	140	29.1
Trimmed	4 oz.	40	8.3
Dry seeds	4 oz.	383	69.2

I

ICE CREAM and **FROZEN CUSTARD** (See also listing by flavor or brand name, e.g., **CHOCOLATE ICE CREAM** or *DREAMSICLE* or *GOOD HUMOR)*			
Sweetened:			
10% fat (USDA)	1 cup (4.7 oz.)	257	27.7
12% fat (USDA)	1 cup (5 oz.)	294	29.3
12% fat (USDA)	2½-oz. slice (⅛ of qt. brick)	147	14.6
12% fat (USDA)	small container (3½ fl. oz.)	128	12.8
16% fat (USDA)	1 cup (5.2 oz.)	329	26.6
Chocolate, 11.7% fat (Dean)	1 cup (5.6 oz.)	352	38.4
Nut, 14% fat (Dean)	1 cup (5.6 oz.)	376	36.3
Strawberry, 10.5% fat (Dean)	1 cup (5.6 oz.)	336	40.0
Vanilla, 10.1% fat (Dean)	1 cup (5.3 oz.)	296	33.8
Dietetic (See **FROZEN DESSERT**)			
ICE CREAM BAR, chocolate-coated:			
(Popsicle Industries)	3 fl. oz.	180	
(Sealtest)	1 bar (2½ fl. oz.)	149	12.1

(USDA): United States Department of Agriculture
(HEW/FAO): Health, Education and Welfare/Food and Agriculture Organization
* Prepared as Package Directs

Food and Description	Measure or Quantity	Calories	Carbo-hydrates (grams)
ICE CREAM CONE, cone only:			
(Comet) any color	1 piece (4 grams)	19	3.9
Rolled sugar (Comet) any color	1 piece (.4 oz.)	49	10.2
ICE CREAM CUP, cup only:			
(Comet) any color	1 piece (5 grams)	20	4.1
Pilot (Comet)	1 piece (4 grams)	19	3.9
ICE CREAM SANDWICH			
(Sealtest)	1 sandwich (3 fl. oz.)	173	26.1
ICE MILK:			
Hardened (USDA)	1 cup (4.6 oz.)	199	29.3
Soft-serve (USDA)	1 cup (6.2 oz.)	266	39.2
2.5% fat (Borden)	1 cup (4.6 oz.)	186	35.2
3.25% fat (Borden)	1 cup (4.7 oz.)	194	36.2
Any flavor (Borden) *Lite Line*	1 cup	198	32.0
5% fat (Dean)	1 cup (4.9 oz.)	227	35.0
Count Calorie, 2.1% fat (Dean)	1 cup (4.8 oz.)	155	17.1
(Sealtest) *Light n' Lively*:			
Buttered almond	1 cup (4.8 oz.)	234	35.8
Caramel nut	1 cup (4.8 oz.)	240	37.4
Chocolate	1 cup (4.8 oz.)	210	38.4
Coffee	1 cup (4.8 oz.)	204	36.8
ICE MILK BAR, chocolate-coated:			
(Popsicle Industries)	3 fl. oz.	133	
(Sealtest)	1 bar (2½ fl. oz.)	132	13.6
ICE STICK, twin pop (Sealtest)	3 fl. oz.	70	17.9
ICES (See individual fruit ice flavors)			
ICING (See **CAKE ICING**)			
INCONNU or **SHEEFISH**, raw:			
Whole (USDA)	1 lb. (weighed whole)	417	0.
Meat only (USDA)	4 oz.	166	0.
INDIAN PUDDING, New England (B&M)	½ cup (4 oz.)	120	27.1

Food and Description	Measure or Quantity	Calories	Carbo-hydrates (grams)
INSTANT BREAKFAST (See individual brand name or company listings)			
IRISH WHISKEY (See **DISTILLED LIQUORS**)			
ITALIAN DINNER, frozen:			
(Banquet)	11-oz. dinner	446	44.6
(Swanson)	13½-oz. dinner	448	54.1

J

JACKFRUIT, fresh (USDA):			
Whole	1 lb. (weighed with seeds & skin)	124	32.3
Flesh only	4 oz.	111	28.8
JACK MACKEREL, raw, meat only (USDA)	4 oz.	162	0.
JACK ROSE MIX (Bar-Tender's)	1 serving (⅝ oz.)	70	17.2
JALAPENO BEAN DIP (Fritos)	1 oz.	34	2.9
JAM, sweetened (See also individual listings by flavor):			
(USDA)	1 oz.	77	19.8
(USDA)	1 T. (.7 oz.)	54	14.0
JAPANESE-STYLE VEGETABLES, frozen (Birds Eye)	⅓ of 10-oz. pkg.	105	5.8

(USDA): United States Department of Agriculture
(HEW/FAO): Health, Education and Welfare/Food and Agriculture Organization
* Prepared as Package Directs

Food and Description	Measure or Quantity	Calories	Carbo-hydrates (grams)
JELLY, sweetened, all flavors (See also individual listings by flavor):			
(USDA)	1 T. (.6 oz.)	49	12.7
(Bama)	1 T. (.7 oz.)	51	12.7
(Crosse & Blackwell)	1 T. (.7 oz.)	51	12.8
(Kraft)	1 oz.	74	18.4
(Ma Brown)	1 oz.	73	17.0
(Polaner)	1 T.	54	13.5
(Smucker's)	1 T. (.7 oz.)	49	12.4
JELLY ROLL (Van de Kamp's):			
Lemon	9-oz. cake	879	
Raspberry	9-oz. cake	589	
JERUSALEM ARTICHOKE:			
Unpared (USDA)	1 lb. (weighed with skin)	207	52.3
Pared (USDA)	4 oz.	75	18.9
JOHANNISBERGER RIESLING WINE:			
(Deinhard) 11% alcohol	3 fl. oz.	72	4.5
(Inglenook) Estate, 12% alcohol	3 fl. oz.	61	.9
(Louis M. Martini) 12.5% alcohol	3 fl. oz.	90	.2
JORDAN ALMOND (See **CANDY**)			
JUICE (See individual flavors)			
JUJUBE or **CHINESE DATE** (USDA):			
Fresh, whole	1 lb. (weighed with seeds)	443	116.4
Fresh, flesh only	4 oz.	119	31.3
Dried, whole	1 lb. (weighed with seeds)	1159	297.1
Dried, flesh only	4 oz.	325	83.5
JUNIOR FOOD (See **BABY FOOD**)			

Food and Description	Measure or Quantity	Calories	Carbo-hydrates (grams)
JUNIORS (Tastykake):			
Chocolate	1 pkg. (2¾ oz.)	397	70.8
Chocolate devil food	1 pkg. (2¾ oz.)	284	45.2
Coconut	1 pkg. (2¾ oz.)	415	83.5
Coconut devil food	1 pkg. (2¾ oz.)	318	60.4
Jelly square	1 pkg. (3¼ oz.)	429	91.7
Koffee Kake	1 pkg. (2½ oz.)	395	59.7
Lemon	1 pkg. (2¾ oz.)	422	84.8
JUNKET (See individual flavors)			

K

KABOOM, cereal	1 cup (1 oz.)	109	24.6
KAFE VIN (Lejon) 19.7% alcohol	3 fl. oz.	183	22.8
KALE:			
Raw, leaves only (USDA)	1 lb. (weighed untrimmed)	154	26.1
Boiled, leaves including stems (USDA)	½ cup (1.9 oz.)	15	2.2
Frozen, chopped (Birds Eye)	½ cup (3.3 oz.)	29	4.2
KARO, syrup			
Dark corn	1 T. (.7 oz.)	60	15.0
Imitation maple	1 T. (.7 oz.)	59	14.7
Light corn	1 T. (.7 oz.)	60	15.0
Pancake & waffle	1 T. (.7 oz.)	60	14.9
KEFIR (Alta-Dena Dairy):			
Plain	1 cup	168	
Fruit	1 cup	208	

KETCHUP (See CATSUP)

(USDA): United States Department of Agriculture
(HEW/FAO): Health, Education and Welfare/Food and Agriculture Organization
* Prepared as Package Directs

Food and Description	Measure or Quantity	Calories	Carbohydrates (grams)
KIDNEY (USDA):			
Beef, raw	4 oz.	147	1.0
Beef, braised	4 oz.	286	.9
Calf, raw	4 oz.	128	.1
Hog. raw	4 oz.	120	1.2
Lamb, raw	4 oz.	119	1.0
KIELBASA (Oscar Mayer)	6-oz. link	530	10.0
KINGFISH, raw (USDA):			
Whole	1 lb. (weighed whole)	210	0.
Meat only	4 oz.	119	0.
KIPPERS (See **HERRING**)			
KIRSCH LIQUEUR (Garnier) 96 proof	1 fl. oz.	83	8.8
KIRSCHWASSER (Leroux) 96 proof	1 fl. oz.	80	0.
KIX, cereal	1½ cups (1 oz.)	112	23.8
KNOCKWURST (Oscar Mayer)	1 link (2.4 oz.)	210	2.2
KOHLRABI (USDA):			
Raw, whole	1 lb. (weighed with skin, without leaves)	96	21.9
Raw, diced	1 cup (4.8 oz.)	40	9.1
Boiled, drained	4 oz.	27	6.0
Boiled, drained	1 cup (5.5 oz.)	37	8.2
KOOL-AID, regular (General Foods)	1 cup (9.3 oz.)	98	25.0
KOOL-POPS (General Foods)	1 bar (1.5 oz.)	32	8.1
KOTTBULLAR (Hormel)	1 oz. (1-lb. can)	48	.9
KRIMPETS (Tastykake):			
Apple spice	1 cake (.9 oz.)	135	25.2
Butterscotch	1 cake (.9 oz.)	123	22.9
Chocolate	1 cake (.9 oz.)	119	21.6
Jelly	1 cake (.9 oz.)	103	21.0
Lemon	1 cake (.9 oz.)	113	21.4
Orange	1 cake (.9 oz.)	114	21.5

Food and Description	Measure or Quantity	Calories	Carbo-hydrates (grams)
KUMMEL LIQUEUR:			
(Garnier) 70 proof	1 fl. oz.	75	4.3
(Hiram Walker) 70 proof	1 fl. oz.	71	3.2
(Leroux) 70 proof	1 fl. oz.	75	4.1
(Old Mr. Boston) 70 proof	1 fl. oz.	78	2.0
KUMQUAT, fresh (USDA):			
Whole	1 lb. (weighed with seeds)	274	72.1
Flesh & skin	4 oz.	74	19.4
Flesh only	5-6 med. kumquats	65	17.1

L

LAKE COUNTRY WINE			
(Taylor):			
White dinner, 12.5% alcohol	3 fl. oz.	78	2.2
Red dinner, 12.5% alcohol	3 fl. oz.	81	2.9
LAKE HERRING, raw (USDA):			
Whole	1 lb.	226	0.
Meat only	4 oz.	109	0.
LAKE TROUT, raw (USDA):			
Drawn	1 lb. (weighed with head, fins & bones)	282	0.
Meat only	4 oz.	191	0.
LAKE TROUT or SISCOWET, raw (USDA):			
Less than 6.5 lb. whole	1 lb. (weighed whole)	404	0.

(USDA): United States Department of Agriculture
(HEW/FAO): Health, Education and Welfare/Food and Agriculture Organization
* Prepared as Package Directs

Food and Description	Measure or Quantity	Calories	Carbohydrates (grams)
Less than 6.5 lb. whole	4 oz. (meat only)	273	0.
More than 6.5 lb. whole	1 lb. (weighed whole)	856	0.
More than 6.5 lb. whole	4 oz. (meat only)	594	0.
LAMB, choice grade (USDA):			
Chop, broiled:			
Loin. One 5-oz. chop (weighed before cooking with bone) will give you:			
Lean & fat	2.8 oz.	280	0.
Lean only	2.3 oz.	122	0.
Rib. One 5-oz. chop (weighed before cooking with bone) will give you:			
Lean & fat	2.9 oz.	334	0.
Lean only	2 oz.	118	0.
Fat, separable, cooked	1 oz.	201	0.
Leg:			
Raw, lean & fat	1 lb. (weighed with bone)	845	0.
Roasted, lean & fat	4 oz.	316	0.
Roasted, lean only	4 oz.	211	0.
Shoulder:			
Raw, lean & fat	1 lb. (weighed with bone)	1082	0.
Roasted, lean & fat	4 oz.	383	0.
Roasted, lean only	4 oz.	232	0.
LAMB'S-QUARTERS (USDA):			
Raw, trimmed	1 lb.	195	33.1
Boiled, drained	4 oz.	36	5.7
LAMB STEW, canned (B&M)	1 cup (8.1 oz.)	192	11.4
LARD:			
(USDA)	1 cup (7.2 oz.)	1849	0.
(USDA)	1 T. (.5 oz.)	117	0.
LASAGNE:			
Canned (Chef Boy-Ar-Dee)	8 oz. (⅕ of 40-oz. can)	279	29.7
Canned (Nalley's)	8 oz.	213	27.2

Food and Description	Measure or Quantity	Calories	Carbohydrates (grams)
Frozen, with meat sauce (Buitoni)	½ of 15-oz. pkg.	255	24.9
Frozen (Celeste)	¼ of 2-lb. pkg.	413	23.1
*Mix, dinner (Chef Boy-Ar-Dee)	8¾-oz. pkg.	273	37.7
Mix (Golden Grain) Stir-N-Serv	7-oz. pkg.	755	130.0
Mix (Hunt's) *Skillet*	1-lb. 1-oz. pkg.	812	114.6
*Mix (Jeno's) Add 'n Heat	30-oz. pkg.	1599	83.3
Seasoning mix (Lawry's)	1.1-oz. pkg.	86	19.6
LEEKS, raw (USDA):			
Whole	1 lb. (weighed untrimmed)	123	26.4
Trimmed	4 oz.	59	12.7
LEMON, fresh, peeled (USDA)	1 med. (2⅛″ dia.)	20	6.1
LEMONADE:			
Chilled (Sealtest)	½ cup (4.4 oz.)	55	13.4
Frozen, concentrate, sweetened:			
(USDA)	6-fl.-oz. can	427	112.0
*Diluted with 4⅓ parts water (USDA)	½ cup (4.4 oz.)	55	14.1
*(Minute Maid)	½ cup (4.2 oz.)	49	12.5
(ReaLemon)	6-oz. can	414	108.0
*(Seneca)	½ cup (4.3 oz.)	56	14.0
*(Snow Crop)	½ cup (4.2 oz.)	49	12.5
Frozen, low calorie (Weight Waters)	½ cup (3.9 oz.)	5	1.3
Mix:			
*(Salada)	6 fl. oz.	79	19.2
*(Wyler's)	6 fl. oz.	64	15.8
*(Wyler's) pink	6 fl. oz.	64	15.8
LEMON CAKE MIX:			
*(Duncan Hines)	¹⁄₁₂ of cake	202	35.0
*(Pillsbury)	¹⁄₁₂ of cake	210	34.0

(USDA): United States Department of Agriculture
(HEW/FAO): Health, Education and Welfare/Food and Agriculture Organization
* Prepared as Package Directs

Food and Description	Measure or Quantity	Calories	Carbo- hydrates (grams)
*Chiffon (Betty Crocker)	¹⁄₁₆ of cake	151	26.8
Coconut (Betty Crocker)	1 oz.	121	22.3
Cream moist cake (Pillsbury)	1 oz.	122	21.8
*Pudding cake (Betty Crocker)	⅛ of cake	227	45.4
LEMON EXTRACT:			
Pure (Ehlers)	1 tsp.	14	
(Virginia Dare) 77% alcohol	1 tsp.	22	0.
LEMON JUICE:			
Fresh:			
(USDA)	1 cup (8.6 oz.)	61	19.5
(USDA)	1 T. (.5 oz.)	4	1.2
(Sunkist)	1 lemon (3.9 oz.)	11	4.0
(Sunkist)	1 T. (.5 oz.)	4	1.0
Canned, unsweetened (USDA)	1 cup (8.6 oz.)	56	18.6
Canned, unsweetened (USDA)	1 T. (.5 oz.)	3	1.1
Plastic container (USDA)	¼ cup (2 oz.)	13	4.3
Plastic container, *ReaLemon*	1 T. (.5 oz.)	3	.8
Frozen, unsweetened:			
Concentrate (USDA)	½ cup (5.1 oz.)	169	54.6
Single strength (USDA)	½ cup (4.3 oz.)	27	8.8
Full strength, already reconstituted:			
(Minute Maid)	½ cup (4.2 oz.)	27	8.5
(Snow Crop)	½ cup (4.2 oz.)	27	8.5
LEMON-LIMEADE, sweetened, concentrate, frozen:			
*(Minute Maid)	½ cup (4.2 oz.)	50	12.7
*(Snow Crop)	½ cup (4.2 oz.)	50	12.7
LEMON-LIME SOFT DRINK:			
Sweetened:			
(Dr. Brown's)	6 fl. oz.	74	18.4
(Hoffman)	6 fl. oz.	74	18.4
(Key Food)	6 fl. oz.	74	18.4
(Kirsch)	6 fl. oz.	70	17.5
(Nedick's)	6 fl. oz.	74	18.4
(Salute)	6 fl. oz.	72	18.2
(Shasta)	6 fl. oz.	73	18.4
(Waldbaum)	6 fl. oz.	74	18.4

Food and Description	*Measure or Quantity*	*Calories*	*Carbo-hydrates (grams)*
(Yukon Club)	6 fl. oz.	74	18.4
Low calorie:			
Diet Rite	6 fl. oz.	2	.4
(Hoffman)	6 fl. oz.	1	.2
(Shasta)	6 fl. oz.	<1	<.1
LEMON PEEL, CANDIED:			
(USDA)	1 oz.	90	22.9
(Liberty)	1 oz.	93	22.6
LEMON PIE:			
(Hostess)	4½-oz. pie	447	56.1
(Mrs. Smith's)	⅙ of 8″ pie (4.2 oz.)	340	45.0
(Tastykake)	4-oz. pie	366	52.0
Chiffon, home recipe (USDA)	⅙ of 9″ pie (3.8 oz.)	338	47.3
Cream, frozen (Banquet)	2½ oz.	179	25.5
Cream, frozen (Morton)	⅙ of 16-oz. pie (2.7 oz.)	194	26.0
Cream, frozen (Mrs. Smith's)	⅙ of 8″ pie (2.8 oz.)	227	31.7
Krunch (Mrs. Smith's)	⅙ of 8″ pie (4.3 oz.)	383	56.7
Meringue, home recipe (USDA)	⅙ of 9″ pie (4.9 oz.)	357	52.8
Meringue, frozen (Mrs. Smith's)	⅙ of 8″ pie (3.7 oz.)	261	40.0
LEMON PIE FILLING:			
(Comstock)	1-lb. 5-oz. can	864	191.8
(Lucky Leaf)	8 oz.	412	95.4
(Wilderness)	22-oz. can	1104	230.2
LEMON PUDDING:			
Canned (Betty Crocker)	½ cup	198	40.1
Canned (Hunt's)	5-oz. can	175	35.3

(USDA): United States Department of Agriculture
(HEW/FAO): Health, Education and Welfare/Food and Agriculture Organization
* Prepared as Package Directs

Food and Description	Measure or Quantity	Calories	Carbo- hydrates (grams)
LEMON PUDDING or PIE FILLING MIX:			
Regular:			
*(Jell-O)	½ cup (5.1 oz.)	178	38.8
*(My-T-Fine)	½ cup (5 oz.)	179	31.7
*(Royal)	⅛ of 9″ pie (including crust, 4.6 oz.)	224	39.8
Instant:			
*(Jell-O)	½ cup (5.3 oz.)	178	30.5
*(Royal)	½ cup (5.1 oz.)	178	28.7
LEMON RENNET CUSTARD MIX:			
Powder:			
(Junket)	1 oz.	116	28.1
*(Junket)	4 oz.	109	14.7
Tablet:			
(Junket)	1 tablet	1	.2
*With sugar (Junket)	4 oz.	101	13.5
LEMON SOFT DRINK:			
Sweetened:			
(Canada Dry)	6 fl. oz.	74	18.6
(Hoffman)	6 fl. oz.	81	20.2
(Kirsch)	6 fl. oz.	64	16.1
(Royal Crown)	6 fl. oz.	89	22.2
Low calorie:			
(Canada Dry)	6 fl. oz.	18	0.
(No-Cal)	6 fl. oz.	2	0.
(Shasta)	6 fl. oz.	<1	<.1
LEMON TURNOVER, frozen			
(Pepperidge Farm)	1 turnover (3.3 oz.)	341	33.1
LENTIL:			
Whole:			
Dry:			
(USDA)	½ lb.	771	136.3
(USDA)	1 cup (6.7 oz.)	649	114.8
(Sinsheimer)	1 oz.	95	17.0
Cooked, drained (USDA)	½ cup (3.6 oz.)	107	19.5
Split, dry (USDA)	½ lb.	782	140.2

Food and Description	Measure or Quantity	Calories	Carbo-hydrates (grams)
LENTIL SOUP, canned:			
With ham (Crosse & Blackwell)	6½ oz. (½ can)	123	17.0
*(Manischewitz)	8 oz. (by wt.)	166	29.3
Mix (Lipton) *Cup-a-Soup*	1.2-oz. pkg.	123	20.9
LETTUCE (USDA):			
Bibb, untrimmed	1 lb. (weighed untrimmed)	47	8.4
Bibb, untrimmed	7.8-oz. head (4″ dia.)	23	4.1
Boston, untrimmed	1 lb. (weighed untrimmed)	47	8.4
Boston, untrimmed	7.8-oz. head (4″ dia.)	23	4.1
Butterhead varieties (See Bibb & Boston)			
Cos (See Romaine)			
Dark green (See Romaine)			
Grand Rapids	1 lb. (weighed untrimmed)	52	10.2
Grand Rapids	2 large leaves (1.8 oz.)	9	1.8
Great Lakes	1 lb. (weighed untrimmed)	56	12.5
Great Lakes, trimmed	1-lb. head (4¾″ dia.)	59	13.2
Iceberg:			
Untrimmed	1 lb. (weighed untrimmed)	56	12.5
Trimmed	1-lb. head (4¾″ dia.)	59	13.2
Leaves	1 cup (2.3 oz.)	9	1.9
Chopped	1 cup (2 oz.)	8	1.7
Chunks	1 cup (2.6 oz.)	10	2.1
Looseleaf varieties (See Salad Bowl)			
New York	1 lb. (weighed untrimmed)	56	12.5

(USDA): United States Department of Agriculture
(HEW/FAO): Health, Education and Welfare/Food and Agriculture Organization
* Prepared as Package Directs

Food and Description	Measure or Quantity	Calories	Carbo-hydrates (grams)
New York	1-lb. head (4¾″ dia.)	59	13.2
Romaine: Untrimmed	1 lb. (weighed untrimmed)	52	10.2
Trimmed, shredded & broken into pieces	½ cup (.8 oz.)	4	.8
Salad Bowl	1 lb. (weighed untrimmed)	52	10.2
Salad Bowl	2 large leaves (1.8 oz.)	9	1.8
Simpson	1 lb. (weighed untrimmed)	52	10.2
Simpson	2 large leaves (1.8 oz.)	9	1.8
White Paris (See Romaine)			
LIEBFRAUMILCH WINE:			
(Anheuser) 10% alcohol	3 fl. oz.	63	.9
(Deinhard) 11% alcohol	3 fl. oz.	60	3.6
(Deinhard) *Hans Christof*, 11% alcohol	3 fl. oz.	60	3.6
(Julius Kayser) Glockenspiel, 10% alcohol	3 fl. oz.	57	1.8
LIFE, cereal (Quaker)	⅔ cup (1 oz.)	107	20.4
LIKE, soft drink, low calorie (Seven-Up)	6 fl. oz.	1	.3
LIMA BEAN (See BEAN, LIMA)			
LIME, fresh, whole: (USDA)	1 lb. (weighed with skin & seeds)	107	36.2
(USDA)	1 med. (2″ dia., 2.4 oz.)	15	4.9
LIMEADE, concentrate, sweetened, frozen: (USDA)	6-fl.-oz. can	408	107.9
*Diluted with 4⅓ parts water (USDA)	½ cup (4.4 oz.)	51	13.6
*(Minute Maid)	½ cup (4.2 oz.)	50	13.0

Food and Description	Measure or Quantity	Calories	Carbo-hydrates (grams)
(ReaLemon)	6-oz. can	414	108.0
*(Snow Crop)	½ cup (4.2 oz.)	50	13.0
*LIMEADE MIX (Wyler's)	6 fl. oz.	64	15.8
LIME ICE, home recipe (USDA)	8 oz. (by wt.)	177	73.9
LIME JUICE:			
Fresh (USDA)	1 cup (8.7 oz.)	64	22.1
Canned or bottled, unsweetened:			
(USDA)	1 cup (8.7 oz.)	64	22.1
(USDA)	1 fl. oz. (1.1 oz.)	8	2.8
Plastic container *ReaLime*	1 T. (.5 oz.)	2	.5
LIME PIE, Key lime, cream, frozen (Banquet)	2½ oz.	204	27.5
*LIME PIE FILLING MIX, Key lime (Royal)	⅛ of 9″ pie (including crust, 4.6 oz.)	222	39.4
LIME SOFT DRINK:			
(Canada Dry)	6 fl. oz.	98	24.6
(Yukon Club)	6 fl. oz.	64	16.1
LINGCOD, raw (USDA):			
Whole	1 lb. (weighed whole)	130	0.
Meat only	4 oz.	95	0.
LIQUEUR (See individual kinds)			
LITCHI NUT (USDA):			
Fresh:			
Whole	4 oz. (weighed in shell, with seeds)	44	11.2
Flesh only	4 oz.	73	18.6

(USDA): United States Department of Agriculture
(HEW/FAO): Health, Education and Welfare/Food and Agriculture Organization
* Prepared as Package Directs

Food and Description	Measure or Quantity	Calories	Carbo-hydrates (grams)
Dried:			
Whole	4 oz. (weighed in shell, with seeds)	145	36.9
Flesh only	2 oz.	157	40.1
LIVER (USDA):			
Beef, raw	1 lb.	635	24.0
Beef, fried	4 oz.	260	6.0
Calf, raw	1 lb.	635	18.6
Calf, fried	4 oz.	296	4.5
Chicken, raw	1 lb.	585	13.2
Chicken, simmered	4 oz.	187	3.5
Goose, raw	1 lb.	826	24.5
Hog, raw	1 lb.	594	11.8
Hog, fried	4 oz.	273	2.8
Lamb, raw	1 lb.	617	13.2
Lamb, broiled	4 oz.	296	3.2
Turkey, raw	1 lb.	626	13.2
Turkey, simmered	4 oz.	197	3.5
LIVER PÂTÉ (See PÂTÉ)			
LIVER SAUSAGE or **LIVER-WURST:**			
Ring (Oscar Mayer)	1 oz.	86	0.
Sliced (Oscar Mayer)	1 slice (.9 oz.)	95	.4
Spread (Underwood)	1 T. (.5 oz.)	45	.5
LOBSTER:			
Raw:			
Whole (USDA)	1 lb. (weighed whole)	107	.6
Meat only (USDA)	4 oz.	103	.6
Cooked, meat only (USDA)	4 oz.	108	.3
Canned, meat only (USDA)	4 oz.	108	.3
Frozen, South African rock lobster tail	2-oz. tail	65	.1
LOBSTER NEWBURG:			
Home recipe (USDA)	4 oz.	220	5.8
Frozen (Stouffer's)	11½-oz. pkg.	671	16.0
LOBSTER PASTE, canned (USDA)	1 oz.	51	.4
LOBSTER SALAD, home recipe (USDA)	4 oz.	125	2.6

Food and Description	Measure or Quantity	Calories	Carbo-hydrates (grams)
LOBSTER SOUP, canned, cream of (Crosse & Blackwell)	6½ oz. (½ can)	92	6.5
LOCHON ORA, Scottish liqueur (Leroux) 70 proof	1 fl. oz.	89	7.4
LOGANBERRY (USDA):			
Fresh:			
Untrimmed	1 lb. (weighed with caps)	267	64.2
Trimmed	1 cup (5.1 oz.)	89	21.5
Canned, solids & liq.:			
Water pack	4 oz.	45	10.7
Juice pack	4 oz.	61	14.4
Light syrup	4 oz.	79	19.5
Heavy syrup	4 oz.	101	25.2
Extra heavy syrup	4 oz.	122	30.8
LOG CABIN, syrup:			
Buttered	1 T. (.7 oz.)	52	12.7
Maple-honey	1 T.	54	14.0
LOGAN (USDA):			
Fresh:			
Whole	1 lb. (weighed with shell & seeds)	147	38.0
Flesh only	4 oz.	69	17.9
Dried:			
Whole	1 lb. (weighed with shell & seeds)	467	120.8
Flesh only	4 oz.	324	83.9
LOQUAT, fresh (USDA):			
Whole	1 lb. (weighed with seeds)	168	43.3
Flesh only	4 oz.	54	14.1

(USDA): United States Department of Agriculture
(HEW/FAO): Health, Education and Welfare/Food and Agriculture Organization
* Prepared as Package Directs

Food and Description	Measure or Quantity	Calories	Carbo-hydrates (grams)
LOVE BIRD COCKTAIL, dry mix (Holland House)	1 serving (.6-oz. pkg.)	69	17.0
LUCKY CHARMS, cereal	1 cup (1 oz.)	110	23.6
LUMBERJACK, syrup (Nalley's)	1 oz.	78	19.6
LUNCHEON MEAT (See also individual listings, e.g. **BOLOGNA**):			
All meat (Oscar Mayer)	1-oz. slice	98	.9
Banquet (Eckrich)	1 slice	54	1.0
Bar-B-Q Loaf (Oscar Mayer)	1-oz. slice	48	2.5
Chicken breast loaf (Eckrich)	1 oz.	32	
Cocktail loaf (Oscar Mayer)	1-oz. slice	62	3.8
Gourmet loaf (Eckrich)	1-oz. slice	38	2.0
Ham & cheese (see **HAM & CHEESE**)			
Honey loaf (Eckrich)	1 slice	42	2.0
Honey loaf (Oscar Mayer)	1-oz. slice	40	.9
Jellied:			
Beef loaf (Oscar Mayer)	1-oz. slice	41	.8
Corned beef loaf (Oscar Mayer)	1-oz. slice	39	.3
Luncheon loaf (Sugardale)	1-oz. slice	77	
Luncheon roll, sausage, all meat (Oscar Mayer)	.8-oz. slice	27	.2
Luxury Loaf (Oscar Mayer)	1-oz. slice (8 per ½ lb.)	40	1.3
Meat loaf (USDA)	1 oz.	57	.9
Minced roll sausage, all meat (Oscar Mayer)	.8-oz. slice	54	.9
Old-fashioned loaf:			
(Eckrich)	1 slice	76	2.0
(Oscar Mayer)	1-oz. slice	62	2.3
(Sugardale)	1-oz. slice	76	
Olive loaf (Oscar Mayer)	1-oz. slice	62	2.6
Peppered loaf (Oscar Mayer)	1-oz. slice	46	2.0
Pickle loaf (Eckrich)	1 slice	86	1.5
Pickle & pimento:			
(Hormel)	1 oz. (6-lb. can)	81	.3
(Oscar Mayer)	1-oz. slice	62	3.8
(Sugardale)	1-oz. slice	78	Tr.
Picnic loaf (Oscar Mayer)	1-oz. slice	64	1.0

Food and Description	Measure or Quantity	Calories	Carbo-hydrates (grams)
Plain loaf (Oscar Mayer)	1-oz. slice	75	1.4
Pure beef (Oscar Mayer)	1-oz. slice	75	1.2
Spiced (Hormel)	1 oz.	70	1.0
LUNG, raw (USDA):			
Beef	1 lb.	435	0.
Calf	1 lb.	481	0.
Lamb	1 lb.	467	0.

MACADAMIA NUT:

Whole (USDA)	1 lb. (weighed in shell)	972	22.4
Shelled (Royal Hawaiian)	¼ cup (2 oz.)	394	9.1

MACARONI. Plain macaroni products are essentially the same in caloric value and carbohydrate content on the same weight basis. The longer they are cooked, the more water is absorbed and this affects the nutritive values.

Dry:			
Elbow-type (USDA)	1 cup (4.8 oz.)	502	102.3
1-inch pieces (USDA)	1 cup (3.8 oz.)	406	82.7
2-inch pieces (USDA)	1 cup (3 oz.)	317	64.7
(USDA)	1 oz.	105	21.3
20% protein (Buitoni)	1 oz.	101	18.2
Cooked (USDA):			
8–10 minutes, firm	1 cup (4.6 oz.)	192	39.1
8–10 minutes, firm	4 oz.	168	34.1
14–20 minutes, tender	1 cup (4.9 oz.)	155	32.2
14–20 minutes, tender	4 oz.	126	26.1

(USDA): United States Department of Agriculture
(HEW/FAO): Health, Education and Welfare/Food and Agriculture
                Organization
* Prepared as Package Directs

Food and Description	Measure or Quantity	Calories	Carbo- hydrates (grams)
MACARONI & BEEF:			
(Buitoni)	8 oz.	222	24.6
In tomato sauce, canned			
(Franco-American)	1 cup	225	25.0
(Swanson)	11¼-oz. dinner	302	35.0
With tomatoes, frozen			
(Stouffer's)	11½-oz. pkg.	410	39.0
MACARONI & CHEESE:			
Home recipe, baked (USDA)	1 cup (7.1 oz.)	430	40.2
Canned:			
(USDA)	1 cup	228	25.7
(Franco-American)	1 cup	219	25.0
(Heinz)	8¼-oz. can	231	27.0
Frozen:			
(Banquet)	20-oz. pkg.	742	82.0
(Banquet) cookin' bag	8 oz.	279	75.9
(Kraft)	12½-oz. pkg.	612	54.2
(Morton) casserole	8-oz. pkg.	295	29.5
(Morton) casserole	20-oz. pkg.	737	73.7
(Stouffer's)	12-oz. pkg.	477	52.1
MACARONI & CHEESE MIX:			
Dry (USDA)	1 oz.	113	17.8
*Cheddar sauce (Betty Crocker)	¾ cup	244	36.7
Dinner (Golden Grain)	¼ of 7¼-oz. pkg.	202	38.0
MACARONI DINNER:			
& beef, frozen:			
(Banquet)	12-oz. dinner	394	55.1
(Morton)	11-oz. dinner	287	37.4
& cheese:			
*(Chef-Boy-Ar-Dee)	4½-oz. pkg.	201	33.8
*(Kraft)	4 oz.	203	26.1
*(Kraft) deluxe	4 oz.	202	27.9
Frozen (Banquet)	12-oz. dinner	326	45.6
Frozen (Morton)	12¾-oz. dinner	384	50.7
Frozen (Swanson)	12¾-oz. dinner	367	48.4
Creole (Heinz)	8¾-oz. can	169	28.4
*Italian-style (Kraft)	4 oz.	119	20.5
*Mexican-style (Kraft)	4 oz.	126	22.6
*Monte Bello with sauce mix (Betty Crocker)	1 cup	350	38.9
MACARONI ENTREE, shells in meat sauce (Buitoni)	4 oz.	117	15.3

Food and Description	Measure or Quantity	Calories	Carbo-hydrates (grams)
MACARONI SALAD, canned (Nalley's)	4 oz.	203	13.9
MACKEREL (USDA):			
Atlantic:			
Raw:			
Whole	1 lb. (weighed whole)	468	0.
Meat only	4 oz.	217	0.
Broiled with butter	4 oz.	268	0.
Canned, solids & liq.	4 oz.	208	0.
Pacific:			
Raw:			
Dressed	1 lb. (weighed with bones & skin)	519	0.
Meat only	4 oz.	180	0.
Canned, solids & liq.	4 oz.	204	0.
Salted	4 oz.	346	0.
Smoked	4 oz.	248	0.
MACKEREL, JACK (See **JACK MACKEREL**)			
MADEIRA WINE (Leacock) 19% alcohol	3 fl. oz.	120	6.3
MAGGI, seasoning	1 T.	22	.1
MAI TAI COCKTAIL:			
(Lemon Hart) 48 proof	3 fl. oz.	180	15.6
(National Distillers) *Duet,* 12.5% alcohol	8-fl.-oz. can	288	28.8
(Party Tyme) 12½% alcohol	2 fl. oz.	65	5.7
Dry mix (Bar-Tender's)	1 serving (5.8 oz.)	69	17.0
Dry mix (Holland House)	1 serving (.6-oz. pkg.)	69	17.0
Dry mix (Party Tyme)	1 serving (½ oz.)	50	11.8
Liquid mix (Holland House)	1½ fl. oz.	50	12.0
Liquid mix (Party Tyme)	2 fl. oz.	44	11.2

(USDA): United States Department of Agriculture
(HEW/FAO): Health, Education and Welfare/Food and Agriculture Organization
* Prepared as Package Directs

Food and Description	Measure or Quantity	Calories	Carbo-hydrates (grams)
MALT, dry (USDA)	1 oz.	104	21.9
MALTED MILK MIX:			
Dry powder (USDA)	1 oz.	116	20.1
Chocolate, instant (Borden)	2 heaping tsps. (.7 oz.)	77	16.0
Chocolate (Carnation)	3 heaping tsps. (.7 oz.)	85	18.3
Chocolate (Horlicks)	3 heaping tsps. (1.1 oz.)	124	26.0
Chocolate, dry (Kraft)	2 heaping tsps. (.4 oz.)	51	10.0
*Chocolate (Kraft)	1 cup (8.7 oz.)	241	29.8
Natural, instant (Borden)	2 heaping tsps. (.7 oz.)	80	13.4
Natural (Carnation)	3 heaping tsps. (.7 oz.)	88	15.6
Natural (Horlicks)	3 heaping tsps. (1.1 oz.)	127	22.3
Natural, dry (Kraft)	2 heaping tsps. (.4 oz.)	52	9.2
*Natural (Kraft)	1 cup (8.6 oz.)	240	27.7
MALTEX, cereal	1 oz.	109	22.7
MALT EXTRACT, dried (USDA)	1 oz.	104	25.3
MALT LIQUOR:			
Big Cat	12 fl. oz.	155	
Champale, 6.25% alcohol	12 fl. oz. (12.6 oz.)	173	11.5
Country Club, 6.8% alcohol	12 fl. oz.	183	2.8
MALT-O-MEAL, cereal	¾ cup (1 oz. dry)	102	22.3
MAMEY or **MAMMEE APPLE,** fresh (USDA)	1 lb. (weighed with skin & seeds)	143	35.2
MANDARIN ORANGE, CANNED, solids & liq.:			
Light syrup (Del Monte)	½ cup (4.5 oz.)	77	20.6
Low calorie (Diet Delight)	½ cup (4.3 oz.)	31	7.4

Food and Description	Measure or Quantity	Calories	Carbo-hydrates (grams)
MANDARIN ORANGE, FRESH (See **TANGERINE**)			
MANGO, fresh (USDA):			
Whole	1 lb. (weighed with seeds & skin)	201	51.1
Whole	1 med. (7 oz.)	88	22.5
Flesh only, diced or sliced	½ cup (2.9 oz.)	54	13.8
MANHATTAN COCKTAIL:			
(Hiram Walker) 55 proof	3 fl. oz.	147	3.0
(National Distillers) *Duet,* 20% alcohol	8-fl.-oz. can	576	11.2
(Party Tyme) 20% alcohol	2 fl. oz.	74	1.5
Dry mix (Bar-Tender's)	1 serving (⅛ oz.)	24	5.6
MANICOTTI, without sauce, frozen (Buitoni)	4 oz.	218	19.9
MAPLE FLAVORING, imitation maple (Ehlers)	1 tsp.	8	
MAPLE RENNET CUSTARD MIX:			
Powder:			
(Junket)	1 oz.	117	27.9
*(Junket)	4 oz.	109	14.7
Tablet:			
(Junket)	1 tablet	1	.2
*& sugar (Junket)	4 oz.	101	13.5
MAPLE SYRUP (See also individual brand names):			
(USDA)	1 T. (.7 oz.)	50	13.0
(Cary's)	1 T. (.8 oz.)	63	15.7
MARASCHINO LIQUEUR:			
(Garnier) 60 proof	1 fl. oz.	94	11.1
(Leroux) 60 proof	1 fl. oz.	88	9.7

(USDA): United States Department of Agriculture
(HEW/FAO): Health, Education and Welfare/Food and Agriculture
           Organization
* Prepared as Package Directs

Food and Description	Measure or Quantity	Calories	Carbohydrates (grams)
MARBLE CAKE MIX:			
Dry (USDA)	1 oz.	120	21.4
*With boiled white icing			
(USDA)	4 oz.	375	70.3
*(Betty Crocker)	1/12 of cake	206	37.2
MARGARINE, salted or			
unsalted:			
(USDA)	1 lb.	3266	1.8
(USDA)	1 cup (8 oz.)	1633	.9
(USDA)	1 T. (.5 oz.)	101	<.1
(Blue Bonnet) regular or soft	1 T. (.5 oz.)	101	.1
(Borden) Danish flavor	1 T. (.5 oz.)	101	<.1
(Fleischmann's) regular or			
soft	1 T. (.5 oz.)	101	.1
(Golden Glow)	1 T. (.4 oz.)	89	.1
(Holiday)	1 T. (.5 oz.)	100	0.
(Imperial) stick	1 T. (.5 oz.)	100	.1
(Imperial) *Sof-Spread*	1 T. (.5 oz.)	100	.1
(Mazola)	1 T. (.5 oz.)	102	.1
(Miracle) corn oil	1 T. (9 grams)	67	<.1
(Nucoa)	1 T. (.5 oz.)	102	.1
(Nucoa) soft	1 T. (.4 oz.)	91	.1
(Parkay) regular	1 T. (.5 oz.)	101	.1
(Parkay) soft cup	1 T. (.5 oz.)	95	.1
(Parkay) corn oil, deluxe	1 T. (.5 oz.)	101	.1
(Parkay) corn oil, soft	1 T. (.5 oz.)	95	.1
(Parkay) safflower oil, soft	1 T. (.5 oz.)	95	.1
(Parkay) squeeze	1 T. (.5 oz.)	101	.1
(Phenix)	1 T. (.5 oz.)	101	.1
(Promise) soft or stick	1 T. (.5 oz.)	100	.1
(Saffola) regular or soft	1 T. (.5 oz.)	101	<.1
MARGARINE, IMITATION,			
diet:			
(Fleischmann's)	1 T. (.5 oz.)	50	0.
(Imperial)	1 T. (.5 oz.)	49	0.
(Mazola)	1 T. (.5 oz.)	51	0.
(Parkay) soft	1 T.	55	0.
MARGARINE, WHIPPED:			
(Blue Bonnet)	1 T. (9 grams)	67	<.1
(Imperial)	1 T. (9 grams)	64	<.1
(Miracle)	1 T. (9 grams)	67	<.1
(Parkay) cup	1 T.	67	<.1

Food and Description	Measure or Quantity	Calories	Carbo-hydrates (grams)
MARGARITA COCKTAIL:			
(National Distillers) *Duet,*			
12.5% alcohol	8-fl.-oz. can	248	20.0
(Party Tyme) 12.5% alcohol	2 fl. oz.	66	5.7
Dry mix (Bar-Tender's)	1 serving (⅝ oz.)	70	17.3
MARGAUX, French red Bordeaux (Barton &			
Guestier) 12% alcohol	3 fl. oz.	62	.4
MARINADE MIX:			
(Adolph's) chicken	1 pkg. (1 oz.)	66	14.8
(Lawry's) lemon pepper	1 pkg. (2.7 oz.)	159	29.7
MARMALADE:			
Sweetened:			
(USDA)	1 T. (.7 oz.)	51	14.0
(Bama)	1 T. (.7 oz.)	54	13.5
(Crosse & Blackwell)	1 T. (.6 oz.)	60	14.9
(Kraft)	1 oz.	78	19.3
(Ma Brown)	1 oz.	73	17.0
(Smucker's)	1 T. (.7 oz.)	53	13.6
Dietetic or low calorie:			
(Dia-Mel)	1 T. (.5 oz.)	6	1.4
(Louis Sherry)	1 T. (.6 oz.)	6	1.5
(S and W) *Nutradiet*	1 T. (.5 oz.)	11	2.6
(Slenderella)	1 T. (.6 oz.)	22	5.6
MARMALADE PLUM			
(USDA):			
Fresh, whole	1 lb. (with skin & seeds)	431	108.9
Fresh, flesh only	4 oz.	142	35.8
MARTINI COCKTAIL:			
Gin:			
(Hiram Walker) 67.5 proof	3 fl. oz.	168	.6
(National Distillers) *Duet,* 21% alcohol	8-fl.-oz. can	560	1.6
(Party Tyme) 24% alcohol	2 fl. oz.	82	0.

(USDA): United States Department of Agriculture
(HEW/FAO): Health, Education and Welfare/Food and Agriculture Organization
* Prepared as Package Directs

Food and Description	Measure or Quantity	Calories	Carbo-hydrates (grams)
Liquid mix (Holland House)	1½ fl. oz.	15	3.8
Liquid mix (Party Tyme)	2 fl. oz.	12	3.2
Vodka:			
(Hiram Walker) 60 proof	3 fl. oz.	147	Tr.
(National Distillers) *Duet*, 20% alcohol	8-fl.-oz. can	536	1.6
(Party Tyme) 21% alcohol	2 fl. oz.	72	0.
*MASA HARINA (Quaker)	2 tortillas (6" dia.)	139	27.8
*MASA TRIGO (Quaker)	2 tortillas (6" dia.)	150	25.5
MATZO:			
Regular (Manischewitz)	1 matzo (1.1 oz.)	114	28.1
American (Manischewitz)	1 matzo (1 oz.)	121	22.6
Diet-10's (Goodman's)	1 sq.	109	23.0
Diet-thins (Manischewitz)	1 matzo (1 oz.)	113	24.5
Egg (Manischewitz)	1 matzo (1.2 oz.)	133	26.6
Egg'n Onion (Manischewitz)	1 matzo (1 oz.)	116	24.6
Midgetea (Goodman's)	1 matzo (.4 oz.)	40	7.4
Onion Tams (Manischewitz)	1 piece (3 grams)	13	1.9
Round tea (Goodman's)	1 matzo (.6 oz.)	70	12.9
Tam Tams (Manischewitz)	1 piece (3 grams)	14	1.7
Tasteas (Manischewitz)	1 matzo (1 oz.)	119	24.2
Thin tea (Manischewitz)	1 matzo (1 oz.)	114	24.8
Unsalted (Goodman's)	1 matzo (1 oz.)	109	23.0
Unsalted (Horowitz-Margareten)	1 matzo (1.2 oz.)	135	28.2
Whole wheat (Manischewitz)	1 matzo (1.2 oz.)	124	24.2
MATZO MEAL (Manischewitz)	1 cup (4.1 oz.)	438	96.2
MAYONNAISE:			
(USDA)	1 cup (7.8 oz.)	1587	4.9
(USDA)	1 T. (.5 oz.)	101	.3
(Bama)	1 T. (.5 oz.)	95	.3
(Bennett's)	1 T. (.5 oz.)	113	.3
(Best-Foods) *Real*	1 cup (7.7 oz.)	1572	3.3
(Hellmann's) *Real*	1 T. (.5 oz.)	102	<.1
(Dia-Mel)	1 T. (.5 oz.)	99	Tr.
(Kraft)	1 T. (.5 oz.)	102	.1

Food and Description	Measure or Quantity	Calories	Carbo-hydrates (grams)
(Kraft) *Salad Bowl*	1 T. (.5 oz.)	102	.2
(Nalley's)	1 oz.	214	.9
(Saffola)	1 T. (.5 oz.)	92	.3
***MAYPO*, cereal, dry, any flavor:**			
Instant	1 oz.	105	19.8
1-minute	1 oz.	107	19.8
MAY WINE (Deinhard) 11% alcohol	3 fl. oz.	60	1.0
MEAL (See CORNMEAL or CRACKER MEAL or MATZO MEAL)			
MEATBALL:			
Cocktail (Cresca)	1 meatball	10	
Dinner, with Kluski noodles, frozen (Tom Thumb)	3-lb. 8-oz. tray	2362	140.5
In sauce, canned (Prince)	1 can (3.7 oz.)	171	8.1
Stew, canned (Chef Boy-Ar-Dee)	¼ of 30-oz. can	179	11.7
(Libby's)	8 oz.	275	24.3
Stew (Morton House)	24-oz. can	885	56.5
With gravy, canned (Chef Boy-Ar-Dee)	¼ of 15¼-oz. can	118	4.6
With gravy & whipped potatoes, frozen (Swanson)	9¼-oz. pkg.	330	28.4
MEAT LOAF DINNER, frozen:			
(Banquet)	11-oz. dinner	412	29.0
(Kraft)	5 oz.	332	16.0
(Morton)	11-oz. dinner	390	28.1
(Swanson)	10-oz. dinner	419	42.2
(Swanson) 3-course	16½-oz. dinner	544	52.8
MEAT LOAF SEASONING MIX (Lawry's)	1 pkg. (3½ oz.)	333	65.2

(USDA): United States Department of Agriculture
(HEW/FAO): Health, Education and Welfare/Food and Agriculture Organization
* Prepared as Package Directs

Food and Description	Measure or Quantity	Calories	Carbo-hydrates (grams)
MEAT, POTTED:			
(Armour Star)	3-oz. can	181	0.
(Hormel)	3-oz. can	158	1.0
(Libby's)	5½-oz. can	328	.5
MEAT TENDERIZER			
(Adolph's):			
Unseasoned	1 tsp. (5 grams)	2	.5
Seasoned	1 tsp. (5 grams)	2	.3
MEDOC WINE (Cruse) 12% alcohol	3 fl. oz.	72	
MELBA TOAST:			
Garlic (Keebler)	1 piece (2 grams)	9	1.5
Garlic, rounds (Old London)	1 piece (2 grams)	10	1.8
Onion, rounds (Old London)	1 piece (2 grams)	10	1.8
Plain (Keebler)	1 piece (2 grams)	9	1.5
Pumpernickel (Old London)	1 piece (5 grams)	17	3.4
Rye:			
(Keebler)	1 piece (2 grams)	8	1.7
(Old London)	1 piece (5 grams)	17	3.4
Unsalted (Old London)	1 piece (5 grams)	18	3.5
Sesame (Keebler)	1 piece (2 grams)	11	1.4
Sesame, rounds (Old London)	1 piece (2 grams)	11	1.6
Wheat (Old London)	1 piece (5 grams)	17	3.4
Wheat, unsalted (Old London)	1 piece (5 grams)	18	3.5
White:			
(Keebler)	1 piece (4 grams)	16	3.3
(Old London)	1 piece (5 grams)	17	3.4
Rounds (Old London)	1 piece (2 grams)	10	1.8
Unsalted (Old London)	1 piece (5 grams)	18	3.5
MELLORINE (Sealtest)	¼ pt. (2.3 oz.)	132	15.8
MELON (See individual listings, e.g. **CATALOUPE, WATERMELON**, etc.)			
MELON BALL, cantaloupe & honeydew, in syrup, frozen (USDA)	½ cup (4.1 oz.)	72	18.2
MENHADEN, Atlantic, canned, solids & liq. (USDA)	4 oz.	195	0.

Food and Description	Measure or Quantity	Calories	Carbo-hydrates (grams)
MEXICAN DINNER:			
Combination, frozen:			
(Banquet)	12-oz. dinner	571	72.1
(Morton)	14-oz. dinner	409	47.6
(Patio)	11-oz. dinner	380	33.0
(Rosarita)	12-oz. dinner	518	
Mexican style, frozen:			
(Banquet)	16-oz. dinner	608	73.5
(Patio) 5-compartment	12-oz. dinner	380	50.0
(Patio) 3-compartment	12-oz. dinner	270	30.0
(Swanson)	16¼-oz. dinner	658	67.3
Skillet Mexicana (Hunt's)	1-lb. 2-oz. pkg.	699	130.0
MEXICAN-STYLE VEGETABLES, frozen			
(Birds Eye)	⅓ of 10-oz. pkg.	144	17.0
MILK AMPLIFIER, syrup			
(Hershey's)	1 oz.	78	18.6
MILK CONDENSED, sweetened, canned:			
(USDA)	1 cup (10.8 oz.)	982	166.2
Dime Brand	1 fl. oz. (1.3 oz.)	125	21.1
Eagle Brand	1 cup (10.6 oz.)	942	150.0
Magnolia Brand	1 T. (.7 oz.)	60	9.5
MILK, DRY:			
Whole (USDA) packed cup	1 cup (5.1 oz.)	728	55.4
Nonfat, instant:			
(USDA) ⅞ cup makes 1 qt.	⅞ cup (3.2 oz.)	330	47.6
(Carnation)	1 cup (2.4 oz.)	244	37.4
*(Carnation)	1 cup (8.6 oz.)	81	12.4
*(Sanalac)	1 cup	80	11.5
(Weight Watchers)	1 packet (3 grams)	10	1.4
Chocolate (Carnation)	1 cup (2.4 oz.)	260	44.1
*Chocolate (Carnation)	1 cup (8.6 oz.)	129	21.9

(USDA): United States Department of Agriculture
(HEW/FAO): Health, Education and Welfare/Food and Agriculture
  Organization
* Prepared as Package Directs

Food and Description	Measure or Quantity	Calories	Carbo-hydrates (grams)
MILK, EVAPORATED,			
canned:			
Regular:			
Unsweetened (USDA)	1 cup (8.9 oz.)	345	24.4
(Borden)	14.5-oz. can	563	39.9
(Carnation)	1 cup (8.9 oz.)	348	25.0
(Pet)	1 cup	352	24.0
Skimmed:			
(Carnation)	1 cup (9 oz.)	192	27.9
(Pet)	1 cup (8.8 oz.)	176	26.4
(Sunshine)	1 cup (8.9 oz.)	200	28.8
MILK, FRESH:			
Whole:			
3.25% fat (Borden)			
homogenized	1 cup (8.6 oz.)	152	11.8
3.5% fat (Dean)	1 cup (8.6 oz.)	151	11.0
3.3% fat (Meadow Gold)	1 cup	166	12.0
3.25% fat (Sealtest)	1 cup (8.6 oz.)	144	10.8
3.5% fat (Sealtest)	1 cup (8.6 oz.)	151	11.0
3.7% fat (Sealtest)	1 cup (8.6 oz.)	157	11.1
Multivitamin (Sealtest)	1 cup (8.6 oz.)	151	11.0
Skim:			
2% fat (Dean)	1 cup (8.7 oz.)	133	12.5
1% fat (Dean)	1 cup (8.7 oz.)	103	11.8
0.5% fat (Dean)	1 cup (8.2 oz.)	91	11.7
0.5% fat (Meadow Gold)	1 cup	87	13.0
(Borden)	1 cup (8.6 oz.)	99	13.6
(Sealtest)	1 cup (8.6 oz.)	79	11.3
Diet (Sealtest)	1 cup (8.6 oz.)	103	13.8
Light n' Lively (Sealtest)	1 cup (8.6 oz.)	114	13.6
Lite Line (Borden)	1 cup (8.6 oz.)	119	14.2
Pro-Line (Borden) 2% fat	1 cup (8.6 oz.)	140	14.2
Skim-line (Borden)	1 cup (8.6 oz.)	99	13.6
Vita Lure (Sealtest) 2% fat	1 cup (8.6 oz.)	137	13.6
Viva (Meadow Gold) 2% fat	1 cup	137	14.0
Buttermilk, cultured, fresh:			
(Dean)	1 cup (8.6 oz.)	95	11.5
0.1% fat (Borden)	1 cup (8.6 oz.)	88	12.4
1.0% fat (Borden)	1 cup (8.6 oz.)	107	12.4
3.5% fat (Borden)	1 cup (8.6 oz.)	159	12.0
Light n' Lively (Sealtest)	1 cup (8.6 oz.)	95	10.5

Food and Description	Measure or Quantity	Calories	Carbohydrates (grams)
Skim milk (Sealtest)	1 cup (8.6 oz.)	71	9.3
Chocolate milk drink, fresh:			
With whole milk:			
1% fat (Dean)	1 cup (8.9 oz.)	166	27.9
3.5% fat (Dean)	1 cup (8.8 oz.)	212	25.5
2% fat (Sealtest)	1 cup (8.6 oz.)	178	26.1
3.4% fat (Sealtest)	1 cup (8.6 oz.)	207	25.9
With skim milk:			
2.0% fat (Meadow Gold)	1 cup	185	27.0
.5% fat (Sealtest)	1 cup (8.6 oz.)	146	26.2
1% fat (Sealtest)	1 cup (8.6 oz.)	158	26.2
2% fat (Sealtest)	1 cup (8.6 oz.)	178	26.1
MILK, HUMAN (USDA)	1 oz. (by wt.)	22	2.7
MILK SHAKE (McDonald's):			
Chocolate	1 serving (9.5 oz.)	318	51.9
Strawberry	1 serving (9.4 oz.)	313	50.4
Vanilla	1 serving (9.7 oz.)	324	55.0
MILLET, whole-grain (USDA)	1 lb.	1483	330.7
MINCEMEAT:			
(Crosse & Blackwell)	1 cup (10.4 oz.)	960	228.8
Condensed (None Such)	9-oz. pkg.	950	224.3
Ready-to-use (None Such)	1 cup (10.6 oz.)	690	157.5
(Wilderness)	22-oz. can	1291	260.4
With brandy & rum (None Such)	1 cup (10.6 oz.)	675	151.5
MINCE PIE:			
Home recipe, 2-crust (USDA)	⅛ of 9″ pie (5.6 oz.)	428	65.1
(Tastykake)	4-oz. pie	373	50.8
Frozen:			
(Banquet)	5 oz.	401	62.8
(Morton)	⅙ of 24-oz. pie	297	43.0
(Mrs. Smith's)	⅙ of 8″ pie (4.2 oz.)	339	51.7

(USDA): United States Department of Agriculture
(HEW/FAO): Health, Education and Welfare/Food and Agriculture Organization
* Prepared as Package Directs

Food and Description	Measure or Quantity	Calories	Carbo-hydrates (grams)
MINESTRONE SOUP:			
Condensed (USDA)	8 oz. (by wt.)	197	26.3
*Prepared with equal volume water (USDA)	1 cup (8.6 oz.)	105	14.2
*(Campbell)	1 cup	82	10.5
(Crosse & Blackwell)	6½ oz. (½ can)	107	17.0
*Mix (Golden Grain)	1 cup	69	11.2
MISO, cereal & soybeans (USDA)	4 oz.	194	26.6
MOCHA EXTRACT (Ehlers)	1 tsp.	2	
*MOCHA NUT PUDDING MIX, instant (Royal)	½ cup (5.1 oz.)	199	30.6
MOLASSES:			
Barbados (USDA)	½ cup (5.4 oz.)	417	108.0
Barbados (USDA)	1 T. (.7 oz.)	51	13.3
Blackstrap (USDA)	½ cup (5.4 oz.)	328	85.0
Blackstrap (USDA)	1 T. (.7 oz.)	40	10.4
Light (USDA)	½ cup (5.4 oz.)	388	100.1
Light (USDA)	1 T. (.7 oz.)	48	12.4
Medium (USDA)	½ cup (5.4 oz.)	357	92.4
Medium (USDA)	1 T. (.7 oz.)	44	11.4
(Brer Rabbit) Gold Label	1 T.	60	14.6
(Brer Rabbit) Green Label	1 T.	53	13.3
Unsulphured (Grandma's)	1 T. (.7 oz.)	60	15.0
MOR (Wilson) canned luncheon meat	3 oz.	266	1.6
MORTADELLA, sausage (USDA)	1 oz.	89	.2
MOSELMAID, German Moselle wine (Deinhard) 11% alcohol	3 fl. oz.	60	1.0
MOUNTAIN WINE (Louis M. Martini) 12.5% alcohol	3 fl. oz.	90	.2
MOXIE, soft drink	6 fl. oz.	89	22.2
MR. PIBB, soft drink	6 fl. oz.	70	18.6
MRS. BUTTERWORTH'S SYRUP	1 T. (.7 oz.)	53	13.0

Food and Description	Measure or Quantity	Calories	Carbo-hydrates (grams)
MUFFIN:			
Blueberry:			
Home recipe (USDA)	3″ muffin (1.4 oz.)	112	16.8
Frozen (Morton)	1.6-oz. muffin	116	20.8
Frozen (Mrs. Smith's)	.9-oz. muffin	116	18.0
Bran:			
Home recipe (USDA)	3″ muffin (1.4 oz.)	104	17.2
With raisins (Thomas')	1.9-oz. muffin	170	26.7
Corn:			
Home recipe, prepared with whole-ground cornmeal (USDA)	1.4-oz. muffin (2⅜″ dia.)	115	17.0
(Drake's)	2-oz. muffin	229	33.7
Frozen (Morton)	1.7-oz. muffin	132	20.4
Frozen (Mrs. Smith's)	1-oz. muffin	157	25.0
(Thomas')	2-oz. muffin	194	26.8
English:			
(Arnold)	2.2-oz. muffin	145	26.7
(Newly Weds)	2.5-oz. muffin	167	33.2
(Thomas')	2.1-oz. muffin	140	28.4
(Wonder)	2-oz. muffin	133	25.5
Golden Egg Toasting (Arnold)	2.5-oz. muffin	162	26.8
Plain, home recipe (USDA)	1.4-oz. muffin (2⅜″ dia.)	118	16.9
Scone (Wonder) *Raisin Round*	1 scone (2 oz.)	147	27.2
Sour dough (Wonder)	2-oz. muffin	133	26.1
Wheat Berry (Wonder)	2-oz. muffin	136	26.6
MUFFIN MIX:			
*Apple cinnamon (Betty Crocker)	2¾″ muffin	159	26.4
*Banana nut (Betty Crocker)	2¾″ muffin	167	24.6
Blueberry:			
*Wild (Betty Crocker)	2¾″ muffin	118	19.3
*(Duncan Hines)	1.2-oz. muffin	89	15.6
*Butter pecan (Betty Crocker)	2¾″ muffin	159	21.3

(USDA): United States Department of Agriculture
(HEW/FAO): Health, Education and Welfare/Food and Agriculture Organization
* Prepared as Package Directs

Food and Description	Measure or Quantity	Calories	Carbo-hydrates (grams)
Corn:			
With enriched flour (USDA)	1 oz.	118	20.4
*Prepared with egg & milk (USDA)	1.4-oz. muffin (2⅜″ dia.)	92	14.2
With cake flour & nonfat dry milk (USDA)	1 oz.	116	20.3
*Prepared with egg & water (USDA)	1.4-oz. muffin (2⅜″ dia.)	119	20.8
(Albers)	1 oz.	118	19.5
*(Betty Crocker)	2¾″ muffin	156	24.8
*(Dromedary)	1.4-oz. muffin	144	20.5
*(Flako)	1.5-oz. muffin (1/12 of pkg.)	133	20.7
(Pillsbury) golden	1 oz.	112	18.8
*Date nut (Betty Crocker)	2¾″ muffin	152	21.8
*Honey bran (Betty Crocker)	2¾″ muffin	154	26.2
*Lemon (Betty Crocker)	1 muffin	149	23.5
*Oatmeal (Betty Crocker)	2¾″ muffin	166	23.8
*Orange (Betty Crocker) Sunkist	2¾″ muffin	153	26.6
*Spice (Betty Crocker)	2¾″ muffin	151	23.4
MULLET, raw (USDA):			
Whole	1 lb. (weighed whole)	351	0.
Meat only	4 oz.	166	0.
MUNG BEAN SPROUT (See BEAN SPROUT)			
MUSCATEL WINE:			
(Gold Seal) 19% alcohol	3 fl. oz.	158	9.4
(Taylor) 19.5% alcohol	3 fl. oz.	147	11.1
MUSHROOM:			
Raw (USDA):			
Whole	½ lb. (weighed untrimmed)	62	9.7
Trimmed, slices	½ cup (1.2 oz.)	10	1.5
Sliced (Shady Oaks)	½ cup (1.3 oz.)	10	1.5
Canned, solids & liq.:			
(USDA)	½ cup (4.3 oz.)	21	2.9
(USDA)	4 oz.	19	2.7

Food and Description	Measure or Quantity	Calories	Carbohydrates (grams)
Solids & liq. (Shady Oaks)	4-oz. can	19	2.0
Sliced, chopped or whole, broiled in butter (B in B)	6-oz. can	50	4.1
Whole, sliced, or stems & pieces (Green Giant)	4-oz. can	24	3.9
(Oxford Royal)	4 oz.	17	2.4
Frozen:			
Whole (Birds Eye)	⅓ pkg. (1.5 oz.)	11	1.9
Whole, in butter sauce, *Sauté*	⅓ of 6-oz. pkg.	30	2.0
MUSHROOM SOUP:			
*Barley (Manischewitz)	1 cup	72	12.2
Bisque (Crosse & Blackwell)	6½ oz. (½ can)	103	8.3
Cream of:			
Condensed (USDA)	8 oz. (by wt.)	252	19.1
*Prepared with equal volume water (USDA)	1 cup (8.5 oz.)	134	10.1
*Prepared with equal volume milk (USDA)	1 cup (8.6 oz.)	216	16.2
*(Campbell)	1 cup	131	8.5
*(Heinz)	1 cup (8½ oz.)	124	10.4
(Heinz) *Great American*	1 cup (8¾ oz.)	131	12.4
*Dietetic (Claybourne)	8 oz. (by wt.)	79	10.7
*Dietetic (Slim-ette)	8 oz. (by wt.)	60	10.7
Low sodium (Campbell)	7¼-oz. can	124	8.9
*Golden (Campbell)	1 cup	80	7.7
MUSHROOM SOUP MIX:			
*(Golden Grain)	1 cup	121	16.0
*(Lipton) beef flavor	1 cup	39	6.3
Cream of (Lipton) *Cup-a-Soup*	1 pkg. (.7 oz.)	86	9.6
Cream of (Wyler's)	1 pkg. (.7 oz.)	78	10.1
MUSKELLUNGE, raw (USDA):			
Whole	1 lb. (weighed whole)	242	0.
Meat only	4 oz.	124	0.

(USDA): United States Department of Agriculture
(HEW/FAO): Health, Education and Welfare/Food and Agriculture Organization
* Prepared as Package Directs

Food and Description	Measure or Quantity	Calories	Carbo-hydrates (grams)
MUSKMELON (See CANTA-LOUPE, CASABA or HONEYDEW)			
MUSKRAT, roasted (USDA)	4 oz.	174	0.
MUSSEL (USDA):			
Atlantic & Pacific, raw, in shell	1 lb. (weighed in shell)	153	7.2
Atlantic & Pacific, raw, meat only	4 oz.	108	3.7
Pacific, canned, drained	4 oz.	129	1.7
MUSTARD, prepared:			
Brown:			
(French's) Spicey	1 tsp.	6	.5
(Gulden's)	¼-oz. packet	6	.4
(Heinz)	1 tsp.	8	.5
German style (Kraft)	1 oz.	30	1.7
Grey Poupon	1 tsp. (5 grams)	5	.2
Horseradish (French's)	1 tsp.	6	.4
Horseradish (Kraft)	1 oz.	29	1.6
Medford (French's)	1 tsp.	5	.4
Salad (Kraft)	1 oz.	23	1.7
Yellow:			
(Gulden's)	¼-oz. packet	5	.4
(Heinz)	1 tsp.	5	.5
(Kraft)	1 oz.	23	1.7
MUSTARD GREENS:			
Raw, whole (USDA)	1 lb. (weighed untrimmed)	98	17.8
Boiled, drained (USDA)	1 cup (7.8 oz.)	51	8.8
Frozen:			
Not thawed (USDA)	4 oz.	23	3.6
Boiled, drained (USDA)	½ cup (3.8 oz.)	21	3.3
Chopped (Birds Eye)	½ cup (3.3 oz.)	19	2.2
MUSTARD SPINACH (USDA):			
Raw	1 lb.	100	17.7
Boiled, drained solids	4 oz.	18	3.2

Food and Description	Measure or Quantity	Calories	Carbo-hydrates (grams)

N

NASSAU DRY WINE (Gallo)
  20% alcohol | 3 fl. oz. | 106 | 7.5

NATURAL CEREAL:
  100% (Quaker) | ¼ cup (1 oz.) | 140 | 17.0
  100%, with fruit (Quaker) | ¼ cup (1 oz.) | 136 | 17.8

NEAR BEER (See BEER, NEAR)

NEAPOLITAN CREAM PIE,
  frozen:
  (Banquet) | 2½ oz. | 188 | 27.2
  (Mrs. Smith's) | ⅛ of 8" pie (2.8 oz.) | 244 | 33.3

NECTARINE, fresh (USDA):
  Whole | 1 lb. (weighed with pits) | 267 | 71.4
  Flesh only | 4 oz. | 73 | 19.4

NEW ZEALAND SPINACH
  (USDA):
  Raw | 1 lb. | 86 | 14.1
  Boiled, drained solids | 4 oz. | 15 | 2.4

NIERSTEINER (Julius Kayser)
  10% alcohol | 3 fl. oz. | 54 | .9

NOODLE. Plain noodle products
  are essentially the same in
  caloric value and carbohydrate
  content on the same weight
  basis. The longer they are
  cooked, the more water is
  absorbed and this affects the
  nutritive values. (USDA):
  Dry, 1½" strips | 1 cup (2.6 oz.) | 283 | 52.6

(USDA): United States Department of Agriculture
(HEW/FAO): Health, Education and Welfare/Food and Agriculture
                    Organization
* Prepared as Package Directs

Food and Description	Measure or Quantity	Calories	Carbohydrates (grams)
Dry	1 oz.	110	20.4
Cooked	1 cup (5.6 oz.)	200	37.3
Cooked	1 oz.	35	6.6
NOODLE & BEEF:			
Canned (Heinz)	8½-oz. can	171	18.1
Canned (Nalley's)	8 oz.	152	11.8
Frozen (Banquet)	2-lb. pkg.	735	102.0
NOODLE, CHOW MEIN, canned:			
(USDA)	1 cup (1.6 oz.)	220	26.1
(Chun King)	1 cup	211	23.2
(Hung's)	1 oz.	148	16.1
(La Choy)	1 cup	258	29.0
NOODLE DINNER:			
*Canton, mix (Betty Crocker)	1 cup	403	33.1
*With cheese, mix (Kraft)	4 oz.	204	21.7
*With chicken, mix (Kraft)	4 oz.	122	18.9
With chicken, frozen (Swanson)	11-oz. dinner	370	46.0
*Romanoff, mix (Kraft)	4 oz.	215	20.0
*Stroganoff, mix (Betty Crocker)	1 cup	500	41.6
NOODLE MIX:			
*Almondine (Betty Crocker)	½ cup	213	26.2
*Almondine *Noodle-Roni*	4 oz.	143	21.7
*Au gratin *Noodle-Roni*	4 oz.	129	22.2
Egg Noodles Plus (Pennsylvania Dutch Brand):			
Beef sauce	½ cup	137	24.1
Butter sauce	½ cup	151	23.1
Cheese sauce	½ cup	147	23.7
Chicken sauce	½ cup	143	24.8
Mushroom sauce	½ cup	137	24.3
Onion sauce	½ cup	140	25.2
*Italiano (Betty Crocker)	½ cup	207	27.6
*Parmesano, *Noodle-Roni*	⅛ of 6-oz pkg.	130	23.0
*Romanoff (Betty Crocker)	½ cup	241	26.4
*Romanoff *Noodle-Roni*	4 oz.	179	22.5
Scallop-A-Roni	½ cup	88	13.4
Twist-A-Roni	½ cup (3.5 oz.)	120	18.0

Food and Description	Measure or Quantity	Calories	Carbo-hydrates (grams)
NOODLE SOUP:			
Beef (See **BEEF SOUP**)			
Chicken (See **CHICKEN SOUP**)			
*With ground beef, canned (Campbell)	1 cup	91	9.2
N-RICH, cream substitute	1 tsp. (3 grams)	10	1.7
NUITS ST. GEORGE, French red Burgundy (Barton & Guestier) 13.5% alcohol	3 fl. oz.	70	.5
NUT, mixed (see also individual kinds):			
Dry roasted:			
(Flavor House)	1 oz.	172	5.4
(Planters)	1 oz.	176	6.2
(Skippy)	1 oz.	168	5.7
Oil roasted:			
With peanuts (Planters)	1 oz.	176	6.2
Without peanuts (Planters)	1 oz.	178	6.0
NUT LOAF (See **BREAD, CANNED**)			
NUTMEG (Ehlers)	1 tsp.	12	
NUTRIMATO (Mott's)	4 oz.	55	10.0

O

OAT FLAKES, cereal (Post)	⅔ cup (1 oz.)	107	19.0
OATMEAL:			
Instant:			
Dry:			
(H-O)	1 cup (2.4 oz.)	258	44.5
(H-O)	1 T. (4 grams)	16	2.8

(USDA): United States Department of Agriculture
(HEW/FAO): Health, Education and Welfare/Food and Agriculture Organization
* Prepared as Package Directs

Food and Description	Measure or Quantity	Calories	Carbohydrates (grams)
(Quaker)	1-oz. packet (¾ cup cooked)	107	19.0
(3 Minute)	1 oz.	109	19.3
Sweet & mellow (H-O)	1.4-oz. packet	149	29.4
With apple & cinnamon (Quaker)	1⅛-oz. packet (¾ cup cooked)	119	24.0
With dates & caramel (H-O)	1.4-oz. packet	147	30.8
With maple & brown sugar (Quaker)	1⅝-oz. packet (¾ cup cooked)	177	36.2
With raisins & spice:			
(H-O)	1.6-oz. packet	167	33.3
(Quaker)	1.5-oz. packet (¾ cup cooked)	154	32.1
*Cooked (3 Minute)	1 cup	175	31.0
Quick:			
Dry:			
(H-O)	1 cup (2.5 oz.)	265	45.8
(H-O)	1 T. (4 grams)	17	2.9
(Ralston)	⅓ cup (1 oz.)	113	19.3
Cooked:			
*(Albers)	1 cup	148	26.0
*(Quaker)	⅔ cup (1 oz. dry)	107	18.8
Regular:			
Dry:			
(USDA)	1 cup (2.5 oz.)	281	49.1
(USDA)	1 T. (4 grams)	18	3.1
Old-fashioned (H-O)	1 cup (2.6 oz.)	280	49.7
Old-fashioned (H-O)	1 T. (5 grams)	18	3.1
*(Ralston)	⅓ cup (1 oz.)	128	20.3
Cooked:			
*(USDA)	1 cup (8.5 oz.)	132	23.3
*Old-fashioned (Quaker)	⅔ cup (1 oz. dry)	107	18.8
OCEAN PERCH (USDA):			
Atlantic:			
Raw, whole	1 lb. (weighed whole)	124	0.
Fried	4 oz.	257	7.7
Frozen, breaded, fried, reheated	4 oz.	362	18.7

Food and Description	Measure or Quantity	Calories	Carbo-hydrates (grams)
Pacific, raw:			
Whole	1 lb. (weighed whole)	116	0.
Meat only	4 oz.	108	0.
Frozen (Gorton)	⅓ of 1-lb. pkg.	133	0.
OCEAN PERCH MEAL, frozen:			
(Banquet)	8¾-oz. dniner	434	49.8
(Weight Watchers)	18-oz. dinner	307	18.4
& broccoli (Weight Watchers)	9½-oz. luncheon	185	7.1
OCTOPUS, raw, meat only (USDA)	4 oz.	83	0.
OESTRICHLER LENCHEN RIESLING, German Rhine wine (Deinhard) 11% alcohol	3 fl. oz.	72	4.5
OIL, salad or cooking:			
(USDA) including olive	½ cup (3.9 oz.)	972	0.
Corn (Fleischmann's)	1 T. (.5 oz.)	126	0.
Corn (Kraft)	1 oz.	251	0.
Corn (Mazola)	1 cup (7.7 oz.)	1989	0.
Corn (Mazola)	1 T. (.5 oz.)	126	0.
Crisco	1 T. (.5 oz.)	124	0.
Peanut (Planters)	1 T. (.5 oz.)	126	0.
Safflower (Kraft)	1 oz.	251	0.
Safflower, *Saff-o-life*	1 T.	124	0.
(Saffola)	1 T. (.5 oz.)	124	0.
(Wesson)	1 T. (.5 oz.)	124	0.
OKRA:			
Raw, whole (USDA)	1 lb. (weighed untrimmed)	140	29.6
Boiled, drained (USDA):			
Whole	½ cup (3.1 oz.)	26	5.3
Pods	8 pods (3″ x ⅝″, 3 oz.)	25	5.1

(USDA): United States Department of Agriculture
(HEW/FAO): Health Education and Welfare/Food and Agriculture Organization
* Prepared as Package Directs

Food and Description	Measure or Quantity	Calories	Carbo-hydrates (grams)
Slices	½ cup (2.8 oz.)	23	4.8
Canned, with tomatoes (King Pharr)	½ cup	26	5.0
Frozen:			
Cut, boiled, drained (USDA)	½ cup (3.2 oz.)	35	8.1
Whole, boiled, drained (USDA)	½ cup (2.4 oz.)	26	6.1
Cut (Birds Eye)	½ cup (3.3 oz.)	36	7.6
Whole (Birds Eye)	½ cup (2.5 oz.)	27	5.7
OLD-FASHIONED COCKTAIL:			
(Hiram Walker) 62 proof	3 fl. oz.	165	3.0
Dry mix (Bar-Tender's)	1 serving (⅙ oz.)	20	4.7
Liquid mix (Holland House)	1½ fl. oz.	54	13.5
OLD MANSE SYRUP	1 T. (.7 oz.)	53	13.2
OLEOMARGARINE (See MARGARINE)			
OLIVE:			
Greek style, with pits, drained (USDA)	1 oz.	308	7.9
Green, pitted & drained:			
(USDA)	1 oz.	33	.4
(USDA)	4 med. or 3 extra large or 2 giant	19	.2
(USDA)	1 olive (1¾⁄16″ x 1¹⁄16″)	6	<.1
(La Manna, Azema & Farnan)	1 med. manzanilla	4	.1
Spanish (Mario's)	1 med.		
Ripe, by variety:			
Ascolano, any size (USDA)	1 oz.	37	.7
Manzanilla, any size (USDA)	1 oz.	37	.7
Mission, any size (USDA)	1 oz.	52	.9
Mission (USDA)	3 small or 2 large	18	.3
Mission, slices (USDA)	½ cup (2.2 oz.)	114	2.0

Food and Description	Measure or Quantity	Calories	Carbohydrates (grams)
Sevillano, any size (USDA)	1 oz.	26	.8
Ripe, by size:			
Select (Lindsay)	1 olive	3	.1
Medium (Lindsay)	1 olive	4	.1
Large (Lindsay)	1 olive	5	.1
Extra large (Lindsay)	1 olive	5	.1
Mammoth (Lindsay)	1 olive	6	.1
Giant (Lindsay)	1 olive	8	.2
Jumbo (Lindsay)	1 olive	10	.2
Colossal (Lindsay)	1 olive	13	.3
Supercolossal (Lindsay)	1 olive	16	.3
Super supreme (Lindsay)	1 olive	18	.3
ONION:			
Raw (USDA):			
Whole	1 lb. (weighed untrimmed)	175	35.9
Whole	3.9-oz. onion (2½" dia.)	38	8.7
Chopped	½ cup (3 oz.)	33	7.5
Chopped	1 T. (.4 oz.)	4	1.0
Grated	1 T. (.5 oz.)	5	1.2
Slices	½ cup (2 oz.)	21	4.9
Boiled, drained (USDA):			
Whole	½ cup (3.7 oz.)	30	6.8
Halves or pieces	½ cup (3.2 oz.)	26	5.8
Boiled, canned, solids & liq. (Durkee) O & C	16-oz. jar	128	30.4
Cream sauce:			
Canned (Durkee) O & C	15½-oz. can	352	36.6
Frozen (Birds Eye)	⅓ pkg. (3 oz.)	132	12.7
Dehydrated, flakes (Gilroy)	1 tsp. (2 grams)	6	1.3
Frozen:			
Chopped (Birds Eye)	¼ cup (1 oz.)	11	2.5
Whole, small (Birds Eye)	½ cup (4 oz.)	51	12.0
French-fried rings:			
(Durkee) O & C	3-oz. can	534	30.9
Frozen (Birds Eye)	2 oz.	166	17.1
Frozen, batter-fried (Mrs. Paul's)	9-oz. pkg.	567	50.5

(USDA): United States Department of Agriculture
(HEW/FAO): Health, Education and Welfare/Food and Agriculture Organization

* Prepared as Package Directs

Food and Description	Measure or Quantity	Calories	Carbo-hydrates (grams)
Frozen, breaded & fried (Mrs. Paul's)	5-oz. pkg.	424	41.3
Pickled, cocktail (Crosse & Blackwell)	1 T. (.5 oz.)	1	.3
ONION BOUILLON:			
Cube (Herb-Ox)	1 cube (4 grams)	10	1.4
Cube (Wyler's)	1 cube (4 grams)	10	1.2
Instant (Herb-Ox)	1 packet (5 grams)	15	2.0
ONION, GREEN, raw (USDA):			
Whole	1 lb. (weighed untrimmed)	157	35.7
Bulb & entire top	1 oz.	10	2.3
Bulb without green top	3 small onions (.9 oz.)	11	2.6
Slices, bulb & white portion of top	½ cup (1.8 oz.)	22	5.2
Tops only	1 oz.	8	1.6
ONION JUICE (McCormick)	1 tsp.	<1	
ONION SOUP:			
Condensed (USDA)	8 oz. (by wt.)	122	9.8
*Prepared with equal volume water (USDA)	1 cup (8.5 oz.)	65	5.3
*(Campbell)	1 cup	41	3.3
(Crosse & Blackwell)	6½ oz. (½ can)	46	4.8
(Hormel)	15-oz. can	144	5.5
ONION SOUP MIX:			
*(Golden Grain)	1 cup	41	7.0
*(Lipton)	1 cup	34	5.7
(Lipton) *Cup-a-Soup*	1 pkg. (.4 oz.)	30	5.4
*(Wyler's)	1 cup	37	7.1
ONION, WELCH, raw (USDA):			
Whole	1 lb. (weighed untrimmed)	100	19.2
Trimmed	4 oz.	39	7.4
OPOSSUM, roasted, meat only (USDA)	4 oz.	251	0.
ORANGE, fresh: All varieties: Orange, whole, medium (USDA)	5.5-oz. orange (3″ dia.)	77	19.0

Food and Description	Measure or Quantity	Calories	Carbo- hydrates (grams)
Sections (USDA)	1 cup (8.5 oz.)	118	29.4
Sections, sweetened, chilled, bottled (Kraft)	4 oz.	61	14.1
California Navel:			
Whole (USDA)	1 lb. (weighed with rind & seeds)	157	39.2
Whole (USDA)	6.3-oz. orange (2⅘" dia.)	62	15.5
Sections (USDA)	1 cup (8.5 oz.)	123	30.6
Wedge, unpeeled (Sunkist)	⅛ orange	10	4.0
Cut, bite-size (Sunkist)	½ cup	62	16.0
California Valencia (USDA):			
Whole	1 lb. (weighed with rind & seeds)	174	42.2
Fruit including peel	6.3-oz. orange (2⅝" dia.)	72	27.9
Sections	1 cup (8.5 oz.)	123	29.9
Florida, all varieties (USDA):			
Whole	1 lb. (weighed with rind & seeds)	158	40.3
Whole	7.4-oz. orange (3" dia.)	73	18.6
Sections	1 cup (8.5 oz.)	113	28.9
ORANGEADE:			
Chilled (Sealtest)	½ cup (4.4 oz.)	64	15.6
Frozen, sweetened:			
*(Minute Maid)	½ cup (4.2 oz.)	63	14.5
*(Snow Crop)	½ cup (4.2 oz.)	63	14.5
*Mix (Salada)	½ cup	53	12.9
ORANGE-APRICOT JUICE DRINK, canned:			
(USDA) 40% fruit juices	1 cup (8.8 oz.)	124	31.6
(Del Monte)	1 cup (8.6 oz.)	118	32.3
ORANGE-BANANA JUICE DRINK, canned (BC)	1 cup	120	

(USDA): United States Department of Agriculture
(HEW/FAO): Health, Education and Welfare/Food and Agriculture Organization
* Prepared as Package Directs

Food and Description	Measure or Quantity	Calories	Carbo-hydrates (grams)
ORANGE CAKE:			
Frosted (Sara Lee)	2 oz.	206	30.0
Mix:			
*(Betty Crocker) layer	1/12 of cake	201	36.8
*Chiffon (Betty Crocker)	1/16 of cake	135	27.1
*(Duncan Hines)	1/12 of cake (2.7 oz.)	201	35.0
(Pillsbury)	1 oz.	120	21.9
ORANGE DRINK:			
Canned (Hi-C)	6 fl. oz. (6.3 oz.)	98	22.4
Chilled (Sealtest)	6 fl. oz.	87	21.3
*Mix (Lipton)	6 fl. oz.	85	21.2
ORANGE EXTRACT (Ehlers)	1 tsp.	14	
ORANGE-GRAPEFRUIT JUICE:			
Canned, unsweetened (USDA)	1 cup (8.7 oz.)	106	24.8
Canned, sweetened (Del Monte)	1/2 cup (4.3 oz.)	55	14.0
Frozen, concentrate:			
Unsweetened (USDA)	6-fl.-oz. can	330	77.9
*Unsweetened, diluted with 3 parts water (USDA)	1/2 cup (4.4 oz.)	55	13.0
*Unsweetened (Minute Maid)	1/2 cup (4.2 oz.)	51	12.4
*Unsweetened (Snow Crop)	1/2 cup (4.2 oz.)	51	12.4
ORANGE-GRAPEFRUIT JUICE DRINK, canned (BC)	6 fl. oz.	90	
ORANGE ICE (Sealtest)	1/4 pt. (3.2 oz.)	130	32.6
ORANGE JUICE:			
Fresh:			
All varieties (USDA)	1/2 cup (4.4 oz.)	56	12.9
California Navel (USDA)	1/2 cup (4.4 oz.)	60	14.0
California Valencia (USDA)	1/2 cup (4.4 oz.)	58	13.0
Florida, early or mid-season (USDA)	1/2 cup (4.4 oz.)	50	11.5
Florida Temple (USDA)	1/2 cup (4.4 oz.)	67	16.0
Florida Valencia (USDA)	1/2 cup (4.4 oz.)	56	13.0

Food and Description	Measure or Quantity	Calories	Carbohydrates (grams)
(Sunkist)	½ cup (4.4 oz.)	52	13.0
Chilled, fresh (Kraft)	½ cup (4.4 oz.)	60	13.8
Chilled (Minute Maid)	½ cup (4.4 oz.)	55	13.1
Chilled, fresh (Sealtest)	½ cup (4.3 oz.)	64	14.4
Canned, sweetened:			
(Del Monte)	½ cup (4.3 oz.)	58	15.0
(Heinz)	5½-fl.-oz. can	91	21.0
(Libby's)	½ cup (4.4 oz.)	56	13.3
(Stokely-Van Camp)	½ cup (4.4 oz.)	65	15.3
Canned, unsweetened:			
(Del Monte)	½ cup (4.3 oz.)	46	11.8
(Heinz)	5½-fl.-oz. can	71	16.5
Dehydrated, crystals:			
(USDA)	4-oz. can	431	100.8
*Reconstituted (USDA)	½ cup (4.4 oz.)	57	13.4
Frozen, concentrate:			
(USDA)	6-fl.-oz. can	337	80.9
*Diluted with 3 parts water (USDA)	½ cup (4.4 oz.)	56	13.3
*(Birds Eye)	½ cup (4 oz.)	51	13.3
*(Lake Hamilton)	½ cup (4.4 oz.)	58	13.3
*(Minute Maid)	½ cup (4.2 oz.)	60	13.7
*(Nature's Best)	½ cup (4.4 oz.)	58	13.3
*(Snow Crop)	½ cup	60	13.7

ORANGE, MANDARIN (See MANDARIN ORANGE & TANGERINE)

ORANGE PEEL, CANDIED

(Liberty)	1 oz.	93	22.6

ORANGE-PINEAPPLE DRINK, canned:

Juice drink (BC)	6 fl. oz.	96	
(Hi-C)	6 fl. oz.	88	21.8
(Wagner)	6 fl. oz.	86	21.6

ORANGE-PINEAPPLE JUICE,

chilled (Kraft)	½ cup (4.4 oz.)	64	14.9

(USDA): United States Department of Agriculture
(HEW/FAO): Health, Education and Welfare/Food and Agriculture Organization

* Prepared as Package Directs

Food and Description	Measure or Quantity	Calories	Carbo-hydrates (grams)
ORANGE-PINEAPPLE PIE			
(Tastykake)	4-oz. pie	374	56.2
***ORANGE PLUS** (Birds Eye)	½ cup (4.4 oz.)	67	16.6
ORANGE RENNET CUSTARD MIX:			
Powder:			
(Junket)	.1 oz.	116	27.7
*(Junket)	4 oz.	108	14.6
Tablet:			
(Junket)	1 tablet (<1 gram)	1	.2
*With sugar (Junket)	4 oz.	101	13.5
ORANGE SHERBET (See SHERBET)			
ORANGE SOFT DRINK:			
Sweetened:			
(Canda Dry)	6 fl. oz. (6.4 oz.)	98	24.6
(Clicquot Club)	6 fl. oz.	103	25.0
(Cott)	6 fl. oz.	103	25.0
(Dr. Brown's)	6 fl. oz.	91	22.6
(Fanta)	6 fl. oz.	92	23.8
(Hoffman)	6 fl. oz.	93	23.2
(Kirsch)	6 fl. oz.	88	21.9
(Mission)	6 fl. oz.	103	25.0
(Nedick's)	6 fl. oz.	91	22.6
(Nehi)	6 fl. oz. (6.6 oz.)	100	24.8
Orangette	6 fl. oz.	94	24.3
(Patio)	6 fl. oz. (6.6 oz.)	96	24.0
(Salute)	6 fl. oz.	101	25.5
(Shasta)	6 fl. oz.	95	24.0
(Waldbaum)	6 fl. oz.	91	22.6
(Yoo-Hoo) high-protein	6 fl. oz. (6.4 oz.)	100	18.9
(Yukon Club)	6 fl. oz.	95	23.8
Low calorie:			
(Canada Dry)	6 fl. oz.	5	.2
Diet Rite	6 fl. oz.	1	.2
(Dr. Brown's)	6 fl. oz.	1	.2
(Hoffman)	6 fl. oz.	1	.2
(No-Cal)	6 fl. oz.	2	0.
(Shasta)	6 fl. oz.	<1	<.1
ORGEAT SYRUP (Julius Wile)	1 fl. oz.	103	26.0

Food and Description	Measure or Quantity	Calories	Carbohydrates (grams)
ORVIETO WINE, Italian white:			
(Antinori) 12% alcohol	3 fl. oz.	84	6.3
(Antinori) *Castello La Scala,* 12½% alcohol	3 fl. oz.	87	6.3
OVALTINE, dry:			
Malt	1 oz.	110	23.0
Swiss chocolate	1 oz.	111	24.0
OXTAIL CONSOMMÉ MIX, instant (Knorr Swiss)	1 tsp.	11	
OXTAIL SOUP (Crosse & Blackwell)	6½ oz. (½ can)	136	7.5
OYSTER:			
Raw:			
Eastern, meat only: (USDA)	13–19 med. oysters (1 cup, 8.5 oz.)	158	8.2
(USDA)	4 oz.	75	3.9
(Epicure)	1 cup	220	13.0
Pacific & Western, meat only (USDA)	4 oz.	103	7.3
Canned, solids & liq. (USDA)	4 oz.	86	5.6
Fried (USDA)	4 oz.	271	21.1
Frozen (Ship Ahoy)	10-oz. pkg.	239	5.0
Smoked, Japanese baby Cresca)	3⅔-oz. can	222	
OYSTER CRACKER (See **CRACKER**)			
OYSTER STEW:			
Home recipe (USDA): 1 part oysters to 1 part milk by volume	1 cup (8.5 oz., 6–8 oysters)	245	14.2

(USDA): United States Department of Agriculture
(HEW/FAO): Health, Education and Welfare/Food and Agriculture Organization
* Prepared as Package Directs

Food and Description	Measure or Quantity	Calories	Carbohydrates (grams)
1 part oysters to 2 parts milk by volume	1 cup (8.5 oz.)	233	10.8
1 part oysters to 3 parts milk by volume	1 cup (8.5 oz.)	206	11.3
*Canned (Campbell)	1 cup	142	11.6
Frozen, commercial:			
Condensed (USDA)	8 oz. (by wt.)	231	15.6
*Prepared with equal volume water (USDA)	1 cup (8.5 oz.)	122	8.2
*Prepared with equal volume milk (USDA)	1 cup (8.5 oz.)	202	14.2

P

Food and Description	Measure or Quantity	Calories	Carbohydrates (grams)
PAGAN PINK WINE (Gallo) 11% alcohol	3 fl. oz.	81	6.8
PAISANO WINE (Gallo) 13% alcohol	3 fl. oz.	53	1.3
PANCAKE, home recipe (USDA)	4" pancake (1 oz.)	62	9.2
PANCAKE & WAFFLE MIX (See also PANCAKE & WAFFLE MIX, DIETETIC):			
*Blueberry (Pillsbury) *Hungry Jack*	4" pancake	120	16.0
Buckwheat:			
(USDA)	1 cup (4.8 oz.)	443	94.9
(USDA)	1 oz.	93	19.9
*Prepared with egg & milk (USDA)	4" pancake (1 oz.)	54	6.4
*(Aunt Jemima)	4" pancake (1.2 oz.)	61	8.0
Buttermilk:			
(USDA)	1 cup (4.8 oz.)	481	102.2
(USDA)	1 oz.	101	21.5
*Prepared with milk (USDA)	4" pancake (1 oz.)	55	8.6
*Prepared with milk & egg (USDA)	4" pancake (1 oz.)	61	8.7
*(Aunt Jemima)	4" pancake (1 oz.)	84	11.2
*(Duncan Hines)	4" pancake (2 oz.)	109	19.4

Food and Description	Measure or Quantity	Calories	Carbo-hydrates (grams)
*(Pillsbury) *Hungry Jack*	4″ pancake	80	9.7
*Complete (Pillsbury) *Hungry Jack*	4″ pancake	73	14.0
Plain:			
(USDA)	1 cup (4.8 oz.)	481	102.2
(USDA)	1 oz.	101	21.5
*Prepared with milk (USDA)	1 pancake (1 oz.)	55	8.6
*Prepared with milk & egg (USDA)	6″ x ½″ pancake (7 T. batter)	164	23.7
*(Aunt Jemina) complete	4″ pancake (1.2 oz.)	60	11.7
*(Aunt Jemima) *Easy Pour*	4″ pancake (1.3 oz.)	78	11.0
*(Aunt Jemima) original	4″ pancake (1 oz.)	60	7.8
(Golden Mix)	1 cup	459	80.8
*(Golden Mix)	4″ pancake	106	12.5
*(Pillsbury):			
Extra light	4″ pancake	90	11.7
Complete, *Hungry Jack*	4″ pancake	73	14.0
Extra light, *Hungry Jack*	4″ pancake	73	10.7
*PANCAKE & WAFFLE MIX, DIETETIC, buttermilk or plain (Tillie Lewis)	4″ pancake (.5 oz. dry)	43	8.6
PANCAKE & WAFFLE SYRUP:			
Cane & maple (USDA)	1 T. (.7 oz.)	50	13.0
Chiefly corn, light & dark (USDA)	1 T. (.7 oz.)	58	15.0
Sweetened (Bama)	1 T. (.7 oz.)	53	13.2
Sweetened (Golden Griddle)	1 T. (.7 oz.)	52	13.1
Sweetened (Polaner)	1 T.	54	13.5
Sweetened (Smucker's)	1 T. (.8 oz.)	62	16.0
Dietetic or low calorie:			
(Diet Delight)	1 T. (.6 oz.)	12	3.1
(Tillie Lewis)	1 T.	13	3.0

(USDA): United States Department of Agriculture
(HEW/FAO): Health, Education and Welfare/Food and Agriculture Organization
* Prepared as Package Directs

Food and Description	Measure or Quantity	Calories	Carbo-hydrates (grams)
PANCAKE BREAKFAST (Swanson)	6-oz. breakfast	463	41.6
PANCREAS, raw (USDA):			
Beef, lean only	4 oz.	160	0.
Calf	4 oz.	183	0.
Hog or hog sweetbread	4 oz.	274	0.
PAPAW, fresh (USDA):			
Whole	1 lb. (weighed with rind & seeds)	289	57.2
Flesh only	4 oz.	96	19.1
PAPAYA, Fresh (USDA):			
Whole	1 lb. (weighed with skin & seeds)	119	30.4
Cubed	1 cup (6.4 oz., ½″ cubes)	71	18.2
PARISIAN-STYLE VEGETABLES, frozen (Birds Eye)	⅓ of 10-oz. pkg.	90	7.4
PARSLEY, fresh (USDA):			
Whole	½ lb.	100	19.3
Chopped	1 T. (4 grams)	2	.3
PARSNIP (USDA):			
Raw, whole	1 lb. (weighed unpared)	293	67.5
Boiled, drained, cut in pieces	½ cup (3.7 oz.)	70	15.8
PARTY FRUIT, soft drink (Kirsch)	6 fl. oz.	88	22.1
PARTY PUNCH, undiluted (Mogen David) 12% alcohol	3 fl. oz.	156	21.4
PARV-A-ZERT (SugarLo)	⅓ pt. (3.5 oz.)	202	26.2
PASHA TURKISH COFFEE, Turkish liqueur (Leroux) 53 proof	1 fl. oz.	97	13.3

Food and Description	Measure or Quantity	Calories	Carbo-hydrates (grams)
PASSION FRUIT, fresh (USDA):			
Whole	1 lb. (weighed with shell)	212	50.0
Pulp & seeds	4 oz.	102	24.0
PASTINAS, dry (USDA):			
Carrot	1 oz.	105	21.5
Egg	1 oz.	109	20.4
Spinach	1 oz.	104	21.2
PASTOSO (Petri)			
13% alcohol	3 fl. oz. (2.9 oz.)	71	1.2
PASTRAMI (Vienna)	1 oz.	57	.4
PASTRY SHELL (See also PIE CRUST):			
Home recipe, baked (USDA)	1 shell (1.5 oz.)	212	18.6
Frozen (Pepperidge Farm)	1 shell (1.8 oz.)	232	14.5
Pot pie, bland (Stella D'oro)	1 shell (1.6 oz.)	205	22.8
Pot pie, bland (Keebler)	4″ shell (1.7 oz.)	236	29.6
Tart, sweet (Keebler)	3″ shell (1 oz.)	158	16.6
PÂTÉ, canned:			
De foie gras (USDA)	1 oz.	131	1.4
De foie gras (USDA)	1 T. (.5 oz.)	69	.7
Liver (Hormel)	1 oz.	78	1.1
Liver (Sell's)	1 T. (.5 oz.)	45	.5
Swiss Parfait with herbs or truffles (Cresca)	1 oz.	73	
PDQ, chocolate	1 T. (.6 oz.)	64	15.0
PEA, GREEN:			
Raw (USDA):			
In pod	1 lb. (weighed in pod)	145	24.8
Shelled	1 lb.	381	65.3
Shelled	½ cup (2.4 oz.)	58	9.9
Boiled, drained (USDA)	½ cup (2.9 oz.)	58	9.9

(USDA): United States Department of Agriculture
(HEW/FAO): Health, Education and Welfare/Food and Agriculture Organization
* Prepared as Package Directs

Food and Description	Measure or Quantity	Calories	Carbo-hydrates (grams)
Canned, regular pack:			
Alaska, Early or June, solids & liq. (USDA)	½ cup (4.4 oz.)	82	15.5
Alaska, Early or June, drained solids (USDA)	½ cup (3 oz.)	76	14.4
Alaska, drained solids (Butter Kernel)	½ cup (4.1 oz.)	69	12.8
Early June, with onion (Green Giant)	¼ of 17-oz. can	67	12.8
Early, *Le Sueur,* solids & liq.	½ of 8.5-oz. can	58	10.6
Early, solids & liq. (Stokely-Van Camp)	½ cup (4.1 oz.)	76	14.3
Sweet, drained solids (Butter Kernel)	½ cup (4.1 oz.)	60	10.4
Sweet, solids & liq.:			
(Green Giant)	½ of 8.5-oz. can	59	10.5
(Libby's)	½ cup (4.3 oz.)	52	11.4
(Stokely-Van Camp)	½ cup (4 oz.)	65	11.9
Solids & liq. (Del Monte)	½ cup (4 oz.)	55	9.8
Seasoned, solids & liq. (Del Monte)	½ cup (4 oz.)	60	10.7
(King Pharr)	½ cup	98	17.0
Canned, dietetic pack:			
Alaska, Early or June, solids & liq. (USDA)	4 oz.	62	11.1
Drained solids (USDA)	4 oz.	88	16.2
Drained liq. (USDA)	4 oz.	25	4.6
Sweet, solids & liq. (Blue Boy)	4 oz.	49	8.0
Solids & liq. (Diet Delight)	½ cup (4.4 oz.)	52	9.0
(S and W) *Nutradiet*	4 oz.	40	7.6
Frozen:			
Not thawed (USDA)	½ cup (2.5 oz.)	53	9.2
Boiled, drained (USDA)	½ cup (3 oz.)	57	9.9
Sweet (Birds Eye)	½ cup (3.3 oz.)	70	12.2
Tender tiny (Birds Eye)	½ cup (3.3 oz.)	70	12.0
In butter sauce, baby peas, *LeSueur*	⅓ of 10-oz. pkg.	78	10.9
In butter sauce, sweet (Green Giant)	⅓ of 10-oz. pkg.	86	11.3
With cream sauce (Birds Eye)	½ cup (2.7 oz.)	125	13.6

Food and Description	Measure or Quantity	Calories	Carbo-hydrates (grams)
With cream sauce (Green Giant)	⅓ of 10-oz. pkg.	66	11.0
With sliced mushroom (Birds Eye)	⅓ of 10-oz. pkg.	66	11.7
PEA, MATURE SEED, dry:			
Raw:			
Whole (USDA)	1 lb.	1542	273.5
Whole (USDA)	1 cup (7.1 oz.)	680	120.6
Split:			
(USDA)	1 lb.	1579	284.4
(USDA)	1 cup (7.2 oz.)	706	127.3
(Sinsheimer)	1 oz.	99	17.5
Cooked, split, drained solids (USDA)	½ cup (3.4 oz.)	112	20.2
PEA POD, edible-podded or Chinese:			
Raw (USDA)	1 lb. (weighed untrimmed)	228	51.7
Boiled, drained solids (USDA)	4 oz.	49	10.8
PEA & CARROT:			
Canned, regular pack, solids & liq. (Del Monte)	½ cup (4 oz.)	46	8.9
Canned, dietetic pack, solids & liq.:			
(Blue Boy)	4 oz.	26	5.9
(Diet Delight)	½ cup (4.2 oz.)	47	8.4
(S and W) *Nutradiet*	4 oz.	36	7.4
Frozen:			
Not thawed (USDA)	4 oz.	62	11.8
Boiled, drained solids (USDA)	½ cup (3.1 oz.)	46	8.8
(Birds Eye)	½ cup (3.3 oz.)	55	8.7
In cream sauce (Green Giant)	⅓ of 10-oz. pkg.	60	10.2

(USDA): United States Department of Agriculture
(HEW/FAO): Health, Education and Welfare/Food and Agriculture Organization
* Prepared as Package Directs

Food and Description	Measure or Quantity	Calories	Carbo-hydrates (grams)
PEA & CELERY, frozen (Birds Eye)	½ cup (3.3 oz.)	55	9.8
PEA & ONION, frozen:			
(Birds Eye)	½ cup (3.3 oz.)	67	12.3
In butter sauce (Green Giant)	⅓ of 9-oz. pkg.	75	10.0
PEA & POTATO, with cream sauce, frozen (Birds Eye)	½ cup (2.7 oz.)	131	14.9
PEA SOUP, GREEN:			
Canned, low sodium:			
(Campbell)	7½-oz. can (by wt.)	140	22.2
*(Claybourne)	8 oz.	98	19.1
Canned, regular pack:			
Condensed (USDA)	8 oz. (by wt.)	240	41.7
*Prepared with equal volume water (USDA)	1 cup (8.6 oz.)	130	22.5
*Prepared with equal volume milk (USDA)	1 cup (8.6 oz.)	208	28.7
*(Campbell)	1 cup	131	21.0
Dry mix:			
*(Golden Grain)	1 cup	76	10.5
*(Lipton)	1 cup	130	23.0
(Lipton) *Cup-a-Soup*	1 pkg. (1.2 oz.)	127	22.1
Frozen, condensed:			
With ham (USDA)	8 oz. (by wt.)	256	36.3
*With ham, prepared with equal volume water (USDA)	8 oz. (by wt.)	129	18.1
PEA SOUP, SPLIT:			
Canned, regular pack:			
Condensed (USDA)	8 oz. (by wt.)	268	38.6
*Prepared with equal volume water (USDA)	1 cup (8.6 oz.)	145	20.6
*With ham (Campbell)	1 cup	160	21.7
*(Manischewitz)	8 oz. (by wt.)	133	22.6
*With ham (Heinz)	1 cup (8 ¾ oz.)	153	23.0
With smoked ham (Heinz) *Great American*	1 cup (9 oz.)	186	24.0
Canned, dietetic:			
*(Slim-ette)	8 oz.	50	9.0
(Tillie Lewis)	1 cup	152	26.1

Food and Description	Measure or Quantity	Calories	Carbo-hydrates (grams)
PEACH:			
Fresh:			
Whole, without skin (USDA)	1 lb. (weighed unpeeled)	150	38.3
Whole (USDA)	4-oz. peach (2″ dia.)	38	9.6
Diced (USDA)	½ cup (4.7 oz.)	51	12.9
Sliced (USDA)	½ cup (3 oz.)	32	8.2
Chilled, bottled (Kraft)	4 oz.	66	17.2
Canned, regular pack, solids & liq.:			
Juice pack (Libby's)	4 oz.	69	18.1
Light syrup (USDA)	4 oz.	66	17.1
Heavy syrup (USDA)	2 med. halves & 2 T. syrup	91	23.5
Heavy syrup, halves (USDA)	½ cup (4.1 oz.)	100	25.7
(Del Monte) cling	½ cup (4.6 oz.)	95	25.1
(Del Monte) freestone	½ cup (4.6 oz.)	108	29.1
(Del Monte) spiced	½ cup (4.5 oz.)	94	29.9
(Hunt's)	½ cup (4.5 oz.)	96	25.7
(Stokely-Van Camp)	½ cup (4 oz.)	89	23.1
(White House)	½ cup (4.5 oz.)	100	25.6
Canned, dietetic or unsweetened pack:			
Water pack, solids & liq. (USDA)	½ cup (4.3 oz.)	38	9.9
(Blue Boy) sliced, solids & liq.	4 oz.	32	7.4
(Diet Delight) cling, halves	½ cup (4.4 oz.)	61	15.0
(Diet Delight) freestone, halves	½ cup (4.4 oz.)	64	15.1
(S and W) *Nutradiet*, cling, halves, un-sweetened	2 halves (3.5 oz.)	28	6.6
(Tillie Lewis) cling	½ of 8-oz. can	43	11.6
(Tillie Lewis) Elberta	¼ of 1-lb. can	43	11.3

(USDA): United States Department of Agriculture
(HEW/FAO): Health, Education and Welfare/Food and Agriculture Organization
* Prepared as Package Directs

Food and Description	Measure or Quantity	Calories	Carbo-hydrates (grams)
(Yes Madame) Elberta, halves & slices	4 oz	34	8.1
Dehydrated:			
Uncooked (USDA)	1 oz.	96	24.9
Cooked, with added sugar, solids & liq. (USDA)	½ cup (5.4 oz.)	184	47.6
Dried:			
Uncooked (USDA)	1 lb.	1188	309.8
Uncooked (USDA)	½ cup (3.1 oz.)	231	60.1
Cooked, unsweetened (USDA)	½ cup (5–6 halves & 3 T. liq., 4.8 oz.)	111	28.9
Cooked, with added sugar (USDA)	½ cup (5–6 halves & 3 T. liq., 5.4 oz.)	181	46.8
Uncooked (Del Monte)	½ cup (3.1 oz.)	199	51.0
Frozen:			
Not thawed, slices, sweetened (USDA)	12-oz. pkg.	299	76.8
Not thawed, slices, sweetened (USDA)	16-oz. can	400	102.6
Quick thaw (Birds Eye)	½ cup (5 oz.)	87	22.3
PEACH CREEK (Annie Green Springs) 8% alcohol	3 fl. oz. (2.9 oz.)	63	6.8
PEACH LIQUEUR:			
(Bols) 60 proof	1 fl. oz.	96	8.9
(Hiram Walker) 60 proof	1 fl. oz.	81	8.0
(Leroux) 60 proof	1 fl. oz.	85	8.9
PEACH NECTAR, canned (Del Monte)	1 cup (8.7 oz.)	140	37.9
PEACH PIE:			
Home recipe (USDA)	⅙ of 9″ pie (5.6 oz.)	403	60.4
(Tastykake)	4-oz. pie	360	52.8
Frozen (Banquet)	5 oz.	320	45.5
Frozen (Mrs. Smith's)	⅙ of 8″ pie (4.2 oz.)	301	41.7
PEACH PIE FILLING:			
(Lucky Leaf)	8 oz.	300	74.0
(Wilderness)	21-oz. can	679	148.3

Food and Description	Measure or Quantity	Calories	Carbohydrates (grams)
PEACH PRESERVE, dietetic or low calorie:			
(Dia-Mel)	1 T.	6	1.4
(Kraft)	1 oz.	35	8.6
(Tillie Lewis)	1 T. (.8 oz.)	11	2.9
PEACH TURNOVER, frozen			
(Pepperidge Farm)	1 turnover (3.3 oz.)	323	33.4
PEANUT:			
Raw (USDA):			
In shell	1 lb. (weighed in shell)	1868	61.6
With skins	1 oz.	160	5.3
Without skins	1 oz.	161	5.0
Roasted:			
Whole (USDA)	1 lb. (weighed in shell)	1769	62.6
Shelled, with skins (USDA)	1 oz.	165	5.8
Salted (USDA)	1 oz.	166	5.3
Halves, salted (USDA)	½ cup (2.5 oz.)	421	13.5
Chopped (USDA)	½ cup (2.4 oz.)	404	13.0
Chopped, salted (USDA)	1 T. (9 grams)	53	1.7
Dry (Flavor House)	·1 oz.	166	5.3
Dry (Franklin)	1 oz.	163	5.4
Dry (Frito-Lay)	1 oz.	168	4.1
Dry (Planters)	1 oz. (jar)	170	5.4
Dry (Skippy)	1 oz.	167	4.4
Oil (Planters) cocktail	¾-oz. bag	133	3.7
Oil (Planters) cocktail	1 oz. (can)	179	5.0
Oil (Skippy)	1 oz.	178	5.2
(Nab)	1 packet (1¼ oz.)	223	6.7
Toasted (Tom Houston)	2 T. (1.1 oz.)	176	5.6
Spanish (Planters):			
Dry roasted	1 oz. (jar)	175	3.4
Oil roasted	1 oz. (can)	182	3.4

(USDA): United States Department of Agriculture
(HEW/FAO): Health, Education and Welfare/Food and Agriculture Organization
* Prepared as Package Directs

Food and Description	Measure or Quantity	Calories	Carbohydrates (grams)
PEANUT BUTTER:			
(Bama) crunchy	1 T. (.6 oz.)	100	3.4
(Jif)	1 T. (.6 oz.)	95	3.4
(The Peanut Kids)	1 oz.	165	5.5
(Peter Pan)	1 T. (.6 oz.)	93	3.0
(Planters)	1 T. (.6 oz.)	100	2.7
(Skippy) chunk	1 T. (.6 oz.)	96	2.2
(Smucker's)	1 T. (.5 oz.)	85	2.9
Imitation (Bama) *Skyway*	1 T. (.6 oz.)	96	4.3
PEAR:			
Fresh (USDA):			
Whole	1 lb. (weighed with stems & core)	252	63.2
Whole	6.4-oz. pear (3″ x 2½″ dia.)	101	25.4
Quartered	1 cup (6.8 oz.)	117	29.4
Slices	½ cup (6.8 oz.)	50	12.5
Canned, regular pack, solids & liq.:			
Juice pack (Libby's)	4 oz.	78	17.8
Light syrup (USDA)	4 oz.	69	17.7
Heavy syrup:			
Halves or slices (USDA)	½ cup (with syrup, 4 oz.)	87	22.3
Solids & liq. (Del Monte)	½ cup (4 oz.)	84	21.6
Solids & liq. (Hunt's)	½ cup (4.5 oz.)	90	23.9
Solids & liq. (Stokely-Van Camp)	½ cup (4 oz.)	87	22.5
Extra heavy syrup (USDA)	4 oz.	104	26.8
(Hunt's)	½ cup (4.5 oz.)	99	23.9
Canned, unsweetened or low calorie:			
Water pack, solids & liq. (USDA)	½ cup (4.3 oz.)	39	10.1
Solids & liq. (Blue Boy) Bartlett	4 oz.	33	9.6
Solids and liq. (Diet Delight)	½ cup (4.4 oz.)	66	16.1
(S and W) *Nutradiet,* quartered, unsweetened	4 oz.	31	7.9
(Tillie Lewis) Bartlett	½ of 8-oz. can	44	12.0
Dried:			
Uncooked (USDA)	1 lb.	1216	305.3
Uncooked (Del Monte)	½ cup (2.8 oz.)	178	46.4

Food and Description	Measure or Quantity	Calories	Carbo- hydrates (grams)
Cooked, without added sugar, solids & liq. (USDA)	4 oz.	143	36.0
Cooked, with added sugar, solids & liq. (USDA)	4 oz.	171	43.1
PEAR, CANDIED (USDA)	1 oz.	86	21.5
PEAR NECTAR, sweetened:			
(Del Monte)	1 cup (8.7 oz.)	140	38.4
(S and W) *Nutradiet*	4 oz. (by wt.)	34	8.2
PECAN:			
In shell (USDA)	1 lb. (weighed in shell)	1652	35.1
Shelled (USDA):			
Whole	1 lb.	3116	66.2
Halves	12–14 (.5 oz.)	96	2.0
Halves	½ cup (1.9 oz.)	371	7.9
Chopped	½ cup (1.8 oz.)	357	7.6
Chopped	1 T. (7 grams)	48	1.0
Dry roasted (Planters)	1 oz.	206	3.5
PECAN PIE:			
Home recipe (USDA)	⅛ of 9″ pie (4.9 oz.)	577	70.8
Frozen (Mrs. Smith's)	⅛ of 8″ pie (4 oz.)	430	58.3
PEPPER, BLACK:			
(USDA)	¼ tsp.	1	.3
(Lawry's) seasoned	1 tsp. (2 grams)	8	1.6
PEPPER, HOT CHILI:			
Green (USDA):			
Raw, whole	4 oz.	31	7.5
Raw, without seeds	4 oz.	42	10.3
Canned, chili sauce	1 oz.	6	1.4
Canned pods, without seeds, solids & liq.	4 oz.	28	6.9

(USDA): United States Department of Agriculture
(HEW/FAO): Health, Education and Welfare/Food and Agriculture Organization
* Prepared as Package Directs

Food and Description	Measure or Quantity	Calories	Carbo-hydrates (grams)
Red:			
Raw, whole (USDA)	4 oz. (weighed with seeds)	105	20.5
Raw, trimmed, pods only (USDA)	4 oz.	54	13.1
Canned, chili sauce (USDA)	1 oz.	6	1.1
Canned, pods, solids & liq. (Del Monte)	¼ cup	11	2.0
Canned, drained (Ortega)	¼ cup (1.8 oz.)	10	1.9
Dried:			
Pods (USDA)	1 oz.	91	17.0
Pods (Chili Products)	1 oz.	88	16.9
Powder with added seasoning (USDA)	1 oz.	96	16.0
Powder with added seasoning (USDA)	1 T. (.5 oz.)	51	8.5
*PEPPER POT SOUP			
(Campbell's)	1 cup	94	8.6
PEPPER, SWEET:			
Green:			
Raw:			
Whole (USDA)	1 lb. (weighed untrimmed)	82	17.9
Without stem & seeds (USDA)	1 med. pepper (2.6 oz.)	13	2.9
Chopped (USDA)	½ cup (2.6 oz.)	16	3.6
Slices (USDA)	½ cup (1.4 oz.)	9	2.0
Strips (USDA)	½ cup (1.7 oz.)	11	2.4
Boiled, strips, drained (USDA)	½ cup (2.4 oz.)	12	2.6
Boiled, drained (USDA)	1 med. pepper (2.6 oz.)	13	2.8
Canned, halves (Cannon)	4 oz.	20	
Red:			
Raw, whole (USDA)	1 lb. (weighed with stems & seeds)	112	25.8
Raw, without stem & seeds (USDA)	1 med. pepper (2.2 oz.)	19	2.4
Canned, diced (Cannon)	4 oz.	31	

Food and Description	Measure or Quantity	Calories	Carbo-hydrates (grams)
PEPPER, STUFFED:			
Home recipe, with beef & crumbs (USDA)	2¾" x 2½" pepper with 1⅛ cups stuffing (6.5 oz.)	314	31.1
Frozen, with veal (Weight Watchers)	12-oz. dinner	224	13.6
PEPPERMINT EXTRACT (Ehlers)	1 tsp.	12	
PEPPERMINT SCHNAPPS (See **SCHNAPPS**)			
PEP WHEAT FLAKES, cereal (Kellogg's)	¾ cup (1 oz.)	103	23.0
PERCH, raw (USDA):			
White, whole	1 lb. (weighed whole)	193	0.
White, meat only	4 oz.	134	0.
Yellow, whole	1 lb. (weighed whole)	161	0.
Yellow, meat only	4 oz.	103	0.
PERNOD (Julius Wile)	1 fl. oz.	79	1.1
PERSIMMON (USDA):			
Japanese or Kaki, fresh:			
With seeds	1 lb. (weighed with skin, calyx & seeds)	286	78.3
With seeds	4.4-oz. persimmon	79	20.1
Seedless	1 lb. (weighed with skin & calyx)	293	75.1
Seedless	4.4-oz. persimmon (2½" dia.)	81	20.7
Native, fresh, whole	1 lb. (weighed with seeds & calyx)	472	124.6
Native, fresh, flesh only	4 oz.	144	38.0

(USDA): United States Department of Agriculture
(HEW/FAO): Health, Education and Welfare/Food and Agriculture Organization
* Prepared as Package Directs

Food and Description	Measure or Quantity	Calories	Carbo-hydrates (grams)
PERX, cream substitute	1 tsp. (5 grams)	8	.6
PETITE MARMITE SOUP, canned (Crosse & Blackwell)	6½ oz. (½ can)	33	3.7
PETTIJOHNS, rolled whole wheat, cooked (Quaker)	⅔ cup (1 oz. dry)	97	20.4
PHEASANT, raw (USDA):			
Ready-to-cook	1 lb. (weighed ready-to-cook)	596	0.
Meat & skin	4 oz.	172	0.
Meat only	4 oz.	184	0.
PICKEREL, chain, raw (USDA):			
Whole	1 lb. (weighed whole)	194	0.
Meat only	4 oz.	95	0.
PICKLE:			
Chowchow (See **CHOWCHOW**)			
Cucumber, fresh or bread & butter:	½ cup (3 oz.)	62	15.2
(USDA)	4 slices or sticks		
(Aunt Jane's)	4 slices or sticks (1 oz.)	21	5.1
(Bond's)	3 pieces	23	5.0
(Del Monte)	3 med. pieces (.9 oz.)	4	1.0
(Fanning's)	14-fl.-oz. bottle	200	51.0
(Heinz)	3 slices	20	4.7
(Lutz & Schramm)	3 slices	30	1.3
Dill:			
(USDA)	4.8-oz. pickle (4" x 1¾")	15	3.0
(Aunt Jane's)	1 pickle (2 oz.)	6	1.2
(Bond's)	1 pickle	1	.2
(Del Monte)	1 large pickle (3.5 oz.)	7	1.4
(Heinz)	1 pickle (4")	7	1.1
Processed (Heinz)	1 pickle (3")	1	.1
L & S Dills	1 large pickle	15	2.0
(Smucker's) baby	1 pickle (2¾")	3	.6
Dill, candied sticks (Smucker's)	.8-oz. pickle	46	11.2
Dill, hamburger (Heinz)	3 slices	1	.1

Food and Description	Measure or Quantity	Calories	Carbo-hydrates (grams)
Dill, hamburger (Smucker's)	3 slices (.4 oz.)	2	.3
Kosher dill (Smucker's)	3½" pickle (1.8 oz.)	8	1.4
Sour:			
Cucumber (USDA)	4.8-oz. pickle (1¾" x 4")	14	2.7
Cucumber (USDA)	1 oz.	3	.6
(Aunt Jane's)	1 pickle (2 oz.)	6	1.1
(Del Monte)	1 large pickle (3.5 oz.)	10	2.0
(Heinz)	1 pickle (2")	1	.2
Sweet:			
Cucumber (USDA):			
Whole	1 oz.	41	10.3
Whole, gherkin	.5-oz. pickle (2½" x ¾")	22	5.5
Chopped	½ cup (2.6 oz.)	108	27.0
Chopped	1 T. (9 grams)	13	3.3
(Aunt Jane's)	1 pickle (1.5 oz.)	62	15.5
(Del Monte)	1 med. pickle (.4 oz.)	14	3.5
(Lutz & Schramm)	1 med. pickle	11	
(Smucker's)	2½" pickle (.4 oz.)	17	4.2
Candied (Aunt Jane's)	1 pickle (1.5 oz.)	72	18.1
Candied, midgets (Smucker's)	2" pickle (9 grams)	14	3.5
Cherry (Del Monte)	½ cup (1.9 oz.)	30	5.3
Chips, fresh pack (Smucker's)	1 piece (5 grams)	10	2.5
Gherkin (Bond's)	1 pickle	19	3.0
Gherkin (Heinz)	1 pickle (2")	16	3.9
Mixed (Heinz)	3 slices	23	5.6
Mixed (Smucker's)	1 piece (8 grams)	12	2.9
Mixed, chopped (Durkee)	½ cup	112	
Mixed, chopped (Durkee)	1 T.	14	
Mustard (Heinz)	1 T.	30	6.8
Relish (See **RELISH**)			

Food and Description	Measure or Quantity	Calories	Carbo-hydrates (grams)
Sticks, fresh pack (Smucker's)	4″ stick (1.1 oz.)	29	7.1
Wax, mild (Del Monte)	½ cup (2.1 oz.)	21	4.6
PIE (See individual kinds)			
PIECRUST (See also **PASTRY SHELL**):			
Home recipe, baked, 9″ pie (USDA)	1 crust (6.3 oz.)	900	78.8
Home recipe, baked, 9″ pie (USDA)	2 crusts (12.7 oz.)	1800	157.7
Frozen:			
(Mrs. Smith's)	8″ shell (5 oz.)	692	48.0
(Mrs. Smith's)	9″ shell (6 oz.)	867	75.0
(Mrs. Smith's)	10″ shell (8 oz.)	1177	100.0
PIECRUST MIX:			
Dry (USDA)	10-oz. pkg. (2 crusts)	1482	140.6
*Prepared with water (USDA)	4 oz.	526	49.9
*Double crust (Betty Crocker)	⅛ of 2 crusts	302	24.1
*Double crust (Pillsbury)	⅛ of 2 crusts	290	27.0
*Graham cracker (Betty Crocker)	⅛ of crust	159	22.3
*(Flako)	⅛ of 9″ shell (.8 oz. dry)	116	11.7
PIE FILLING (See individual kinds)			
PIESPORTER RIESLING (Julius Kayser) 10% alcohol	3 fl. oz.	57	1.7
PIGEON (See **SQUAB**)			
PIGEONPEA (USDA):			
Raw, immature seeds in pods	1 lb.	207	37.7
Dry seeds	1 lb.	1551	288.9
PIGNOLIA (See **PINE NUT**)			
PIGS FEET, pickled:			
(USDA)	4 oz.	226	0.
(Hormel)	1-pt. can	442	.2

Food and Description	Measure or Quantity	Calories	Carbo-hydrates (grams)
PIKE, raw (USDA):			
Blue, whole	1 lb. (weighed whole)	180	0.
Blue, meat only	4 oz.	102	0.
Northern, whole	1 lb. (weighed whole)	104	0.
Northern, meat only	4 oz.	100	0.
Walleye, whole	1 lb. (weighed whole)	240	0.
Walleye, meat only	4 oz.	105	0.
PILI NUT (USDA):			
In shell	1 lb. (weighed in shell)	546	6.9
Shelled	4 oz.	759	9.5
PILLSBURY INSTANT BREAKFAST:			
Chocolate or strawberry	1 pouch	130	27.0
Chocolate malt	1 pouch	130	26.0
Vanilla	1 pouch	130	28.0
PIMENTO, canned:			
Solids & liq. (USDA)	1 med. pod (1.3 oz.)	10	2.2
Solids & liq. (Stokely-Van Camp)	½ cup (4.1 oz.)	31	6.3
Whole pods, slices or pieces (Dromedary)	1 oz.	8	1.2
Drained (Ortega)	¼ cup (1.7 oz.)	6	1.3
PIMM'S CUP, *slings* (Julius Wile):			
#1-Gin	1 fl. oz.	69	3.3
#2-Scotch or #3-Brandy	1 fl. oz.	68	3.0
#4-Rum & brandy	1 fl. oz.	59	.9
#5-Canadian rye	1 fl. oz.	60	1.0
#6-Vodka	1 fl. oz.	63	1.8
PINA COLADA (Party Tyme)	½-oz. pkg.	50	13.2
PINEAPPLE:			
Fresh:			

(USDA): United States Department of Agriculture
(HEW/FAO): Health, Education and Welfare/Food and Agriculture Organization
* Prepared as Package Directs

Food and Description	Measure or Quantity	Calories	Carbo-hydrates (grams)
Whole (USDA)	1 lb. (weighed untrimmed)	123	32.3
Chunks (Dole)	½ cup (3.5 oz.)	52	13.7
Diced (USDA)	½ cup (2.8 oz.)	41	10.7
Slices (USDA)	3-oz. slice (¾" x 3½")	44	11.5
(Del Monte)	½ cup (2.5 oz.)	42	10.8
Canned, regular pack:			
Juice pack:			
Solids & liq. (USDA)	4 oz.	66	17.1
Slices (Del Monte)	2 med. slices & 2½ T. juice (3.7 oz.)	66	15.5
Chunks or crushed (Dole)	½ of 8-oz. can	64	16.5
Light syrup, solids & liq. (USDA)	4 oz.	67	17.5
Heavy syrup:			
(Del Monte)	½ cup (5 oz.)	100	26.8
Crushed, solids & liq. (USDA)	½ cup (4.6 oz.)	97	25.4
Crushed (Dole)	½ cup (includes 2½ T. syrup)	84	21.7
Slices, solids & liq. (USDA)	½ cup (4.9 oz.)	103	27.0
Slices, solids & liq. (USDA)	4 oz.	84	22.0
Slices (USDA)	2 small or 1 large slice & 2 T. syrup	90	23.7
Slices (Dole)	2 med. slices & 2½ T. syrup	84	21.7
Spears (Dole)	2 spears & 2 T. syrup	52	
(Stokely-Van Camp)	½ cup (4 oz.)	84	22.3
Tidbits, solids & liq. (USDA)	½ cup (4.6 oz.)	95	25.0
Tidbits (Dole)	½ cup (includes 2½ T. syrup)	84	21.7
Extra heavy syrup, solids & liq. (USDA)	4 oz.	102	26.5
Canned, unsweetened, low calorie or dietetic:			
Water pack, except crushed (USDA)	4 oz.	44	11.6

Food and Description	Measure or Quantity	Calories	Carbo-hydrates (grams)
Chunks, low calorie (Diet Delight)	½ cup (4.4 oz.)	65	15.6
Chunks, low calorie, solids & liq. (S and W) *Nutradiet*	4 oz.	56	12.6
Crushed, solids & liq. (Diet Delight)	½ cup (4.4 oz.)	77	18.5
Slices:			
Solids & liq. (Diet Delight)	½ cup (4.4 oz.)	65	15.6
In pineapple juice (Dole)	2 med. slices & 2½ T. juice (3.7 oz.)	66	15.5
(Libby's)	4 oz.	48	11.6
(S and W) *Nutradiet*	2½ slices (3.5 oz.)	56	13.1
(White Rose)	4 oz.	67	16.2
Tidbits:			
(Diet Delight)	½ cup (4.4 oz.)	65	15.6
In pineapple juice (Dole)	½ cup (includes 2 T. juice)	77	
(S and W) *Nutradiet*, unsweetened	4 oz.	78	19.2
Solids & liq. (Tillie Lewis)	½ cup (4.4 oz.)	76	18.3
Frozen:			
Chunks sweetened, not thawed (USDA)	½ cup (4.3 oz.)	105	27.3
Chunks in heavy syrup (Dole)	11 chunks & 2½ T. syrup (4 oz.)	87	25.1
PINEAPPLE & APRICOT JUICE DRINK			
(Del Monte)	1 cup (8.6 oz.)	132	32.6
PINEAPPLE CAKE MIX:			
*(Betty Crocker) layer	1/12 of cake	199	36.1
*Upside down (Betty Crocker) *Dole*	1/9 of cake	270	42.3

(USDA): United States Department of Agriculture
(HEW/FAO): Health, Education and Welfare/Food and Agriculture Organization
* Prepared as Package Directs

Food and Description	Measure or Quantity	Calories	Carbo-hydrates (grams)
*(Duncan Hines)	1/12 of cake (2.7 oz.)	201	35.0
*(Pillsbury)	1/12 of cake	210	34.0
PINEAPPLE, CANDIED			
(Liberty)	1 oz.	93	22.6
PINEAPPLE-CHERRY DRINK			
(Del Monte) *Merry*	1/2 cup (4.3 oz.)	52	12.2
PINEAPPLE FLAVORING:			
Imitation (Ehlers)	1 tsp.	12	
Imitation (French's)	1 tsp.	14	
PINEAPPLE & GRAPEFRUIT JUICE, unsweetened, frozen (Dole)	6-fl.-oz. can	334	
PINEAPPLE & GRAPEFRUIT JUICE DRINK, canned:			
(Del Monte)	1/2 cup (4.3 oz.)	62	15.7
Pink (Del Monte)	1/2 cup (4.3 oz.)	64	16.2
(Dole)	1/2 cup (4.4 oz.)	67	16.9
(Wagner)	1/2 cup	57	14.4
Ping (Stokely-Van Camp)	1/2 cup	61	
Pink grapefruit (Dole)	1/2 cup	62	
PINEAPPLE JUICE:			
Canned, unsweetened:			
(Del Monte)	1/2 cup (4.3 oz.)	60	16.2
(Dole)	1/2 cup (4.4 oz.)	69	16.8
(Heinz)	5½-fl.-oz. can	101	23.5
(Libby's)	1/2 cup (4.4 oz.)	68	17.0
(S and W) *Nutradiet*	4 oz.	67	16.2
(Stokely-Van Camp)	1/2 cup (4 oz.)	63	15.5
Frozen, concentrate:			
Unsweetened, undiluted (USDA)	6-fl.-oz. can	387	95.7
*Unsweetened, diluted with 3 parts water (USDA)	1/2 cup (4.4 oz.)	64	15.9
Unsweetened (Dole)	6-fl.-oz. can (7.7 oz.)	389	96.3
PINEAPPLE & ORANGE JUICE:			
(Kraft)	1/2 cup	56	12.6
Unsweetened, frozen (Dole)	6-fl.-oz. can	334	

Food and Description	Measure or Quantity	Calories	Carbo- hydrates (grams)
PINEAPPLE & ORANGE JUICE DRINK, canned:			
(USDA) 40% fruit juices	½ cup (4.4 oz.)	67	16.7
(Del Monte)	½ cup (4.3 oz.)	62	15.8
PINEAPPLE-PEAR JUICE DRINK, canned (Del Monte)	½ cup (4.3 oz.)	68	17.0
PINEAPPLE PIE:			
Home recipe:			
(USDA)	⅛ of 9" pie (5.6 oz.)	400	60.2
Chiffon (USDA)	⅛ of 9" pie (3.8 oz.)	311	42.2
Custard (USDA)	⅛ of 9" pie (5.4 oz.)	334	48.8
(Tastykake)	4-oz. pie	389	57.8
With cheese (Tastykake)	4-oz. pie	436	59.4
Frozen (Mrs. Smith's)	⅛ of 8" pie (4.2 oz.)	300	41.7
PINEAPPLE PIE FILLING (Lucky Leaf)	8 oz.	240	50.0
PINEAPPLE PRESERVE:			
Sweetened (Bama)	1 T. (.7 oz.)	54	13.5
Sweetened (Smucker's)	1 T. (.7 oz.)	52	13.3
(Tillie Lewis)	1 T. (.5 oz.)	10	2.4
PINEAPPLE SOFT DRINK:			
(Canada Dry)	6 fl. oz.	79	19.8
(Hoffman)	6 fl. oz.	89	22.3
(Kirsch)	6 fl. oz.	89	22.3
(Nedick's)	6 fl. oz.	89	22.3
(Yoo-Hoo) high-protein	6 fl. oz. (6.4 oz.)	100	18.9
PINE NUT (USDA):			
Pignolias, shelled	4 oz.	626	13.2
Piñon, whole	4 oz. (weighed in shell)	418	13.5
Piñon, shelled	4 oz.	720	23.2

(USDA): United States Department of Agriculture
(HEW/FAO): Health, Education and Welfare/Food and Agriculture Organization
* Prepared as Package Directs

Food and Description	Measure or Quantity	Calories	Carbo- hydrates (grams)
PINOT CHARDONNAY WINE (Louis M. Martini) 12.5% alcohol	3 fl. oz.	90	.2
PINOT NOIR WINE: (Inglenook) Estate, 12% alcohol	3 fl. oz. (2.9 oz.)	58	.3
(Louis M. Martini) 12.5% alcohol	3 fl. oz.	90	.2
PISTACHIO NUT: In shell (USDA)	4 oz. (weighed in shell)	337	10.8
Shelled (USDA)	½ cup (2.2 oz.)	368	11.8
Shelled (USDA)	1 T. (8 grams)	46	1.5
***PISTACHIO NUT PUDDING MIX**, instant (Royal)	½ cup (5.1 oz.)	179	28.2
PITANGA, fresh (USDA): Whole	1 lb. (weighed whole)	187	45.9
Flesh only	4 oz.	58	14.2
PIZZA PIE: (Celeste) *Bambino*	10-oz. pie	634	66.8
Cheese (Buitoni)	4 oz.	270	36.6
Cheese (Celeste)	20-oz. pie	1284	142.4
Cheese, little (Chef Boy-Ar-Dee)	2½-oz. pie	162	22.7
Cheese (Jeno's)	13-oz. pie	881	104.8
Cheese (Jeno's) Serv-A-Slice	1 slice (1.7 oz.)	116	12.7
Cheese (Jeno's) snack tray	½-oz. pizza	30	4.8
Cheese (Kraft)	14-oz pie	826	98.9
Cheese, *Pee Wee* (Kraft)	2½-oz. pie	169	20.1
Hamburger (Jeno's)	13½-oz. pie	922	110.8
Pepperoni (Buitoni)	4 oz.	288	38.7
Pepperroni (Chef Boy-Ar-Dee)	⅛ of 14-oz pie	150	18.1
Pepperoni (Jeno's)	13¼-oz. pie	1010	111.4
Pepperoni (Jeno's) Serv-A-Slice	1 slice (1.8 oz.)	145	14.4
Pepperoni (Jeno's) snack tray	½-oz. pie	37	4.7
Sausage (Buitoni)	4 oz.	281	34.1
Sausage (Celeste)	23-oz. pie	1600	152.0

Food and Description	Measure or Quantity	Calories	Carbo- hydrates (grams)
Sausage (Celeste) *Bambino*	9-oz. pie	642	71.2
Sausage (Chef Boy-Ar-Dee)	⅛ of 13¼-oz pie	141	17.9
Sausage (Jeno's)	13½-oz. pie	903	108.6
Sausage (Jeno's) Serv-A-Slice	1 slice (2 oz.)	143	14.3
Sausage (Jeno's) snack tray	½-oz. pie	35	4.6
Sausage (Kraft)	14½-oz. pie	999	99.5
PIZZA PIE MIX:			
*With cheese (Chef Boy-Ar-Dee)	⅛ of 15½-oz. pie	187	26.5
*With cheese (Kraft)	4 oz.	265	26.1
*With sausage (Chef Boy-Ar-Dee)	⅛ of 17-oz. pie	222	27.0
PIZZA SAUCE, canned:			
(Buitoni)	4 oz.	76	10.0
(Chef Boy-Ar-Dee)	5¼ oz. (½ of 10½-oz. can)	116	7.0
(Contadina)	1 cup (8 oz.)	144	23.2
PLANTAIN, raw (USDA):			
Whole	1 lb. (weighed with skin)	389	101.9
Flesh only	4 oz.	135	35.4
PLUM:			
Damson, fresh (USDA):			
Whole	1 lb. (weighed with pits)	272	73.5
Flesh only	4 oz.	75	20.2
Japanese and hybrid, fresh (USDA):			
Whole	1 lb. (weighed with pits)	205	52.4
Whole	2.1-oz. plum (2″ dia.)	27	6.9
Diced	½ cup (2.9 oz.)	39	10.1
Halves	½ cup (3.1 oz.)	42	10.8
Slices	½ cup (3 oz.)	40	10.3

(USDA): United States Department of Agriculture
(HEW/FAO): Health, Education and Welfare/Food and Agriculture Organization
* Prepared as Package Directs

Food and Description	Measure or Quantity	Calories	Carbo-hydrates (grams)
Prune-type, fresh (USDA):			
Whole	1 lb. (weighed with pits)	320	84.0
Halves	½ cup (2.8 oz.)	60	15.8
Canned, purple, regular pack, solids & liq.:			
Light syrup (USDA)	4 oz.	71	18.8
Heavy syrup:			
(USDA) with pits	½ cup (4.5 oz.)	106	27.6
(USDA) without pits	½ cup (4.2 oz.)	100	25.9
(Del Monte)	½ cup (4.1 oz.)	112	30.4
Extra heavy syrup (USDA)	4 oz.	116	30.3
Canned, unsweetened or low calorie, solids & liq.:			
Greengage, water pack	4 oz	37	9.8
Purple:			
Water pack, solids & liq. (USDA)	4 oz.	52	13.5
(Diet Delight)	½ cup (4.4 oz.)	80	19.7
(S and W) *Nutradiet*, low calorie	4 oz.	57	13.8
Prune (Tillie Lewis)	½ of 8-oz. can	61	16.2
PLUM PIE (Tastykake)	4-oz. pie	364	53.8
PLUM PRESERVE (Smucker's)	1 T. (.7 oz.)	49	12.5
PLUM PUDDING:			
(Crosse & Blackwell)	4 oz.	340	62.4
(Richardson & Robbins)	½ cup (4 oz.)	300	68.0
POHA (See **GROUND-CHERRY**)			
POKE SHOOTS (USDA):			
Raw	1 lb.	104	16.8
Boiled, drained solids	4 oz.	23	3.5
POLISH-STYLE SAUSAGE:			
(Oscar Mayer) all meat	1 oz. (from 8-oz. link)	81	.5
(Wilson)	3 oz.	245	1.0
POLLOCK (USDA):			
Raw, drawn	1 lb. (weighed with head, tail, fins & bones)	194	0.
Cooked, creamed	4 oz.	145	4.5

Food and Description	Measure or Quantity	Calories	Carbo-hydrates (grams)
POMEGRANATE, raw (USDA):			
Whole	1 lb. (weighed whole)	160	41.7
Pulp only	4 oz.	71	18.6
POMMARD WINE, French red Burgundy:			
(Barton & Guestier) 13% alcohol	3 fl. oz.	67	.4
(Chanson) *St. Vincent,* 11½% alcohol	3 fl. oz.	60	6.3
(Cruse) 12% alcohol	3 fl. oz.	72	
POMPANO, raw (USDA):			
Whole	1 lb. (weighed whole)	422	0.
Meat only	4 oz.	188	0.
POPCORN:			
Unpopped (USDA)	1 oz.	103	20.4
Popped (USDA):			
Plain	1 oz.	109	21.7
Plain, large kernel	1 cup (6 grams)	23	4.6
Butter or oil & salt added	1 oz.	129	16.8
Butter or oil & salt added	1 cup (9 grams)	41	5.3
Sugar-coated	1 cup (1.2 oz.)	134	29.9
(Jiffy Pop)	2½ oz. (½ pkg.)	244	29.8
(Tom Houston)	1 cup (.5 oz.)	68	8.9
Balls (Pophitt)	1 oz.	91	
Buttered (Wise)	1-oz. bag	137	17.5
Butter flavor (Jiffy Pop)	2½ oz. (½ pkg.)	247	29.4
Caramel-coated:			
With peanuts (Old London)	1 cup (1.3 oz.)	142	30.2
Without peanuts (Old London)	1¾-oz. bag	195	43.6
Cheese-flavored (Old London)	¾-oz. bag	110	12.2
Cheese-flavored (Wise)	⅝-oz. bag	90	9.6
Cracker Jack	¾-oz. bag	90	16.7

(USDA): United States Department of Agriculture
(HEW/FAO): Health, Education and Welfare/Food and Agriculture
           Organization
* Prepared as Package Directs

Food and Description	Measure or Quantity	Calories	Carbo-hydrates (grams)
Cracker Jack	1⅜-oz. box	165	30.5
Cracker Jack	3-oz. box	360	66.5
Seasoned (Old London)	1¼-oz. bag	175	22.4
POPOVER, home recipe (USDA)	1 average popover (2 oz.)	128	14.7
*POPOVER MIX (Flako)	2.3-oz. popover (⅛ of pkg.)	163	22.7
POPSICLE (Popsicle Industries):			
Fruit flavors	3 fl. oz. (3.4 oz.)	70	16.4
Chocolate	3 fl. oz.	106	
POP-UP (See **TOASTER CAKE**)			
PORGY, raw (USDA):			
Whole	1 lb. (weighed whole)	208	0.
Meat only	4 oz.	127	0.
PORK, medium-fat:			
Fresh (USDA):			
Boston butt:			
Raw	1 lb. (weighed with bone & skin)	1220	0.
Roasted, lean & fat	4 oz.	400	0.
Roasted, lean only	4 oz.	277	0.
Chop:			
Broiled, lean & fat	1 chop (4 oz., weighed with bone)	295	0.
Broiled, lean & fat	1 chop (3 oz., weighed with bone)	332	0.
Broiled, lean only	1 chop (3 oz., weighed without bone)	230	0.
Fat, separable, cooked	1 oz.	219	0.
Ham (See also **HAM**):			
Raw	1 lb. (weighed with bone & skin)	1188	0.

Food and Description	Measure or Quantity	Calories	Carbo-hydrates (grams)
Roasted, lean & fat	4 oz.	424	0.
Roasted, lean only	4 oz.	246	0.
Loin:			
Raw	1 lb. (weighed with bone)	1065	0.
Roasted, lean & fat	4 oz.	411	0.
Roasted, lean only	4 oz.	288	0.
Picnic:			
Raw	1 lb. (weighed with bone & skin)	1083	0.
Simmered, lean & fat	4 oz.	424	0.
Simmered, lean only	4 oz.	240	0.
Spareribs:			
Raw, with bone	1 lb. (weighed with bone)	976	0.
Braised, lean & fat	4 oz.	499	0.
Cured, light commercial cure:			
Bacon (See **BACON**)			
Bacon butt (USDA):			
Raw	1 lb. (weighed with bone & skin)	1227	0.
Roasted, lean & fat	4 oz.	374	0.
Roasted, lean only	4 oz.	276	0.
Ham (See also **HAM**):			
Raw (USDA)	1 lb. (weighed with bone & skin)	1100	0.
Roasted, lean & fat (USDA)	4 oz.	328	0.
Roasted, lean only (USDA)	4 oz.	212	0.
Fully cooked, boneless:			
Parti-Style (Armour Star)	4 oz.	167	.1
(Wilson) rolled	4 oz.	222	0.
Picnic:			
Raw (USDA)	1 lb. (weighed		

(USDA): United States Department of Agriculture
(HEW/FAO): Health, Education and Welfare/Food and Agriculture Organization
* Prepared as Package Directs

Food and Description	Measure or Quantity	Calories	Carbo- hydrates (grams)
	with bone & skin)	1060	0.
Raw (Wilson) smoked	4 oz.	279	0.
Roasted, lean & fat (USDA)	4 oz.	366	0.
Roasted, lean only (USDA)	4 oz.	239	0.
Canned (Hormel)	4 oz. (3-lb. can)	206	.2
Cured, long-cure, country-style Virginia ham, raw:			
(USDA)	1 lb. (weighed with bone & skin)	1535	1.2
(USDA)	1 lb. (weighed without bone & skin)	1765	1.4

PORK & BEANS (See **BEAN, BAKED**)

PORK, CANNED, chopped
luncheon meat:

(USDA)	1 oz.	83	.4
Chopped (USDA)	1 cup (4.8 oz.)	400	1.8
Diced (USDA)	1 cup (5 oz.)	415	1.8
(Hormel)	1 oz.	70	.3

PORK DINNER, loin of pork,
frozen (Swanson)

	10-oz. dinner	460	40.5

PORK & GRAVY, canned
(USDA)

	4 oz.	290	7.1

PORK RINDS, fried, *Baken-ets*
(See also other brand names)

	1 oz.	139	.2

PORK SAUSAGE:

Uncooked (USDA)	1 oz.	141	Tr.
(Armour Star)	1-oz. sausage	133	0.
(Hormel) country-style	1 oz.	107	.4
Little Sizzlers (Hormel)	1 sausage (.8 oz.)	105	.2
Midget (Hormel)	1 link (.8 oz.)	90	.2
Smoked (Hormel)	1 oz.	97	.3
Little Friers (Oscar Mayer)	1 link (1 oz.)	129	.2
(Wilson)	1 oz.	135	0.

Food and Description	Measure or Quantity	Calories	Carbohydrates (grams)
Canned, drained (USDA)	1 oz.	108	.5
Cooked, *Little Friers* (Oscar Mayer)	1 link (.4 oz.)	44	.2
PORK, SWEET & SOUR, frozen (Chun King)	7½-oz. serving (½ pkg.)	220	26.0
PORT WINE:			
(Gallo) 16% alcohol	3 fl. oz.	94	7.8
(Gallo) ruby, 20% alcohol	3 fl. oz.	112	8.7
(Gallo) tawny, Old Decanter, 20% alcohol	3 fl. oz.	112	8.4
(Gallo) white, 20% alcohol	3 fl. oz.	111	8.4
(Gold Seal) 19% alcohol	3 fl. oz.	158	9.4
(Great Western) Solera, 18% alcohol	3 fl. oz.	138	11.8
(Great Western) Solera, tawny, 18% alcohol	3 fl. oz.	135	11.0
(Great Western) white, 18% alcohol	3 fl. oz.	135	12.3
(Italian Swiss Colony-Gold Medal) 19.7% alcohol	3 fl. oz.	130	8.7
(Louis M. Martini) 19½% alcohol	3 fl. oz.	165	2.0
(Louis M. Martini) tawny, 19½% alcohol	3 fl. oz.	165	2.0
(Robertson's) ruby, 20% alcohol	3 fl. oz.	138	9.9
(Robertson's) tawny, *Dry Humour*, 21% alcohol	3 fl. oz.	145	9.9
(Robertson's) tawny, *Game Bird*, 21% alcohol	3 fl. oz.	145	9.9
(Robertson's) *Rebello Valente*, 20½% alcohol	3 fl. oz.	141	9.9
(Taylor) 19.5% alcohol	3 fl. oz.	150	10.9
(Taylor) tawny, 19.5% alcohol	3 fl. oz.	144	10.0
***POST TOASTIES*,** cereal	1 cup (1 oz.)	108	24.0

(USDA): United States Department of Agriculture
(HEW/FAO): Health, Education and Welfare/Food and Agriculture
               Organization
* Prepared as Package Directs

Food and Description	Measure or Quantity	Calories	Carbo-hydrates (grams)
*POSTUM, instant	1 cup	16	3.7
POTATO:			
Raw (USDA):			
Whole	1 lb. (weighed unpared)	279	62.8
Pared, chopped	1 cup (5.2 oz.)	112	25.1
Pared, diced	1 cup (5.5 oz.)	119	26.8
Pared, slices	1 cup (5.2 oz.)	113	25.5
Cooked (USDA):			
Au gratin or scalloped, with cheese	½ cup (4.3 oz.)	127	17.9
Au gratin or scalloped, without cheese	½ cup (4.3 oz.)	177	16.6
Baked, peeled after baking	2½" dia. potato (3 raw to 1 lb.)	92	20.9
Boiled, peeled after boiling	1 med. (3 raw to 1 lb.)	103	23.3
Boiled, peeled before boiling:			
Whole	1 med. (3 raw to 1 lb.)	79	17.7
Diced	½ cup (2.8 oz.)	51	11.3
Mashed	½ cup (3.7 oz.)	68	15.1
Riced	½ cup (4 oz.)	74	16.5
Sliced	½ cup (2.8 oz.)	52	11.6
French-fried in deep fat (USDA)	10 pieces (2" x ½" x ½", 2 oz.)	156	20.5
French fries (McDonald's)	1 serving (2.4 oz.)	215	27.5
Hash-browned, after holding overnight	½ cup (3.4 oz.)	223	28.4
Mashed, milk added	½ cup (3.5 oz.)	64	12.7
Mashed, milk & butter added	½ cup (3.5 oz.)	92	12.1
Pan-fried from raw	½ cup (3 oz.)	228	27.7
Scalloped (See Au Gratin)			
Canned:			
Solids & liq. (USDA)	1 cup (8.8 oz.)	110	24.5
Solids & liq. (USDA)	4 oz.	50	11.1
Solids & liq. (Del Monte)	1 cup (5.3 oz.)	46	10.3
White (Butter Kernel)	3–4 small potatoes	96	22.0
Solids & liq. (Stokely-Van Camp)	1 cup (8.2 oz.)	102	22.4

Food and Description	Measure or Quantity	Calories	Carbohydrates (grams)
Dehydrated, mashed:			
Flakes, without milk (USDA):			
Dry	½ cup (.8 oz.)	84	19.3
*Prepared with water, milk & fat	½ cup (3.8 oz.)	100	15.5
Flakes (Borden) *Country Store*	¼ cup (1.1 oz.)	60	13.3
Granules, without milk (USDA):			
Dry	½ cup (3.5 oz.)	352	80.4
*Prepared with water, milk & fat	½ cup (3.7 oz.)	101	15.1
Granules, with milk (USDA):			
Dry	½ cup (3.5 oz.)	358	77.7
*Prepared with water & fat	½ cup (3.7 oz.)	83	13.8
Frozen:			
Au gratin (Stouffer's)	11½-oz. pkg.	304	35.6
Au gratin (Swanson)	8-oz. pkg.	241	16.8
Bake-A-Tata (Holloway House):			
With cheese	1 potato (5 oz.)	226	27.4
With sour cream	1 potato (5 oz.)	200	28.0
Diced for hash-browning, not thawed (USDA)	4 oz.	83	19.7
Diced, hash-browned (USDA)	4 oz.	254	32.9
French-fried:			
Not thawed (USDA)	9-oz. pkg.	434	66.6
Heated (USDA)	10 pieces (2″ x ½″ x ½″, 2 oz.)	125	19.2
(Birds Eye)	17 pieces (3 oz.)	144	22.0
Crinkle-cut (Birds Eye)	17 pieces (3 oz.)	144	22.0
Fanci-fries (Birds Eye)	¼ pkg. (3 oz.)	173	21.0
(Mrs. Paul's)	4 oz.	250	38.8
Mashed, heated (USDA)	4 oz.	105	17.8
Potato puffs, French-fried (Birds Eye)	⅓ pkg. (2.7 oz.)	149	14.6

(USDA): United States Department of Agriculture
(HEW/FAO): Health, Education and Welfare/Food and Agriculture Organization
* Prepared as Package Directs

Food and Description	Measure or Quantity	Calories	Carbo- hydrates (grams)
Scalloped (Swanson)	8-oz. pkg.	257	12.9
Shredded for hash-browns (Birds Eye)	⅓ pkg. (3 oz.)	63	14.7
Stuffed, baked (Holloway House):			
With cheese	1 potato (6 oz.)	296	38.2
With sour cream & chives	1 potato (6 oz.)	296	38.2
Tiny Taters (Birds Eye)	⅙ pkg. (2.7 oz.)	109	11.6
POTATO CHIP:			
(USDA)	10 chips (2″ dia., 2 oz.)	114	10.0
(Lay's)	1 oz.	158	13.3
(Nalley's)	1 oz.	158	13.9
(Pringle's)	10 chips (.5 oz.)	73	7.7
Ruffles	1 oz.	158	14.1
(Wise)	⅞-oz. pkg.	131	13.8
Barbecue flavored (Wise)	1 oz.	152	15.0
Onion-garlic chips (Wise)	⅞-oz. pkg.	135	13.2
Ridgies (Wise)	⅞-oz. pkg.	137	13.3
POTATO MIX:			
*Au gratin (Betty Crocker)	½ cup	160	20.8
*Au gratin (French's)	½ cup	95	15.0
*Au gratin (Pillsbury)			
Hungry Jack	½ cup	170	21.0
Buds, instant (Betty Crocker)	½ cup	134	17.1
*Hash brown (Pillsbury)			
Hungry Jack	½ cup	140	25.0
*Mashed, country style (French's)	½ cup	137	16.5
*Mashed, instant (French's)	½ cup	114	16.0
*Mashed (Pillsbury)			
Hungry Jack	½ cup	170	18.0
*Scalloped (Betty Crocker)	½ cup	150	22.2
*Scalloped (French's)	½ cup	109	20.0
*Scalloped (Pillsbury)			
Hungry Jack	½ cup	140	21.0
*POTATO PANCAKE MIX:			
(French's)	3-oz. pkg.	284	62.0
*(French's)	¼ pkg. (3 small pancakes)	90	15.5

Food and Description	Measure or Quantity	Calories	Carbo-hydrates (grams)
POTATO SALAD:			
Home recipe, with cooked salad dressing, seasonings (USDA)	4 oz.	112	18.5
Home recipe, with mayonnaise & French dressing, hard-cooked eggs, seasonings (USDA)	4 oz.	164	15.2
Canned (Nalley's)	4 oz.	178	20.2
POTATO SOUP, Cream of:			
*Canned (Campbell)	1 cup	105	13.1
Frozen:			
Condensed (USDA)	8 oz. (by wt.)	197	22.7
*Prepared with equal volume water (USDA)	1 cup (8.5 oz.)	106	11.8
*Prepared with equal volume milk (USDA)	1 cup (8.6 oz.)	186	18.4
POTATO SOUP MIX:			
*(Lipton)	1 cup	100	18.9
(Wyler's)	1 oz.	88	17.0
POTATO STICK:			
(USDA)	1 oz.	154	14.4
(Wise) Julienne	½-oz. pkg.	78	7.6
(Wise) Julienne	⅝-oz. pkg.	98	9.5
(Wise) Julienne	¾-oz. pkg.	117	11.4
(Wise) Julienne	⅞-oz. pkg.	137	13.3
POUILLY-FUISSÉ WINE,			
French white Burgundy:			
(Barton & Guestier) 12½% alcohol	3 fl. oz.	64	.3
(Chanson) St. Vincent, 12% alcohol	3 fl. oz.	84	6.3
(Cruse) 12% alcohol	3 fl. oz.	72	
POUILLY-FUMÉ, French white			
Loire Valley (Barton & Guestier) 12% alcohol	3 fl. oz.	60	.1

(USDA): United States Department of Agriculture
(HEW/FAO): Health, Education and Welfare/Food and Agriculture Organization
* Prepared as Package Directs

Food and Description	Measure or Quantity	Calories	Carbo-hydrates (grams)
POUND CAKE:			
Home recipe, old-fashioned (USDA)	1.1-oz. slice (3½" x 3" x ½")	142	14.1
All butter (Drake's) Jr.	1 slice (1.2 oz.)	110	19.2
Plain (Drake's)	1 slice (1.6 oz.)	153	25.1
Plain (Sara Lee)	1 oz.	110	13.0
Raisin (Drake's)	1 slice (1½ oz.)	210	34.0
Frozen (Morton)	1 oz.	117	14.8
POUND CAKE MIX:			
*(Betty Crocker)	1/12 of cake	210	28.0
*(Dromedary)	1" slice (2.9 oz.)	313	40.7
*(Pillsbury) *Bundt*	1/12 of cake	300	45.0
PREAM, cream substitute	1 tsp. (2 grams)	11	1.1
PRESERVE (See also individual listings by flavor):			
(USDA)	1 oz.	77	19.8
(USDA)	1 T. (.7 oz.)	54	14.0
(Mrs. Brown)	1 oz.	76	17.0
(Crosse & Blackwell)	1 T. (.8 oz.)	59	14.8
(Kraft)	1 oz.	78	19.3
(Polaner)	1 T.	54	13.5
(Smucker's)	1 T. (.7 oz.)	52	12.9
PRETZEL:			
(USDA)	1 oz.	111	21.5
(USDA)	10 small sticks (6 grams)	12	2.3
(Keebler) Log	1 piece (4 grams)	16	3.4
(Keebler) Stix	1 piece (<1 gram)	2	.4
(Keebler) Twist	1 piece (6 grams)	23	4.3
(Nab) Pretzelette	1 packet (1¼ oz.)	132	26.5
(Nab) *Very-Thin* Sticks	1 packet (¾ oz.)	79	16.7
(Nabisco) Pretzelette	1 piece (2 grams)	6	1.3
(Nabisco) *Mister Salty* Dutch	1 piece (.4 oz.)	51	11.2
(Nabisco) *Mister Salty* 3-ring	1 piece (3 grams)	12	2.3
(Nabisco) *Mister Salty* Veri-Thin	1 piece (5 grams)	20	4.1
(Nabisco) *Mister Salty* Veri-Thin Stick	1 piece (<1 gram)	1	.2
(Old London) nuggets	2-oz. bag	211	44.1
(Old London) rings	1½-oz. pkg.	156	32.9

Food and Description	Measure or Quantity	Calories	Carbo-hydrates (grams)
(Rold Gold) rods	1 oz.	100	21.4
(Rold Gold) twists	1 oz.	100	21.7
(Sunshine) extra thin	1 piece (5 grams)	20	4.0
PRICKLY PEAR, fresh (USDA)	1 lb. (weighed with rind & seeds)	84	21.8
PRINCE BLANC WINE, French white Bordeaux (Barton & Guestier) 12% alcohol	3 fl. oz.	62	.6
PRINCE NOIR WINE, French red Bordeaux (Barton & Guestier) 12% alcohol	3 fl. oz.	61	.4
PRODUCT 19, cereal (Kellogg's)	1 cup (1 oz.)	107	23.4
PRUNE:			
Dried, "softenized" (USDA):			
Small, uncooked	1 prune (5 grams)	11	3.0
Medium, whole, with pits	1 cup (6.6 oz.)	405	107.2
Medium	1 prune (7 grams)	15	4.0
Large	1 prune (9 grams)	20	5.2
Dried, "softenized," cooked:			
Unsweetened (USDA)	1 cup (17–18 med. with ⅓ cup liq.)		
With sugar (USDA)	1 cup (16–18 prunes with ⅓ cup liq., 11.1 oz.)	504	132.1
Canned, cooked (Sunsweet)	1 cup	300	72.0
Canned, stewed (Del Monte)	1 cup (9.4 oz.)	316	83.5
Dehydrated:			
(USDA)	4 oz.	390	103.5
Cooked with sugar, solids & liq. (USDA)	½ cup (4.4 oz.)	227	59.3

(USDA): United States Department of Agriculture
(HEW/FAO): Health, Education and Welfare/Food and Agriculture
   Organization
* Prepared as Package Directs

Food and Description	Measure or Quantity	Calories	Carbo-hydrates (grams)
PRUNE JUICE, canned:			
(Bennett's)	½ cup (4.5 oz.)	99	24.0
(Del Monte) unsweetened	½ cup (4.3 oz.)	58	15.6
(Heinz)	5½-fl.-oz. can	119	28.3
(Mott's) super	4 oz. (by wt.)	99	24.0
RealPrune	½ cup (4.5 oz.)	74	18.1
(Sunsweet) unsweetened	½ cup	82	20.0
PRUNE WHIP, home recipe (USDA)	1 cup (4.8 oz.)	211	49.8
PUDDING or **PUDDING MIX** (See individual kinds)			
PUFF (See **CRACKER** or individual kinds of hors d'oeuvres, such as *CHICKEN PUFF)*			
PUFFA PUFFA RICE, cereal (Kellogg's)	1 cup (1 oz.)	120	24.0
PUFFED OAT CEREAL (USDA):			
Regular	1 oz.	113	21.3
Sugar-coated	1 oz.	112	24.3
PUFFED RICE CEREAL (See **RICE, PUFFED**)			
PULIGNY MONTRACHET WINE, French white Burgundy:			
(Barton & Guestier) 12% alcohol	3 fl. oz.	61	.3
(Chanson) 12% alcohol	3 fl. oz.	84	6.3
PUMPKIN:			
Fresh, whole (USDA)	1 lb. (weighed with rind & seeds)	83	20.6
Fresh, flesh only (USDA)	4 oz.	29	7.4
Canned (Del Monte)	½ cup (4.3 oz.)	39	9.6
Canned (Stokely-Van Camp)	½ cup (4.1 oz.)	38	9.0
PUMPKIN PIE:			
Home recipe (USDA)	⅛ of 9″ pie (5.4 oz.)	321	37.2

Food and Description	Measure or Quantity	Calories	Carbo-hydrates (grams)
(Tastykake)	4-oz. pie	368	50.5
Frozen (Banquet)	5 oz.	306	46.5
Frozen (Mrs. Smith's)	⅛ of 8″ pie (4 oz.)	242	35.0
PUMPKIN SEED, dry (USDA):			
Whole	4 oz. (weighed in hull)	464	12.6
Hulled	4 oz.	627	17.0
*PUNCH DRINK MIX:			
(Hi-C) Florida punch	6 fl. oz. (6.3 oz.)	98	23.6
(Salada)	6 fl. oz.	80	19.4
PURPLE PASSION, soft drink (Canada Dry)	6 fl. oz.	89	22.2
PURSLANE, including stems (USDA):			
Raw	1 lb.	95	17.2
Boiled, drained	4 oz.	17	3.2
PUSSYCAT MIX (Bar-Tender's)	1 serving (⅔ oz.)	75	18.5

Q

QUAIL, raw (USDA):			
Ready-to-cook	1 lb. (weighed with bones)	686	0.
Meat & skin only	4 oz.	195	0.
QUANGAROOS, cereal (Quaker)	1 cup (1 oz.)	112	24.5

QUIK (See individual kinds)

(USDA): United States Department of Agriculture
(HEW/FAO): Health, Education and Welfare/Food and Agriculture Organization
* Prepared as Package Directs

Food and Description	Measure or Quantity	Calories	Carbohydrates (grams)
QUINCE, fresh (USDA):			
Untrimmed	1 lb. (weighed with skin & seeds)	158	42.3
Flesh only	4 oz.	65	17.4
QUINCE JELLY (Smucker's)	1 T. (.7 oz.)	50	12.7
QUININE SOFT DRINK or **TONIC WATER:** Sweetened:			
(Canada Dry)	6 fl. oz. (6.4 oz.)	70	17.4
(Dr. Brown's)	6 fl. oz.	66	16.5
(Fanta)	6 fl. oz.	62	15.7
(Hoffman)	6 fl. oz.	66	16.5
(Kirsch)	6 fl. oz.	71	17.8
(Schweppes)	6 fl. oz.	66	16.5
(Shasta)	6 fl. oz.	57	14.4
(Yukon Club)	6 fl. oz.	67	16.7
Low calorie (No-Cal)	6 fl. oz.	2	0.
QUISP, cereal (Quaker)	1⅛ cups (1 oz.)	122	23.1

R

RABBIT (USDA):			
Domesticated, ready-to-cook	1 lb. (weighed with bones)	581	0.
Domesticated, stewed, flesh only	4 oz.	245	0.
Wild, ready-to-cook	1 lb. (weighed with bones)	490	0.
RACCOON, roasted, meat only (USDA)	4 oz.	289	0.
RADISH (USDA): Common, raw:			
Without tops	½ lb. (weighed untrimmed)	34	7.4
Trimmed, whole	4 small radishes (1.4 oz.)	7	1.4

Food and Description	Measure or Quantity	Calories	Carbo-hydrates (grams)
Trimmed, sliced	½ cup (2 oz.)	10	2.1
Oriental, raw, without tops	½ lb. (weighed unpared)	34	7.4
Oriental, raw, trimmed & pared	4 oz.	22	4.8
RAISIN:			
Dried:			
Whole, pressed down (USDA)	½ cup (2.9 oz.)	237	63.5
Chopped (USDA)	½ cup (2.9 oz.)	234	62.7
Ground (USDA)	½ cup (4.7 oz.)	387	103.7
Cinnamon-coated (Del Monte)	½ cup (2.5 oz.)	213	56.6
Seeded, Muscat (Del Monte)	½ cup (2.5 oz.)	222	58.5
Seedless, natural, California Thompson:			
(Sun Maid)	½ cup (3 oz.)	250	66.0
(Sun Maid)	1 T. (.4 oz.)	31	8.2
Cooked, added sugar, solids & liq. (USDA)	½ cup (4.3 oz.)	260	68.8
RAISIN PIE:			
Home recipe, 2 crusts (USDA)	⅙ of 9" pie (5.6 oz.)	427	67.9
(Tastykake)	4-oz. pie	391	60.8
Frozen (Mrs. Smith's)	⅙ of 8" pie (4.2 oz.)	322	46.7
RAISIN PIE FILLING:			
(Lucky Leaf)	8 oz.	292	67.8
(Wilderness)	22-oz. can	773	180.7
RAJA FISH (See SKATE)			
RALSTON, cereal, dry	¼ cup (1 oz.)	106	20.2

(USDA): United States Department of Agriculture
(HEW/FAO): Health, Education and Welfare/Food and Agriculture Organization
* Prepared as Package Directs

Food and Description	Measure or Quantity	Calories	Carbo- hydrates (grams)
RASPBERRY:			
Black:			
Fresh:			
(USDA)	½ lb. (weighed with caps & stems)	160	34.6
(USDA) without caps & stems	½ cup (2.4 oz.)	49	10.5
Canned, water pack, unsweetened, solids & liq. (USDA)	4 oz.	58	12.1
Red:			
Fresh:			
(USDA)	½ lb. (weighed with caps & stems)	126	29.9
(USDA) without caps & stems	½ cup (2.5 oz.)	41	9.8
Canned, water pack, unsweetened or low calorie:			
Solids & liq. (USDA)	4 oz.	40	10.0
Solids & liq. (Blue Boy)	4 oz.	48	11.2
Frozen, sweetened:			
Not thawed (USDA)	10-oz. pkg.	278	69.9
Not thawed (USDA)	½ cup (4.4 oz.)	122	30.5
Quick thaw (Birds Eye)	½ cup (5 oz.)	148	37.2
RASPBERRY DRINK MIX			
(Wyler's)	1 rounded T. (.8 oz.)	86	21.4
RASPBERRY LIQUEUR,			
(Leroux) 50 proof	1 fl. oz.	74	8.3
RASPBERRY PIE FILLING:			
(Comstock)	1 cup (10.6 oz.)	424	103.6
(Lucky Leaf)	8 oz.	324	79.0
RASPBERRY PRESERVE or JAM:			
(Bama)	1 T. (.7 oz.)	54	13.5
Sweetened (Kraft)	1 oz.	36	8.8
Sweetened (Smucker's)	1 T. (.7 oz.)	53	13.3
Low calorie (Diet Delight)	1 T. (.6 oz.)	24	5.8
Low calorie (Louis Sherry)	1 T. (.5 oz.)	6	1.5

Food and Description	Measure or Quantity	Calories	Carbo-hydrates (grams)
Low calorie (S and W) Nutradiet	1 T. (.5 oz.)	10	2.4
Low calorie (Slenderella)	1 T. (.7 oz.)	25	6.4
RASPBERRY RENNET CUSTARD MIX:			
Powder:			
(Junket)	1 oz.	115	28.0
*(Junket)	4 oz.	108	14.7
Tablet:			
(Junket)	1 tablet	1	.2
*With sugar (Junket)	4 oz.	101	13.5
RASPBERRY SOFT DRINK:			
Sweetened:			
(Clicquot Club)	6 fl. oz.	98	24.0
(Dr. Brown's)	6 fl. oz.	86	21.5
(Hoffman)	6 fl. oz.	89	22.3
(Key Food)	6 fl. oz.	87	21.9
(Kirsch)	6 fl. oz.	88	22.1
(Shasta)	6 fl. oz.	89	22.3
(Waldbaum)	6 fl. oz.	87	21.9
(Yukon Club)	6 fl. oz.	90	22.5
Low calorie (Canada Dry)	6 fl. oz. (6.4 oz.)	1	0.
Low calorie (No-Cal) black	6 fl. oz.	3	<.1
RASPBERRY SYRUP:			
Sweetened (Smucker's)	1 T. (.6 oz.)	45	11.6
Low calorie (No-Cal)	1 tsp. (5 grams)	<1	0.
RASPBERRY TUNOVER, frozen (Pepperidge Farm)	1 turnover (3.3 oz.)	337	36.9
RAVIOLI:			
Canned:			
Beef or meat:			
(Buitoni)	8 oz.	188	26.9
(Chef Boy-Ar-Dee)	8 oz. (⅕ of 40-oz. can)	211	30.2
(Nalley's)	8 oz.	399	62.4
(Prince)	1 can (3.7 oz.)	136	18.7

(USDA): United States Department of Agriculture
(HEW/FAO): Health, Education and Welfare/Food and Agriculture Organization
* Prepared as Package Directs

Food and Description	Measure or Quantity	Calories	Carbo-hydrates (grams)
Cheese:			
(Buitoni)	8 oz.	218	27.3
(Chef Boy-Ar-Dee)	½ of 15-oz. can	262	31.5
(Prince)	1 can (3.7 oz.)	123	18.5
Chicken (Nalley's)	8 oz.	458	82.4
Frozen:			
Beef (Kraft)	12½-oz. pkg.	411	49.9
Beef (Celeste)	7 ravioli (4 oz.)	259	37.5
Cheese (Buitoni)	4 oz.	313	48.6
Cheese (Celeste)	7 ravioli (4 oz.)	264	38.3
Cheese, dinner			
(Celeste)	½ of 15-oz. pkg.	255	38.3
Cheese (Kraft)	12½-oz. pkg.	407	48.1
Meat, without sauce			
(Buitoni)	4 oz.	278	41.6
Raviolettes (Buitoni)	4 oz.	324	56.3
REDFISH (See **DRUM, RED** & **OCEAN PERCH,** Atlantic)			
REDHORSE, SILVER, raw (USDA):			
Drawn	1 lb. (weighed eviscerated)	204	0.
Flesh only	4 oz.	111	0.
RED & GRAY SNAPPER, raw:			
Whole (USDA)	1 lb. (weighed whole)	219	0.
Meat only (USDA)	4 oz.	105	0.
REINDEER, raw, lean only (USDA)	4 oz.	144	0.
RELISH:			
Barbecue (Crosse & Blackwell)	1 T. (.7 oz.)	22	5.4
Barbecue (Heinz)	1 T.	35	8.5
Corn (Crosse & Blackwell)	1 T. (.6 oz.)	15	3.6
Hamburger (Crosse & Blackwell)	1 T. (.6 oz.)	20	4.7
Hamburger (Del Monte)	1 T. (.9 oz.)	33	8.9
Hamburger (Heinz)	1 T.	15	3.6
Hot dog (Crosse & Blackwell)	1 T. (.7 oz.)	22	5.4
Hot dog (Del Monte)	1 T. (.9 oz.)	28	6.9

Food and Description	Measure or Quantity	Calories	Carbo-hydrates (grams)
Hot dog (Heinz)	1 T.	17	3.9
Hot pepper (Crosse & Blackwell)	1 T. (.7 oz.)	22	5.4
India (Crosse & Blackwell)	1 T. (.7 oz.)	26	6.3
India (Heinz)	1 T.	17	3.9
Piccalilli (Crosse & Blackwell)	1 T. (.7 oz.)	26	6.3
Piccalilli (Heinz)	1 T.	23	5.3
Picnic, tangy (Crosse & Blackwell)	1 T.	24	6.0
Sweet:			
(Aunt Jane's)	1 rounded tsp. (.4 oz.)	14	3.4
(Crosse & Blackwell)	1 T. (.7 oz.)	26	6.3
(Del Monte)	1 T. (.9 oz.)	36	9.2
(Heinz)	1 T.	28	6.6
(Smucker's)	1 T. (.6 oz.)	23	5.6
RENNIN CUSTARD PRODUCTS (See individual flavors)			
RHINESKELLER WINE, (Italian Swiss Colony) 12% alcohol	3 fl. oz.	66	3.0
RHINE WINE:			
(Deinhard) Rheinritter, 11% alcohol	3 fl. oz.	60	3.6
(Gallo) 12% alcohol	3 fl. oz.	50	.8
(Gallo) Rhine Garten, 12% alcohol	3 fl. oz.	59	3.0
(Gold Seal) 12% alcohol	3 fl. oz.	82	.4
(Great Western) 12.5% alcohol	3 fl. oz.	72	
(Great Western) Dutchess, 12% alcohol	3 fl. oz.	80	2.6
(Inglenook):			
Navalle, 12% alcohol	3 fl. oz.	76	4.3
Vintage, 12% alcohol	3 fl. oz.	63	1.7
(Italian Swiss Colony) 11% alcohol	3 fl. oz.	59	.6

(USDA): United States Department of Agriculture
(HEW/FAO): Health, Education and Welfare/Food and Agriculture Organization
* Prepared as Package Directs

Food and Description	Measure or Quantity	Calories	Carbo-hydrates (grams)
(Louis M. Martini)			
12.5% alcohol	3 fl. oz.	90	.2
(Taylor) 12.5% alcohol	3 fl. oz.	69	Tr.
RHUBARB:			
Fresh:			
Partly trimmed (USDA)	1 lb. (weighed with part leaves, ends & trimmings)	54	12.6
Trimmed (USDA)	4 oz.	18	4.2
Diced (USDA)	½ cup (2.2 oz.)	10	2.3
Cooked, sweetened, solids & liq. (USDA)	½ cup (4.2 oz.)	169	43.2
Frozen, sweetened:			
Cooked, added sugar (USDA)	½ cup (4.4 oz.)	177	44.9
(Birds Eye)	½ cup (4 oz.)	84	21.4
RHUBARB PIE, home recipe (USDA)	⅙ of 9″ pie (5.6 oz.)	400	60.4
RICE:			
Brown:			
Raw (USDA)	½ cup (3.7 oz.)	374	80.5
Parboiled, long-grain, dry (Uncle Ben's)	1 oz.	105	22.3
Cooked:			
(Carolina)	4 oz.	135	28.9
Parboiled, without butter (Uncle Ben's)	⅔ cup (4.3 oz.)	153	28.6
White:			
Instant or Precooked:			
Dry, long-grain (USDA)	½ cup (1.9 oz.)	296	45.4
Cooked:			
Long-grain (USDA)	½ cup (2.5 oz.)	76	16.9
(Carolina)	⅔ cup (3.3 oz.)	101	22.5
(Minute Rice) no butter or salt	⅔ cup (4 oz.)	124	26.5
Long-grain (Uncle Ben's Quick)	⅔ cup (4 oz.)	105	24.1
Parboiled:			
Dry, long-grain (Uncle Ben's Converted)	1 oz.	101	23.1
Cooked:			
(Aunt Caroline)	⅔ cup (4.1 oz.)	124	27.3

Food and Description	Measure or Quantity	Calories	Carbo-hydrates (grams)
Long-grain (Uncle Ben's Converted)	⅔ cup (4.3 oz.)	121	27.6
Regular:			
Raw (USDA)	½ cup (3.5 oz.)	359	79.6
Cooked:			
Extra long-grain (Carolina)	⅔ cup (4.8 oz.)	149	33.2
(Mahatma)	⅔ cup (4.8 oz.)	149	33.2
(River Brand) fluffy	⅔ cup (4.8 oz.)	149	33.2
(Water Maid)	⅔ cup (4.8 oz.)	149	33.2
White & wild, frozen (Green Giant)	⅓ of 12-oz. pkg.	104	21.0
RICE BRAN (USDA)	1 oz.	78	14.4
RICE CHEX, cereal (Ralston Purina)	1⅛ cups (1 oz.)	111	24.7
RICE FLAKES (USDA) added nutrients	1 cup (1.1 oz.)	117	26.3
RICE, FRIED:			
Canned:			
(La Choy)	1 cup	274	55.0
Chicken (Chun King)	1 cup	257	56.0
Meatless (Chun King)	1 cup	186	46.6
Frozen:			
Chicken (Chun King)	1 cup	309	35.4
Shrimp (Temple)	1 cup	297	51.0
RICE KRISPIES (Kellogg's)	1 cup (1 oz.)	108	24.7
RICE MIX:			
Beef:			
*Rice-A-Roni	⅛ of 1-oz. pkg.	129	27.0
*(Uncle Ben's)	½ cup (4.2 oz.)	103	21.6
*Brown & wild (Uncle Ben's) without butter	½ cup (4.3 oz.)	99	20.3
Chicken:			
*Rice-A-Roni	⅛ of 8-oz. pkg.	153	33.0
*(Uncle Ben's) no butter	½ cup (3.6 oz.)	100	20.5
*(Village Inn)	½ cup	125	24.4

(USDA): United States Department of Agriculture
(HEW/FAO): Health, Education and Welfare/Food and Agriculture Organization
* Prepared as Package Directs

Food and Description	*Measure or Quantity*	*Calories*	*Carbo-hydrates (grams)*
*Chinese, fried, *Rice-A-Roni*	4 oz.	226	27.8
*Curry (Uncle Ben's) no butter	½ cup (4.2 oz.)	100	21.9
*Drumstick (Minute Rice)	½ cup (4.1 oz.)	152	22.4
*Ham with pineapple, *Rice-A-Roni*	4 oz.	113	15.9
*Keriyaki dinner (Betty Crocker)	½ cup	208	19.5
*Long & wild grain (Uncle Ben's) no butter	½ cup (4 oz.)	97	21.0
*Milanese (Betty Crocker)	½ cup	172	24.2
*Oriental, dinner (Jeno's)	⅕ of 40-oz. pkg.	320	23.1
*Pilaf (Uncle Ben's) no butter	½ cup (3.3 oz.)	97	21.1
*Provence (Betty Crocker)	½ cup	184	28.9
*Rib Roast (Minute Rice)	½ cup (4.1 oz.)	149	24.2
Spanish:			
*(Minute Rice)	½ cup (5.6 oz.)	132	23.0
**Rice-A-Roni*	⅙ of 7½-oz. pkg.	125	26.0
*(Uncle Ben's)	½ cup (4.4 oz.)	115	24.0
*Turkey, *Rice-A-Roni*	4 oz.	204	29.5
*Wild, *Rice-A-Roni*	4 oz.	158	24.0
RICE & PEAS with **MUSHROOMS,** frozen:			
(Birds Eye)	⅓ pkg. (2.3 oz.)	113	21.9
(Green Giant)	⅓ of 12-oz. pkg.	100	17.5
RICE POLISH (USDA)	1 oz.	75	16.4
RICE, PUFFED, cereal:			
(Checker)	½ oz.	56	14.4
(Kellogg's)	1 cup (.5 oz.)	55	12.8
(Malt-O-Meal)	½ oz.	52	12.0
(Quaker)	1¼ cup (.5 oz.)	56	12.5
(Van Brode) dietetic	1 oz.	109	25.2
RICE PUDDING, home recipe, with raisins (USDA)	½ cup (4.7 oz.)	193	35.2
RICE, SPANISH:			
Home recipe (USDA)	4 oz.	99	18.8
Canned:			
(Heinz)	8¾-oz. can	196	35.6
(Nalley's)	4 oz.	150	32.4
(Van Camp)	½ cup (3.9 oz.)	96	18.2

Food and Description	Measure or Quantity	Calories	Carbo- hydrates (grams)
RICE, SPANISH, SEASONING MIX (Lawry's)	1½-oz. pkg.	125	20.7
RICE WINE (HEW/FAO):			
Chinese, 20.7% alcohol	3 fl. oz. (3 oz.)	114	3.3
Japanese, 10.6% alcohol	3 fl. oz. (3.1 oz.)	215	39.4
RIESLING WINE:			
(Inglenook) Estate, 12% alcohol	3 fl. oz.	60	.7
(Willm) 11–14% alcohol	3 fl. oz.	66	3.6
RIPPLE WINE (Gallo):			
Red, 11% alcohol	3 fl. oz.	56	3.4
White, 11% alcohol	3 fl. oz.	55	3.2
ROAST 'N BOAST, beef	1½-oz. pkg.	129	26.0
ROCKFISH (USDA):			
Raw, meat only	1 lb.	440	0.
Oven-steamed, with onions	4 oz.	121	2.2
ROCK & RYE LIQUEUR:			
(Garnier) 60 proof	1 fl. oz.	70	6.2
(Hiram Walker) 60 proof	1 fl. oz.	87	9.5
(Leroux) 60 proof	1 fl. oz.	74	8.3
(Leroux) Irish Moss, 70 proof	1 fl. oz.	110	13.0
(Old Mr. Boston) 60 proof	1 fl. oz.	94	5.8
ROE (USDA):			
Raw, carp, cod, haddock, herring, pike or shad	4 oz.	147	1.7
Raw, salmon, sturgeon, turbot	4 oz.	235	1.6
Baked or broiled, cod & shad	4 oz.	143	2.2
Canned, cod, haddock or herring, solids & liq.	4 oz.	134	.3
ROLAIDS (Warner-Lambert)	1 piece	4	1.4

(USDA): United States Department of Agriculture
(HEW/FAO): Health, Education and Welfare/Food and Agriculture Organization
* Prepared as Package Directs

Food and Description	Measure or Quantity	Calories	Carbo-hydrates (grams)
ROLL & BUN:			
Barbeque (Arnold)	1 bun (1.6 oz.)	132	22.6
Brown & serve (Wonder)	1 roll (1 oz.)	85	13.0
Butter crescent (Pepperidge Farm)	1.2-oz. roll	127	18.1
Butterflip (Pepperidge Farm)	.6-oz. roll	58	8.4
Cinnamon nut (Pepperidge Farm)	1 roll (1 oz.)	92	12.1
Club (Pepperidge Farm)	1 roll (1.6 oz.)	114	22.5
Deli Twists (Arnold)	1 roll (1.2 oz.)	115	17.4
Diet Size (Arnold)	.5-oz. roll	40	6.2
Dinner (Arnold)	1 roll (¾ oz.)	71	10.5
Dinner (Pepperidge Farm)	1 roll (.7 oz.)	61	9.9
Dutch Egg, sandwich buns (Arnold)	1 bun (1.7 oz.)	143	22.4
Finger (Arnold) handi-pan	1 roll (.7 oz.)	61	9.6
Finger, poppy (Pepperidge Farm)	1 roll (.7 oz.)	59	9.5
Frankfurter or hot dog:			
(Arnold)	1 bun (1.4 oz.)	121	20.6
New England (Arnold)	1 roll (1.6 oz.)	130	22.0
(Pepperidge Farm)	1 roll (1.4 oz.)	117	20.1
(Wonder)	1 roll (2 oz.)	262	28.4
French, brown & serve:			
Twin (Pepperidge Farm)	1 roll (5.2 oz.)	363	72.6
Triple (Pepperidge Farm)	1 roll (3.5 oz.)	255	50.0
Golden Twist, brown & serve (Pepperidge Farm)	1 roll (1.2 oz.)	122	15.0
Hamburger:			
(Pepperidge Farm)	1 roll (1.4 oz.)	112	19.4
(Wonder)	1 roll (2 oz.)	162	28.4
Hard (USDA)	1 roll (1.8 oz.)	156	29.8
Hard (Levy's)	1 roll (2.5 oz.)	130	27.4
Hearth (Pepperidge Farm)	1 roll (.8 oz.)	59	10.9
Honey, frozen (Morton)	1 bun (2.2 oz.)	170	24.8
Kaiser, brown & serve (Arnold)	1 roll (1.7 oz.)	132	23.2
Parker (Arnold)	1 roll (.7 oz.)	63	9.8
Parkerhouse (Pepperidge Farm)	1 roll (.7 oz.)	57	9.2
Parkerhouse (Sara Lee)	1 oz.	83	12.0
Party Pan (Pepperidge Farm)	1 roll (.4 oz.)	34	5.5
Finger, poppy (Arnold)	1 roll (.6 oz.)	61	9.4

Food and Description	Measure or Quantity	Calories	Carbohydrates (grams)
Raisin (USDA)	1 bun (1 oz.)	78	16.0
Sesame crisp (Pepperidge Farm)	1 roll (.9 oz.)	73	12.4
Whole-wheat (USDA)	1 roll (1.3 oz.)	98	19.9
ROLL DOUGH:			
Frozen, unraised (USDA)	1 oz.	76	13.4
Frozen, baked (USDA)	1 oz.	88	15.9
Refrigerated:			
Crescent (Borden)	1 roll (1 1 oz.)	104	14.6
Crescent (Pillsbury)	1 roll	95	13.5
Dinner, buttermilk (Pillsbury) *Hungry Jack*	1 roll	115	15.0
Parkerhouse (Pillsbury)	1 roll	60	11.0
Pan roll (Pillsbury)	1 roll	75	11.5
Snowflake (Pillsbury)	1 roll	70	11.5
***ROLL MIX** (Pillsbury):*			
Caramel	1 roll	250	38.0
Cinnamon	1 roll	240	37.0
Honey	1 roll	250	39.0
Hot	1 roll	95	15.5
Orange	1 roll	240	37.0
ROMAN MEAL CEREAL	¾ cup (1.3 oz., dry)	130	25.7
ROOT BEER DRINK MIX (Wyler's)	6 fl. oz.	69	17.2
ROOT BEER SOFT DRINK:			
Sweetened:			
(Canada Dry) *Rooti*	6 fl. oz.	79	19.8
(Cott)	6 fl. oz.	85	21.0
(Dad's)	6 fl. oz.	79	19.6
(Dr. Brown's)	6 fl. oz.	77	19.4
(Fanta)	6 fl. oz.	77	19.8
(Hires)	6 fl. oz.	75	18.8
(Key Food)	6 fl. oz.	77	19.4
(Kirsch)	6 fl. oz.	71	17.7
(Mission)	6 fl. oz.	85	21.0

(USDA): United States Department of Agriculture
(HEW/FAO): Health, Education and Welfare/Food and Agriculture Organization
* Prepared as Package Directs

Food and Description	Measure or Quantity	Calories	Carbo-hydrates (grams)
(Nedick's)	6 fl. oz.	77	19.4
(Nehi)	6 fl. oz. (6.6 oz.)	94	23.2
(Patio)	6 fl. oz. (6.6 oz.)	83	20.8
(Salute)	6 fl. oz.	92	23.2
Draft (Shasta)	6 fl. oz.	84	21.3
(Waldbaum)	6 fl. oz.	77	19.4
(Yukon Club)	6 fl. oz.	81	20.1
Low calorie:			
(Canada Dry)	6 fl. oz.	5	.8
(Dad's)	6 fl. oz.	<1	.2
(No-Cal)	6 fl. oz.	<1	<.1
Draft (Shasta)	6 fl. oz.	<1	<.1
ROSE APPLE, raw (USDA):			
Whole	1 lb. (weighed with caps & seeds)	170	43.2
Flesh only	4 oz.	64	16.1
ROSÉ WINE:			
(Antinori) 12% alcohol	3 fl. oz.	84	6.3
Chateau Ste. Roseline, 11–14% alcohol	3 fl. oz.	84	6.3
(Chanson) Rosé des Anges, 12% alcohol	3 fl. oz.	84	6.3
(Cruse) 12% alcohol	3 fl. oz.	72	
(Gallo) 13% alcohol	3 fl. oz.	55	1.8
(Gallo) Gypsy, 20% alcohol	3 fl. oz.	112	12.0
(Great Western) 12.5% alcohol	3 fl. oz.	88	4.7
(Great Western) Isabella, 12.5% alcohol	3 fl. oz.	81	3.8
(Inglenook) Gamay, Estate, 12% alcohol	3 fl. oz. (2.9 oz.)	60	.5
(Inglenook) Navalle, 12% alcohol	3 fl. oz. (2.9 oz.)	62	1.3
(Inglenook) Vintage, 12% alcohol	3 fl. oz. (2.9 oz.)	61	.9
(Italian Swiss Colony-Gold Medal) Grenache, 12.4% alcohol	3 fl. oz.	69	2.2
(Italian Swiss Colony) Grenache, 12% alcohol	3 fl. oz.	61	.5
(Louis M. Martini) Gamay, 12.5% alcohol	3 fl. oz.	90	.2

Food and Description	Measure or Quantity	Calories	Carbohydrates (grams)
(Mogen David) 12% alcohol	3 fl. oz.	75	8.9
Nectarosé, vin rosé d' Anjou, 12% alcohol	3 fl. oz.	70	2.6
(Taylor) 12.5% alcohol	3 fl. oz.	69	Tr.
ROSÉ WINE, SPARKLING (Chanson)	3 fl. oz.	72	3.6
RUDESHEIMER SCHLOSSBERG (Deinhard) 11% alcohol	3 fl. oz.	72	4.5
RUM (See DISTILLED LIQUOR)			
RUM & COLA, canned (Party Tyme) 10% alcohol	2 fl. oz.	55	5.2
RUSK:			
Dutch (Hekman's)	1 piece	55	
Holland (Nabisco)	1 piece (.4 oz.)	49	9.0
RUTABAGA:			
Raw, without tops (USDA)	1 lb. (weighed with skin)	177	42.4
Raw, diced (USDA)	½ cup (2.5 oz.)	32	7.7
Boiled, drained, diced (USDA)	½ cup (3 oz.)	30	7.1
Boiled, drained, mashed (USDA)	½ cup (4.3 oz.)	43	10.0
Canned (King Pharr)	½ cup	52	
RYE, whole grain (USDA)	1 oz.	95	20.8
RYE FLOUR (See FLOUR)			
RYE WAFER, whole grain:			
(USDA)	1 oz.	98	21.6
(USDA)	2 wafers (1⅞" x 3½")	45	9.9
RYE WHISKEY (See DISTILLED LIQUOR)			

(USDA): United States Department of Agriculture
(HEW/FAO): Health, Education and Welfare/Food and Agriculture Organization
* Prepared as Package Directs

Food and Description	Measure or Quantity	Calories	Carbohydrates (grams)
RYE WHISKEY EXTRACT (Ehlers)	1 tsp.	14	
RY-KRISP (See CRACKER)			
RY-KING or *WASA BREAD:*			
Brown	1 slice (.4 oz.)	40	8.7
Golden	1 slice (10 grams)	34	7.4
Lite	1 slice (8 grams)	28	6.0
Seasoned	1 slice (9 grams)	33	7.1

S

Food and Description	Measure or Quantity	Calories	Carbohydrates (grams)
SABLEFISH, raw (USDA):			
Whole	1 lb. (weighed whole)	362	0.
Meat only	4 oz.	215	0.
SABRA, Israeli liqueur (Leroux) 60 proof	1 fl. oz.	91	10.4
SACCHARIN (Dia-Mel)	1 tablet	0	0.
SAFFLOWER SEED KERNELS, dry (USDA)	1 oz.	174	3.5
SAINT-EMILLION WINE, French Bordeaux: (Barton & Guestier)			
12% alcohol	3 fl. oz.	63	.7
(Cruse) 11.5% alcohol	3 fl. oz.	69	
SAINT JOHN'S-BREAD FLOUR (See FLOUR, Carob)			
SAINT-JULIEN WINE (Cruse) 11.5% alcohol	3 fl. oz.	69	
SAKE WINE, 19.8% alcohol (HEW/FAO)	3 fl. oz. (3.1 oz.)	116	4.3
SALAD DRESSING (See also **SALAD DRESSING, LOW CALORIE**):			
(Bama)	1 T. (.5 oz.)	59	1.9

SALAD DRESSING (*Continued*) [297]

Food and Description	Measure or Quantity	Calories	Carbo-hydrates (grams)
Blue or blue cheese:			
(Kraft) Imperial	1 T. (.5 oz.)	68	.9
(Lawry's)	1 T. (.5 oz.)	57	.8
Roka (Kraft)	1 T. (.5 oz.)	55	.8
(Wish-Bone) chunky	1 T. (.5 oz.)	74	.8
Boiled, home recipe (USDA)	1 T. (.6 oz.)	26	2.4
Caesar (Kraft) golden	1 T. (.5 oz.)	63	.8
Caesar (Kraft) Imperial	1 T. (.5 oz.)	77	.6
Caesar (Lawry's)	1 T. (.5 oz.)	70	.5
Canadian (Lawry's)	1 T. (.5 oz.)	72	.6
Coleslaw (Bernstein's)	1 T. (.5 oz.)	60	4.9
Coleslaw (Kraft)	1 T. (.5 oz.)	62	3.4
Cuisine (Kraft)	1 oz.	98	4.7
French:			
Home recipe (USDA)	1 T. (.6 oz.)	101	.6
(Bennett's)	1 T. (.5 oz.)	56	1.8
(Bernstein's)	1 T. (.5 oz.)	56	1.5
(Hellmann's-Best Foods) Family	1 T. (.6 oz.)	65	2.9
(Heinz)	1 T.	78	2.0
(Kraft)	1 T. (.5 oz.)	65	1.9
(Kraft) Casino	1 T. (.5 oz.)	60	3.0
(Kraft) Catalina	1 T. (.5 oz.)	60	3.5
(Kraft) *Miracle*	1 T. (.5 oz.)	57	2.5
(Lawry's) San Francisco	1 T. (.5 oz.)	53	.8
(Marzetti's) blue	1 T. (.5 oz.)	70	3.4
(Nalley's)	½ oz.	55	1.8
(Wish-Bone) Deluxe	1 T. (.5 oz.)	59	2.3
(Wish-Bone) Garlic	1 T. (.5 oz.)	66	3.4
Fruit (Kraft)	1 T. (.5 oz.)	52	3.0
Garlic:			
(Hellmann's) *Old Homestead*	1 T. (.6 oz.)	68	3.3
(Kraft) Salad Bowl	1 oz.	105	3.9
(Lawry's) San Francisco	1 T.	53	.8
(Wish-Bone) creamy	1 T. (.5 oz.)	76	.7
Green Goddess:			
(Bernstein's)	1 T. (.5 oz.)	45	1.1
(Kraft)	1 T. (.5 oz.)	75	.7

(USDA): United States Department of Agriculture
(HEW/FAO): Health, Education and Welfare/Food and Agriculture Organization
* Prepared as Package Directs

Food and Description	Measure or Quantity	Calories	Carbohydrates (grams)
(Lawry's)	1 T. (.5 oz.)	59	.7
(Wish-Bone)	1 T. (.5 oz.)	63	1.2
Hawaiian (Lawry's)	1 T. (.6 oz.)	77	5.8
Heinz Salad Dressing	1 T.	63	2.0
Herb & garlic (Kraft)	1 T. (.5 oz.)	87	.5
Italian:			
(Hellmann's) True	1 T. (.5 oz.)	84	1
(Kraft)	1 T. (.5 oz.)	88	.7
(Lawry's)	1 T. (.5 oz.)	80	.9
(Marzetti) creamy	1 T. (.5 oz.)	73	1.8
(Wish-Bone)	1 T. (.5 oz.)	75	.7
(Wish-Bone) Rosé	1 T. (.5 oz.)	58	.4
Mayonnaise (See **MAYONNAISE**)			
Mayonnaise-type salad dressing (USDA)	1 T. (.5 oz.)	65	2.2
Miracle Whip (Kraft)	1 T. (.5 oz.)	69	1.8
Oil & vinegar (Kraft)	1 T. (.5 oz.)	65	.6
Onion, California (Wish-Bone)	1 T. (.5 oz.)	76	1.0
Potato salad (Marzetti)	1 T. (.5 oz.)	62	2.9
Ranch style (Marzetti)	1 T. (.5 oz.)	66	5.3
Red wine & vinegar (Lawry's)	1 T. (.6 oz.)	61	4.8
Rich 'n Tangy (Dutch Pantry)	1 T. (.6 oz.)	68	4.4
Romano Caesar (Marzetti)	1 T. (.5 oz.)	69	1.3
Roquefort (Bernstein's)	1 T. (.5 oz.)	50	.7
Roquefort (Kraft) refrigerated	1 T. (.5 oz.)	45	1.1
Royal Scandia (Bernstein's)	1 T. (.5 oz.)	56	.8
Russian:			
(Kraft) pourable	1 T. (.5 oz.)	55	4.3
(Wish-Bone)	1 T. (.5 oz.)	54	7.0
Salad Bowl (Kraft)	1 T. (.5 oz.)	53	2.2
Salad Secret (Kraft)	1 T. (.5 oz.)	56	1.8
Sherry (Lawry's)	1 T. (.5 oz.)	55	1.6
Slaw (Marzetti)	1 T. (.5 oz.)	73	3.2
Spin Blend (Hellmann's)	1 T. (.5 oz.)	56	2.7
Sweet & Sour (Kraft)	1 T. (.5 oz.)	28	6.5
Tang (Nalley's)	½ oz.	50	2.4
Thousand Island:			
(Best Foods) pourable	1 T. (.5 oz.)	56	2.3
(Kraft)	1 T. (.5 oz.)	71	1.9
(Kraft) pourable	1 T. (.5 oz.)	56	2.3

Food and Description	Measure or Quantity	Calories	Carbo- hydrates (grams)
(Kraft) refrigerated	1 T. (.5 oz.)	73	2.1
(Lawry's)	1 T. (.5 oz.)	69	2.3
(Marzetti)	1 T. (.5 oz.)	70	2.3
(Wish-Bone)	1 T. (.5 oz.)	71	2.5
Tomato 'n Spice (Dutch Pantry)	1 T. (.6 oz.)	66	3.1
Vinaigrette	1 T. (.5 oz.)	41	.8
SALAD DRESSING, DIETETIC or LOW CALORIE:			
Bleu or blue:			
(Frenchette) chunky	1 T. (.5 oz.)	20	1.3
(Kraft)	1 T. (.5 oz.)	13	.5
(Marzetti)	1 T. (.5 oz.)	23	1.7
(Slim-ette)	1 T. (.5 oz.)	12	.1
(Tillie Lewis)	1 T. (.5 oz.)	13	.5
Caesar (Frenchette)	1 T. (.5 oz.)	32	1.5
Caesar (Tillie Lewis)	1 T.	12	.2
Catalina (Kraft)	1 T. (.5 oz.)	15	2.6
Chef style (Kraft)	1 T. (.5 oz.)	16	2.6
Chef's (Slim-ette)	1 T. (.5 oz.)	14	.2
Chefs (Tillie Lewis)	1 T. (.5 oz.)	2	.4
Coleslaw (Kraft)	1 T. (.5 oz.)	28	3.4
Diet Mayo 7 (Bennett's)	1 T. (.5 oz.)	23	2.0
French:			
(Bennett's)	1 T. (.5 oz.)	21	3.1
(Frenchette)	1 T. (.5 oz.)	9	2.3
(Kraft)	1 T. (.5 oz.)	21	2.0
(Marzetti)	1 T. (.5 oz.)	11	2.6
(Tillie Lewis)	1 T. (.5 oz.)	6	1.2
(Wish-Bone)	1 T. (.6 oz.)	23	3.3
(Wish-Bone) Garlic	1 T.	16	2.7
Gourmet (Frenchette)	1 T. (.5 oz.)	21	2.2
Green Goddess (Frenchette)	1 T. (.5 oz.)	21	1.4
Green Goddess (Slim-ette)	1 T. (.5 oz.)	12	.5
Italian:			
(USDA)	1 T. (.5 oz.)	8	.4
(Bennett's)	1 T. (.5 oz.)	7	.9
(Bernstein's)	1 T. (.4 oz.)	4	.7

USDA): United States Department of Agriculture
HEW/FAO): Health, Education and Welfare/Food and Agriculture Organization
Prepared as Package Directs

Food and Description	Measure or Quantity	Calories	Carbo-hydrates (grams)
(Bernstein's) with cheese	1 T. (.4 oz.)	5	.7
Italianette (Frenchette)	1 T. (.5 oz.)	7	1.3
(Kraft)	1 T. (.5 oz.)	10	.7
(Marzetti)	1 T. (.5 oz.)	8	1.5
(Slim-ette)	1 T. (.5 oz.)	6	.3
(Tillie Lewis)	1 T. (.5 oz.)	<1	.2
(Wish-Bone)	1 T. (.5 oz.)	16	.6
May-lo-naise (Tillie Lewis)	1 T. (.5 oz.)	16	1.0
Mayonette Gold (Frenchette)	1 T. (.5 oz.)	32	1.9
Remoulade (Tillie Lewis)	1 T. (.5 oz.)	10	.8
Russian (Wish-Bone)	1 T. (.5 oz.)	24	4.6
Slaw (Frenchette)	1 T. (.5 oz.)	28	2.8
Slaw (Marzetti)	1 T. (.5 oz.)	27	2.8
Supreme (McCormick)	1 oz.	80	2.0
Thousand Island:			
(Frenchette)	1 T. (.5 oz.)	22	3.0
(Kraft)	1 T. (.5 oz.)	28	2.3
(Marzetti)	1 T. (.5 oz.)	21	3.0
(Wish-Bone)	1 T. (.5 oz.)	25	2.6
Vinaigrette (Bernstein's)	1 T. (.4 oz.)	1	<.1
Whipped (Tillie Lewis)	1 T. (.5 oz.)	16	1.0
SALAD DRESSING MIX, regular & low calorie:			
Bacon (Lawry's)	1 pkg. (.8 oz.)	69	11.9
Bleu or blue cheese:			
*(Good Seasons)	1 T. (.5 oz.)	89	1.3
*(Good Seasons) thick, creamy	1 T. (.5 oz.)	96	.9
(Lawry's)	1 pkg. (.7 oz.)	79	4.5
Caesar garlic cheese (Lawry's)	1 pkg. (.8 oz.)	71	8.7
*Cheese garlic (Good Seasons)	1 T. (.5 oz.)	84	.8
*French, old-fashioned (Good Seasons)	1 T. (.5 oz.)	83	.5
*French (Good Seasons) thick, creamy	1 T. (.5 oz.)	97	1.9
French, old-fashioned (Lawry's)	1 pkg. (.8 oz.)	72	16.8
*French, Riviera (Good Seasons)	1 T. (.6 oz.)	90	2.4
*Garlic (Good Seasons)	1 T. (.5 oz.)	84	.8
Green Goddess (Lawry's)	1 pkg. (.8 oz.)	69	12.7
Italian:			
*(Good Seasons)	1 T. (.5 oz.)	84	.8

Food and Description	Measure or Quantity	Calories	Carbo-hydrates (grams)
*(Good Seasons) cheese or mild	1 T. (.5 oz.)	89	1.3
*(Good Seasons) thick, creamy	1 T. (.5 oz.)	94	1.0
(Lawry's)	1 pkg. (.6 oz.)	44	9.6
(Lawry's) cheese	1 pkg. (.8 oz.)	69	9.4
*Low calorie (Good Seasons)	1 T.	9	2.1
*Onion (Good Seasons)	1 T. (.5 oz.)	84	.8
*Thousand Island (Good Seasons)	1 T. (.6 oz.)	80	1.7
SALAD FRUIT, unsweetened, (S and W) *Nutradiet*	4 oz.	43	9.8
SALAD SEASONING:			
(Durkee)	1 tsp.	4	.7
With cheese (Durkee)	1 tsp.	10	.4
SALAMI:			
Dry (USDA)	1 oz.	128	.3
Cooked (USDA)	1 oz.	88	.4
(Vienna)	1 oz.	74	.5
Beef (Sugardale)	1-oz. slice	76	Tr.
Cotto (Oscar Mayer)	1 slice (.8 oz.)	55	.4
Cotto (Wilson)	1 oz.	84	.4
Hard (Oscar Mayer)	1 slice (.4 oz.)	41	<.1
SALISBURY STEAK:			
Canned, with mushrooms (Morton House)	12¾-oz. can	480	20.4
Frozen:			
(Banquet) buffet	3-lb. pkg.	1524	46.5
(Banquet) cookin' bag	5 oz.	239	7.2
(Holloway House)	1 steak (7 oz.)	320	18.9
(Swanson) with potato	6-oz. pkg.	360	30.5
Dinner, frozen:			
(Morton)	11-oz. dinner	343	25.0
(Morton) 3-course	15½-oz. dinner	642	70.4
(Swanson) *Hungry Man*	17-oz. dinner	943	63.1
(Swanson) 3-course	16-oz. dinner	517	46.9

(USDA): United States Department of Agriculture
(HEW/FAO): Health, Education and Welfare/Food and Agriculture Organization
* Prepared as Package Directs

Food and Description	Measure or Quantity	Calories	Carbo-hydrates (grams)
SALMON:			
Atlantic (USDA):			
Raw, whole	1 lb. (weighed whole)	640	0.
Raw, meat only	4 oz.	246	0.
Canned, solids & liq., including bones	4 oz.	230	0.
Chinook or King:			
Raw, steak (USDA)	1 lb. (weighed with bones)	886	0.
Raw, meat only (USDA)	4 oz.	252	0.
Canned, solids & liq., including bones (USDA)	4 oz.	238	0.
Chum, canned, solids & liq., including bones (USDA)	4 oz.	158	0.
Coho, canned, solids & liq.:			
Including bones (USDA)	4 oz.	174	0.
Steak (Icy Point)	3¾-oz. can	162	0.
Pink or Humpback:			
Raw, steak (USDA)	1 lb. (weighed with bones)	475	0.
Raw, meat only (USDA)	4 oz.	135	0.
Canned, solids & liq.:			
Including bones (USDA)	4 oz.	160	0.
(Del Monte)	7¾-oz. can	268	0.
(Icy Point)	7¾-oz. can	310	0.
(Pink Beauty)	7¾-oz. can	310	0.
Sockeye or Red or Blueback, canned, solids & liq.:			
Including bones (USDA)	4 oz.	194	0.
Including bones (Bumble Bee)	1 cup (6 oz.)	286	0.
(Del Monte)	1 cup (8 oz.)	313	0.
(Icy Point)	3¾-oz. can	181	0.
(Pillar Rock)	7¾-oz. can	376	0.
Unspecified kind of salmon, baked or broiled (USDA)	4.2-oz. steak (approx. 4″ x 3″ x ½″)	218	0.
Frozen, steak (Ship Ahoy)	12-oz. pkg.	405	0.
SALMON RICE LOAF, home recipe (USDA)	4 oz.	138	8.3
SALMON, SMOKED:			
(USDA)	4 oz.	200	0.

Food and Description	Measure or Quantity	Calories	Carbohydrates (grams)
Lox, drained (Vita)	4-oz. jar	136	.2
Nova, drained (Vita)	4-oz. can	221	1.0
SALSIFY (USDA):			
Raw, without tops, freshly harvested	1 lb. (weighed untrimmed)	51	71.0
Raw, without tops, after storage	1 lb. (weighed untrimmed)	324	71.0
Boiled, drained solids, freshly harvested	4 oz.	14	17.1
Boiled, drained solids, after storage	4 oz.	79	17.1
SALT:			
Table (USDA)	1 tsp. (6 grams)	0	0.
Garlic (French's)	1 tsp. (6 grams)	4	.7
Garlic (Lawry's)	1 tsp. (4 grams)	5	1.0
Imitation, butter flavored (Durkee)	1 tsp. (4 grams)	3	Tr.
Lite Salt (Morton)	1 tsp. (6 grams)	0	0.
Onion (French's)	1 tsp. (5 grams)	5	1.0
Seasoned (Lawry's)	1 tsp. (5 grams)	1	.1
Substitute (Adolph's)	1 tsp. (6 grams)	Tr.	Tr.
Substitute, seasoned (Adolph's)	1 tsp. (5 grams)	5	1.2
SALT PORK, raw (USDA):			
With skin	1 lb. (weighed with skin)	3410	0.
Without skin	1 oz.	222	0.
SALT STICK (See **BREAD STICK**)			
SANCERRE WINE, French white, Loire Valley: (Barton & Guestier)			
12% alcohol	3 fl. oz.	61	.3
(Chanson) 12½% alcohol	3 fl. oz.	87	6.3

(USDA): United States Department of Agriculture
(HEW/FAO): Health, Education and Welfare/Food and Agriculture Organization
* Prepared as Package Directs

Food and Description	Measure or Quantity	Calories	Carbo-hydrates (grams)
SAND DAB, raw (USDA):			
Whole	1 lb. (weighed whole)	118	0.
Meat only	4 oz.	90	0.
SANDWICH SPREAD:			
(USDA)	1 T. (.5 oz.)	57	2.4
(Hellmann's-Best Foods)	1 T. (.5 oz.)	62	2.4
(Kraft)	1 oz.	105	5.6
(Nalley's)	1 oz.	100	7.0
(Tillie Lewis) dietetic	1 T.	9	.2
Chicken salad (Carnation)	1.5 oz. (⅕ can)	99	4.2
Ham & cheese (Carnation)	1.5 oz. (⅕ can)	80	4.0
Pimento (Kraft)	1 oz.	117	.8
SAPODILLA, fresh (USDA):			
Whole	1 lb. (weighed whole)	323	79.1
Flesh only	4 oz.	101	24.7
SAPOTES or MARMALADE PLUM, raw (USDA):			
Whole	1 lb. (weighed whole)	431	108.9
Flesh only	4 oz.	142	35.8
SARDINE:			
Atlantic, canned in oil, solids & liq. (USDA)	4 oz.	353	.7
Atlantic, tomato sauce, solids & liq. (Del Monte)	1½ large sardines	138	1.4
Moroccan, skinless & boneless, canned (Cresca):			
In olive oil	3¾-oz. can	341	
In water	3½-oz. can	165	
Norwegian, canned (Underwood):			
In mustard sauce	3¾-oz. can	196	2.3
In oil, drained solids	3¾-oz. can	232	.2
In tomato sauce	3¾-oz. can	169	4.3
Pacific (USDA):			
Raw	4 oz.	181	0.
Canned in brine or mustard, solids & liq.	4 oz.	222	1.9
Canned in tomato sauce, solids & liq.	4 oz.	223	1.9

Food and Description	Measure or Quantity	Calories	Carbo-hydrates (grams)
SARSAPARILLA SOFT DRINK:			
(Hoffman)	6 fl. oz.	83	22.2
(Yukon Club)	6 fl. oz.	89	22.2
SAUCE, regular and dietetic:			
A1	1 T. (.6 oz.)	12	2.7
Barbecue:			
(Chun King) Hawaiian	1 T.	16	3.5
(Contadina) oven	1 T. (.6 oz.)	14	3.6
(French's)	1 T.	9	2.1
(General Foods) original *Open Pit*	1 T. (.6 oz.)	26	6.3
(Heinz) with onion	1 T.	19	4.2
(Kraft)	1 oz.	34	7.9
(Kraft) garlic	1 oz.	32	7.6
(Kraft) hickory smoke	1 oz.	34	7.9
(Kraft) hot	1 oz.	31	7.0
Brown (La Choy)	1 T.	80	19.5
Cheese (Kraft) *Deluxe Dinner*	1 oz.	77	2.0
Chili (See **CHILI SAUCE**)			
Chili, barbecue (Gebhardt)	1 oz.	14	3.0
Chili, hot dog (Gebhardt)	1 oz.	39	2.0
Chutney (Spice Islands)	1 T. (.7 oz.)	35	
Creole (Contadina)	1 T. (.6 oz.)	7	1.2
Enchilada (Gebhardt)	1 oz.	17	2.0
Enchilada (Rosarita)	1 oz.	8	1.2
Escoffier Sauce Diable	1 T. (.6 oz.)	19	4.2
Escoffier Sauce Robert	1 T. (.6 oz.)	20	4.6
Famous (Durkee)	1 T. (.6 oz.)	69	3.2
57 (Heinz)	1 T.	14	2.6
Hard (Crosse & Blackwell)	1 T.	64	8.3
Hollandaise (Cresca)	1 oz.	39	
Horseradish (Marzetti)	1 T. (.5 oz.)	58	2.3
Hot (Gebhardt)	¼ tsp.	<1	
H.P. (Lea & Perrins)	1 T.	20	4.8
Marinara (Buitoni)	4 oz.	67	8.0
Marinara (Chef Boy-Ar-Dee)	3¾ oz. (¼ of 15-oz. can)	68	10.9

(USDA): United States Department of Agriculture
(HEW/FAO): Health, Education and Welfare/Food and Agriculture Organization
* Prepared as Package Directs

Food and Description	Measure or Quantity	Calories	Carbo- hydrates (grams)
Meat (Spice Islands)	1 T. (.7 oz.)	25	
Meat Loaf (Contadina)	1 T. (.6 oz.)	8	1.7
Mint (Crosse & Blackwell)	1 T. (.5 oz.)	16	4.0
Mushroom (Contadina)	1 T. (.6 oz.)	11	1.2
Savory (Heinz)	1 T.	20	4.5
Seafood (Bernstein's)	1 T. (.5 oz.)	19	4.6
Seafood cocktail (Crosse & Blackwell)	1 T. (.6 oz.)	22	4.9
Seafood cocktail (Del Monte)	1 T. (.6 oz.)	20	5.2
Shedd's Old Style	1 T.	48	1.5
Sloppy Joe (Contadina)	1 T. (.6 oz.)	9	2.0
Soy (Chun King)	1 T.	6	.3
Spaghetti (See **SPAGHETTI SAUCE**)			
Steak (Crosse & Blackwell)	1 T. (.7 oz.)	21	4.8
Steak Supreme (Heublein)	1 T. (.6 oz.)	20	4.3
Sweet & sour (Kraft)	1 oz.	55	13.0
Tabasco (See individual listing)			
Tartar:			
(Hellmann's-Best Foods)	1 T. (.5 oz.)	71	.2
(Kraft)	1 oz.	145	1.4
White, home recipe:			
Thin (USDA)	1 cup (8.8 oz.)	302	18.0
Medium (USDA)	1 cup (9 oz.)	413	22.4
Thick (USDA)	1 cup (8.7 oz.)	489	27.2
Worcestershire:			
(Crosse & Blackwell)	1 T.	15	3.6
(Heinz)	1 T.	11	2.5
(Lea & Perrins)	1 T. (.6 oz.)	12	3.0
SAUCE MIX:			
*A la King, without chicken (Durkee)	1 cup (1.1-oz. pkg.)	136	12.8
*Bordelaise (Betty Crocker)	¼ cup	33	5.2
Cheese:			
*(Betty Crocker)	¼ cup	87	1.1
*(Durkee)	1 cup (1.1-oz. pkg.)	337	18.9
*(French's)	¼ cup	81	5.8
*(Kraft) cheddar	1 oz.	52	1.9
*(McCormick)	1 oz.	40	2.0
Hollandaise:			
*(Betty Crocker)	¼ cup	84	4.0

Food and Description	Measure or Quantity	Calories	Carbo-hydrates (grams)
*(Durkee)	⅔ cup (1¼-oz. pkg.)	156	7.8
*(French's)	1 T.	16	.6
*(Kraft)	1 oz.	54	2.0
*(McCormick)	1 oz.	36	2.0
Miracle (Mrs. Paul's)	½-oz. pkg.	10	2.1
*Mushroom (Betty Crocker)	¼ cup	36	5.0
*Newburg (Betty Crocker)	¼ cup	68	5.9
Seafood cocktail (Lawry's)	.6-oz. pkg.	43	9.7
Sloppy Joe (See **SLOPPY JOE MIX**)			
Sour cream:			
*(Durkee)	⅔ cup (1-oz. pkg.)	215	23.5
*(French's)	1 T.	25	1.7
*(Kraft)	1 oz.	61	4.1
*(McCormick)	1 oz.	20	1.2
*Stroganoff (French's)	⅓ cup	104	9.3
*Sweet-sour (Durkee)	1 cup	230	44.6
Tartar (Lawry's)	.6-oz. pkg.	64	9.8
*Teri-yaki (Durkee)	⅔ cup (1¼-oz. pkg.)	66	15.9
*White, medium (Durkee)	1 cup (1-oz. pkg.)	316	23.4
*White, supreme (McCormick)	.6-oz. pkg.	11	2.0
SAUERKRAUT, canned:			
Solids & liq. (USDA)	1 cup (8.3 oz.)	42	9.4
Drained solids (USDA)	1 cup (5 oz.)	31	6.2
Solids & liq. (Del Monte)	1 cup (8 oz.)	36	7.5
Solids & liq. (Steinfield's Western Acres)	½ of 8-oz. can	25	6.0
SAUERKRAUT JUICE, canned (USDA)	½ cup (4.3 oz.)	12	2.8
SAUGER, raw (USDA):			
Whole	1 lb. (weighed whole)	133	0.
Meat only	4 oz.	95	0.

(USDA): United States Department of Agriculture
(HEW/FAO): Health, Education and Welfare/Food and Agriculture Organization
* Prepared as Package Directs

Food and Description	Measure or Quantity	Calories	Carbo-hydrates (grams)
SAUSAGE (See also individual kinds):			
Beef, *Cow-Boy Jo's*	⅝ oz.	81	.9
Breakfast (Oscar Mayer)	1 link (.7 oz.)	67	.5
Brown & serve, before browning (USDA)	1 oz.	111	.8
Brown & serve, after browning (USDA)	1 oz.	120	.8
Brown 'n serve (Hormel)	1 piece (.8 oz.)	78	.2
Cocktail (Cresca)	1 oz.	71	
New England Brand (Wilson)	1 oz.	52	.2
In sauce (Prince)	1 can (3.7 oz.)	187	4.2
SAUTERNES:			
(Barton & Guestier) French white Bordeaux, 13% alcohol	3 fl. oz.	95	7.6
(Barton & Guestier) haut, French white Bordeaux, 13% alcohol	3 fl. oz.	99	8.7
(Gallo) 12% alcohol	3 fl. oz.	50	.9
(Gallo) haut, 12% alcohol	3 fl. oz.	67	2.1
(Gold Seal) dry, 12% alcohol	3 fl. oz.	82	.4
(Gold Seal) semi-soft, 12% alcohol	3 fl. oz.	87	2.6
(Great Western) Aurora, 12.5% alcohol	3 fl. oz.	81	4.7
(Italian Swiss Colony) 12% alcohol	3 fl. oz. (2.9 oz.)	59	1.2
(Louis M. Martini) dry, 12.5% alcohol	3 fl. oz.	90	.2
(Mogen David) cream, 12% alcohol	3 fl. oz.	45	6.2
(Mogen David) dry, American, 12% alcohol	3 fl. oz.	30	1.8
(Taylor) 12.5% alcohol	3 fl. oz.	31	2.9
SCALLION (See **ONION, GREEN**)			
SCALLOP:			
Raw, muscle only (USDA)	4 oz.	92	3.7
Steamed (USDA)	4 oz.	127	

Food and Description	Measure or Quantity	Calories	Carbohydrates (grams)
Frozen:			
Breaded, fried, reheated (USDA)	4 oz.	220	11.9
Breaded, fried (Mrs. Paul's)	7-oz. pkg.	441	45.5
Crisps (Gorton)	½ of 7-oz. pkg.	155	8.0
SCHAV SOUP (Manischewitz)	8 oz. (by wt.)	11	2.1
SCHNAPPS, PEPPERMINT:			
(DeKuyper) 60 proof	1 fl. oz. (1.1 oz.)	79	7.5
(Garnier) 60 proof	1 fl. oz.	83	8.4
(Hiram Walker) 60 proof	1 fl. oz.	78	7.2
(Leroux) 60 proof	1 fl. oz.	87	9.2
(Old Mr. Boston) 42 proof	1 fl. oz.	60	4.5
(Old Mr. Boston) 60 proof	1 fl. oz.	78	4.2
SCONE (Hostess)	1 pkg.	180	33.9
*SCOTCH BROTH (Campbell)	1 cup	84	9.8
SCOTCH WHISKY (See DISTILLED LIQUOR)			
SCRAPPLE (Oscar Mayer)	1 oz.	202	7.0
SCREWDRIVER:			
Dry mix (Bar-Tender's)	1 serving (⅝ oz.)	70	17.4
Dry mix (Holland House)	1 serving (.6 oz. pkg.)	69	17.0
SCUP (See PORGY)			
SEABASS, WHITE, raw, meat only (USDA)	4 oz.	109	0.
SEAFOOD PLATTER, fried (Mrs. Paul's)	9-oz. pkg.	518	57.6
SEGO, diet food:			
*Instant mix with whole milk	1 cup	224	17.6
Liquid diet	10-oz. can	225	35.0

(USDA): United States Department of Agriculture
(HEW/FAO): Health, Education and Welfare/Food and Agriculture Organization
* Prepared as Package Directs

Food and Description	Measure or Quantity	Calories	Carbo-hydrates (grams)
SEKT SPARKLING WINE (Deinhard)	3 fl. oz.	72	3.6
SENEGALESE SOUP (Crosse & Blackwell)	6½ oz. (½ can)	61	6.8
SESAME SEEDS, dry (USDA):			
Whole	1 oz.	160	6.1
Hulled	1 oz.	165	5.0
SESAME TAHINI (A. Sahadi)	1 T. (8 grams)	57	.8
SEVEN-UP, soft drink	6 fl. oz.	73	18.0
SHAD (USDA):			
Raw, whole	1 lb. (weighed whole)	370	0.
Raw, meat only	4 oz.	193	0.
Cooked, home recipe:			
Baked with butter or margarine & bacon slices	4 oz.	228	0.
Creole	4 oz.	172	1.8
Canned, solids & liq.	4 oz.	172	0.
SHAD, GIZZARD, raw (USDA):			
Whole	1 lb. (weighed whole)	299	0.
Meat only	4 oz.	227	0.
SHAKE 'N BAKE, seasoned mix:			
Chicken-coating	2⅜-oz. pkg.	276	40.0
Fish-coating	2-oz. pkg.	224	33.0
Hamburger-coating	2-oz. pkg.	158	21.6
Pork-coating	2⅜-oz. pkg.	260	46.3
SHALLOT, raw (USDA):			
With skin	1 oz.	18	4.2
With skin removed	1 oz.	20	4.8
SHEEFISH (See **INCONNU**)			
SHEEPSHEAD, Atlantic, raw (USDA):			
Whole	1 lb. (weighed whole)	159	0.
Meat only	4 oz.	128	0.

Food and Description	Measure or Quantity	Calories	Carbo-hydrates (grams)
SHERBET (See also individual brands):			
Orange (USDA)	1 cup (6.8 oz.)	259	59.4
Orange (USDA)	⅓ pint (4.6 oz.)	173	39.7
(Borden)	¼ pint (3 oz.)	120	25.9
(Dean) 1.7% fat	¼ pt. (3.3 oz.)	137	30.6
(Meadow Gold)	¼ pt.	120	13.7
(Sealtest)	¼ pt. (3.1 oz.)	120	26.5
SHERBET & FRUIT ICE MIX (Junket)	6 serving pkg. (4 oz.)	388	108.8
SHERRY:			
(Gallo) 20% alcohol	3 fl. oz.	88	2.7
(Gallo) 16% alcohol	3 fl. oz.	76	3.3
(Gold Seal) 19% alcohol	3 fl. oz.	139	4.6
(Great Western) Solera, 18% alcohol	3 fl. oz.	120	8.5
Cocktail (Gold Seal) 19% alcohol	3 fl. oz.	122	1.6
Cocktail (Petri)	3 fl. oz.	102	
Cream:			
(Gallo) 20% alcohol	3 fl. oz.	111	8.4
(Gallo) Old Decanter, Livingston, 20% alcohol	3 fl. oz.	117	12.8
(Gold Seal) 19% alcohol	3 fl. oz.	158	9.4
(Great Western) Solera, 18% alcohol	3 fl. oz.	138	11.6
(Louis M. Martini) 19.5% alcohol	3 fl. oz.	138	1.2
(Taylor) 19.5% alcohol	3 fl. oz.	150	11.3
(Williams & Humbert) Canasta, 20½% alcohol	3 fl. oz.	150	5.4
Dry:			
(Gallo) 20% alcohol	3 fl. oz.	84	1.8
(Gallo) Old Decanter, very dry, 20% alcohol	3 fl. oz.	87	2.1
(Great Western) Solera, 18% alcohol	3 fl. oz.	105	4.2

Food and Description	Measure or Quantity	Calories	Carbo-hydrates (grams)
(Italian Swiss Colony-Gold Medal) 19.7% alcohol	3 fl. oz.	104	1.7
(Louis M. Martini) 19.5% alcohol	3 fl. oz.	138	1.2
(Taylor) 19.5% alcohol	3 fl. oz.	104	2.8
(Williams & Humbert) Carlito Amontillado, 20½% alcohol	3 fl. oz.	120	4.5
(Williams & Humbert) Cedro, 20½% alcohol	3 fl. oz.	120	4.5
(Williams & humbert) Dos Cortados, 20½% alcohol	3 fl. oz.	120	4.5
(Williams & Humbert) Pando, 17% alcohol	3 fl. oz.	120	4.5
Dry Sack (Williams & Humbert) 20½% alcohol	3 fl. oz.	120	4.5
Medium:			
(Great Western) cooking, 18% alcohol	3 fl. oz.	111	6.4
(Italian Swiss Colony-Gold Medal) 19.7% alcohol	3 fl. oz.	106	2.6
(Taylor) 19.5% alcohol	3 fl. oz.	132	7.1
SHERRY FLAVORING (French's)	1 tsp.	17	
SHORTENING (See FAT)			
SHREDDED OATS, cereal (USDA) with added nutrients	1 oz.	107	20.4
SHREDDED WHEAT, cereal:			
(Kellogg's) cinnamon or sugar frosted, *Mini-Wheats*	4 biscuits (1 oz.)	107	23.6
(Nabisco)	1 biscuit (.9 oz.)	86	18.7
(Nabisco) *Spoon Size*	1 biscuit (1 gram)	4	.9
(Quaker)	2 biscuits (1.3 oz.)	135	28.7
SHRIMP:			
Raw:			
Whole (USDA)	1 lb. (weighed in shell)	285	4.7

Food and Description	Measure or Quantity	Calories	Carbo-hydrates (grams)
Meat only (USDA)	4 oz.	103	1.7
Canned:			
Wet pack, solids & liq. (USDA)	4 oz.	91	.9
Dry pack or drained (USDA)	4 oz.	132	.8
Solids & liq. (Bumble Bee)	4½-oz. can	90	.9
Cocktail, tiny, drained, (Icy Point)	4½-oz. can	148	.8
Cocktail, tiny, drained (Pink Beauty)	4½-oz. can	148	.8
Cocktail, tiny, drained (Snow Mist)	4½-oz. can	148	.8
Cooked, French-fried (USDA)	4 oz.	255	11.3
Frozen:			
Raw:			
Breaded (Chicken of the Sea)	4 oz.	158	22.6
Breaded (Gorton)	¼ of 1-lb. pkg.	158	23.0
Peeled (Ship Ahoy)	8-oz. pkg.	207	1.5
Recipe Shrimp (Henderson's)	20-oz. pkg.	284	3.4
Cooked (Sau-Sea)	4 oz.	73	0.
Cooked (Weight Watchers)	½ of 8-oz. pkg.	67	1.3
Fried (Mrs. Paul's)	6-oz. pkg.	316	32.6
SHRIMP COCKTAIL:			
(Sau-Sea)	4-oz. jar	107	20.6
(Sea Snack)	4-oz. jar	110	14.8
SHRIMP DINNER, frozen:			
(Morton)	7¾-oz. dinner	374	41.8
(Swanson)	8-oz. dinner	358	41.5
SHRIMP PASTE, canned (USDA)	1 oz.	51	.4
SHRIMP PUFF, frozen (Durkee)	1 piece (.5 oz.)	44	3.0

(USDA): United States Department of Agriculture
(HEW/FAO): Health, Education and Welfare/Food and Agriculture Organization
* Prepared as Package Directs

Food and Description	Measure or Quantity	Calories	Carbohydrate (grams)
SHRIMP SOUP, Cream of:			
*(Campbell)	1 cup	171	12.8
Canned (Crosse & Blackwell)	½ can (6½ oz.)	92	6.3
Frozen:			
Condensed (USDA)	8 oz. (by wt.)	302	16.2
*Prepared with equal volume water (USDA)	1 cup (8.5 oz.)	158	8.4
*Prepared with equal volume milk (USDA)	1 cup (8.6 oz.)	243	15.2
SIDE CAR COCKTAIL, liq. mix (Holland House)	1½ fl. oz.	66	16.5
SIMBA, soft drink	6 fl. oz.	77	19.3
SIP 'N SLIM COCKTAIL, liq. mix (Holland House)	1½ fl. oz.	14	3.8
SKATE, raw, meat only (USDA)	4 oz.	111	0.
SLENDER, dry (Carnation):			
Chocolate	1-oz. pkg.	104	15.3
Coffee	1-oz. pkg.	104	16.1
Strawberry, wild	1-oz. pkg.	104	16.0
Vanilla, French	1-oz. pkg.	104	15.9
SLOE GIN (See **GIN, SLOE**)			
SLOPPY JOE:			
Canned, with beef (Morton House)	15-oz. can	706	52.1
Frozen (Banquet) cookin' bag	5 oz.	251	36.0
SLOPPY JOE SEASONING MIX:			
(French's)	1½-oz. pkg.	117	26.0
*With meat & tomato paste (Durkee)	3 cups (½-oz. pkg.)	1453	60.4
(Lawry's)	1½-oz. pkg.	139	27.7
(McCormick)	1⁵⁄₁₆-oz. pkg.	112	
*(Wyler's)	¾ cup	25	4.3

Food and Description	Measure or Quantity	Calories	Carbo- hydrates (grams)
SMELT, Atlantic, jack & bay (USDA):			
Raw, whole	1 lb. (weighed whole)	244	0.
Raw, meat only	4 oz.	111	0.
Canned, solids & liq.	4 oz.	227	0.
SMOKIE SAUSAGE:			
(Eckrich):			
Smoked, skinless	2 oz.	94	1.0
Smokee, from 1-lb. pkg.	1.6-oz. link	152	1.5
Smokee, from 12-oz. pkg.	1.2-oz. link	110	1.0
Smokette	1 piece	79	1.0
(Hormel)	1 piece (.8 oz.)	75	.4
(Oscar Mayer) 8 per ¾ lb.	1 link (1.5 oz.)	131	1.0
Cheese (Oscar Mayer)	1.5-oz. link	131	.9
Little Smokies (Oscar Mayer)	1 link (9 grams)	29	.2
(Wilson)	1 oz.	84	.5
SNACK (See **CRACKER, POPCORN, POTATO CHIP,** etc.)			
SNAIL, raw:			
(USDA)	4 oz.	102	2.3
Giant African (USDA)	4 oz.	83	5.0
SNAPPER (See **RED SNAPPER**)			
SNO BALL (Hostess)	1 cake (1.5 oz.)	162	27.2
SOAVE WINE, Italian white (Antinori) 12% alcohol	3 fl. oz.	84	6.3
SODA or **SOFT DRINK** (See individual kinds listed by flavor or brand name)			
SOFT SWIRL (Jell-O):			
All flavors except chocolate	½ cup (3.8 oz.)	168	25.8
Chocolate	½ cup (4 oz.)	190	27.4

USDA): United States Department of Agriculture
HEW/FAO): Health, Education and Welfare/Food and Agriculture
          Organization
* Prepared as Package Directs

Food and Description	Measure or Quantity	Calories	Carbohydrates (grams)
SOLE, raw (USDA):			
Whole	1 lb. (weighed whole)	118	0.
Meat only	4 oz.	90	0.
SORGHUM (USDA):			
Grain	1 oz.	94	20.7
Syrup	1 T. (.7 oz.)	54	12.2
SORREL (See **DOCK**)			
SOUP (See individual listings by kind)			
SOUP BASE, chicken (Wyler's)	1 tsp. (6 grams)	28	3.1
SOURSOP, raw (USDA):			
Whole	1 lb. (weighed with skin & seeds)	200	50.3
Flesh only	4 oz.	74	18.5
SOUSE (USDA)	1 oz.	51	3
SOUTHERN COMFORT, 100 proof	1 fl. oz.	96	3.9
SOYBEAN (USDA):			
Young seeds:			
Raw	1 lb. (weighed in pods)	322	31.7
Boiled, drained	4 oz.	134	11.9
Canned, solids & liq.	4 oz.	85	7.1
Canned, drained solids	4 oz.	117	8.4
Mature seeds, dry:			
Raw	1 lb.	1828	152.6
Raw	1 cup (7.4 oz.)	846	70.4
Cooked	4 oz.	147	12.2
Roasted (Soy Town)	1 oz.	152	5.1
Roasted, sunflower oil (Soy Town)	1 oz.	145	5.1
SOYBEAN CURD or **TORFU:**			
(USDA)	4 oz.	82	2.7
(USDA)	4.2-oz. cake (2¾" x 2½" x 1")	86	2.9

Food and Description	Measure or Quantity	Calories	Carbo-hydrates (grams)
SOYBEAN FLOUR (See **FLOUR**)			
SOYBEAN GRITS, high fat (USDA)	1 cup (4.9 oz.)	524	46.0
SOYBEAN MILK (USDA):			
Fluid	4 oz.	37	2.5
Powder	1 oz.	122	7.9
SOYBEAN PROTEIN (USDA)	1 oz.	91	4.3
SOYBEAN PROTEINATE (USDA)	1 oz.	88	2.2
SOYBEAN SPROUT (See **BEAN SPROUT**)			
SOY SAUCE (See **SAUCE**)			
SPACE FOOD (Pillsbury)	1 oz.	118	19.8
SPAGHETTI. Plain spaghetti products are essentially the same in caloric value and carbohydrate content on the same weight basis. The longer the cooking, the more water is absorbed and this affects the nutritive value (USDA):			
Dry	1 oz.	105	21.3
Dry, broken	1 cup (2.5 oz.)	262	53.4
Cooked:			
8–10 minutes, "al dente"	1 cup (5.1 oz.)	216	43.9
8–10 minutes, "al dente"	4 oz.	168	34.1
14–20 minutes, tender	1 cup (4.9 oz.)	155	32.2
14–20 minutes, tender	4 oz.	126	26.1
SPAGHETTI DINNER:			
With meatballs *(Chef Boy-Ar-Dee)	8¾-oz. pkg.	362	62.0

(USDA): United States Department of Agriculture
(HEW/FAO): Health, Education and Welfare/Food and Agriculture Organization

* Prepared as Package Directs

Food and Description	Measure or Quantity	Calories	Carbo-hydrates (grams)
*With meat sauce (Chef Boy-Ar-Dee)	7-oz. pkg.	285	50.3
*With meat sauce (Kraft) Deluxe Dinner	4 oz.	151	23.1
*With mushroom sauce (Chef Boy-Ar-Dee)	7-oz. pkg.	273	51.5
Frozen:			
(Banquet)	11½-oz. dinner	450	62.9
(Morton)	11-oz. dinner	390	53.0
(Swanson)	12-oz. dinner	323	44.4
SPAGHETTI & FRANKFURTERS in TOMATO SAUCE, canned:			
SpaghettiOs (Franco-American)	1 cup	253	25.7
(Heinz)	8½-oz. can	308	28.2
SPAGHETTI & GROUND BEEF in TOMATO SAUCE, canned:			
(Buitoni)	8 oz.	266	23.6
(Chef Boy-Ar-Dee)	7½ oz. (½ of 15-oz. can)	192	26.4
(Franco-American)	1 cup	272	25.5
(Nalley's)	8 oz.	220	28.6
SPAGHETTI & MEATBALLS in TOMATO SAUCE:			
Home recipe (USDA)	1 cup (8.7 oz.)	332	38.7
Canned:			
(USDA)	1 cup (8.8 oz.)	258	28.5
(Austex)	15½-oz. can	437	48.5
(Buitoni)	8 oz.	258	21.1
(Chef Boy-Ar-Dee)	8 oz. (⅕ of 40-oz. can)	213	27.2
(Franco-American)	1 cup	264	24.3
SpaghettiOs (Franco-American)	1 cup	215	23.0
(Hormel)	15-oz. can	348	20.0
(Libby's)	8 oz.	191	29.3
Frozen (Buitoni)	8 oz.	262	31.2
Frozen (Buitoni)	4 oz.	131	15.6
SPAGHETTI with MEAT SAUCE:			
Canned (Heinz)	8½-oz. can	207	26.3

Food and Description	Measure or Quantity	Calories	Carbo- hydrates (grams)
Frozen:			
(Banquet) cookin' bag	8 oz.	311	31.3
(Kraft)	12½-oz. pkg.	343	48.9
(Morton)	8-oz. casserole	289	28.9
(Swanson)	8-oz. pkg.	233	28.5
SPAGHETTI MIX:			
*American style (Kraft)	4 oz.	121	22.2
*Italian style (Kraft)	4 oz.	119	20.1
SPAGHETTI SAUCE:			
Clam, red (Buitoni)	4 oz.	106	1.4
Clam, white (Buitoni)	4 oz.	140	2.2
Italian, frozen (Celeste)	½ cup (4 oz.)	68	9.2
Italian (Contadina)	½ cup (4.4 oz.)	76	12.0
Marinara (See **SAUCE,** Marinara)			
Meat:			
(Buitoni)	4 oz.	111	5.0
(Chef Boy-Ar-Dee)	¼ of 15-oz. can	93	10.1
With ground meat (Chef Boy-Ar-Dee)	⅐ of 29-oz. jar	136	10.2
(Heinz)	½ cup	110	15.4
(Prince)	½ cup (4.9 oz.)	144	11.0
Meatball (Chef Boy-Ar-Dee)	⅓ of 15-oz. can	202	21.2
Meatless or plain:			
(Buitoni)	4 oz.	76	9.5
(Chef Boy-Ar-Dee)	¼ of 16-oz. jar	73	12.4
(Heinz)	½ cup	98	15.4
(Prince)	½ cup (4.6 oz.)	88	13.0
(Ronzoni)	4 oz.	110	
Mushroom:			
(Buitoni)	4 oz.	69	7.6
(Chef Boy-Ar-Dee)	¼ of 15-oz. can	68	11.4
(Heinz)	½ cup	97	13.8
With meat (Heinz)	½ cup	106	14.0
SPAGHETTI SAUCE MIX:			
*(Durkee)	2½ cups (1½-oz. pkg.)	224	52.1

(USDA): United States Department of Agriculture
(HEW/FAO): Health, Education and Welfare/Food and Agriculture Organization
* Prepared as Package Directs

Food and Description	Measure or Quantity	Calories	Carbo-hydrates (grams)
*(Kraft)	4 oz.	60	9.0
*(McCormick)	4 oz.	80	13.0
(Wyler's)	1½-oz. pkg.		25.0
*Italian (French's)	½ cup	90	10.7
Italian (French's)	1½-oz. pkg.	108	22.6
*Prepared without oil (Spatini)	½ cup (4.2 oz.)	50	9.0
*Prepared with oil (Spatini)	½ cup (4.2 oz.)	76	9.6
With meatballs (Lawry's)	3½-oz. pkg.	330	65.9
*With mushrooms (Durkee)	2⅔ cups (1.2 oz. pkg.)	208	48.1
*With mushrooms (French's)	½ cup	73	9.8
With mushrooms (Lawry's)	1½-oz. pkg.	147	22.6
*(Wyler's)	½ cup	21	3.9
SPAGHETTI with TOMATO SAUCE:			
Twists (Buitoni)	8 oz.	142	24.1
(Van Camp)	1 cup (7.8 oz.)	168	33.8
SPAGHETTI in TOMATO SAUCE with CHEESE:			
Home recipe (USDA)	1 cup (8.8 oz.)	260	37.0
Canned:			
(USDA)	1 cup (8.8 oz.)	190	38.5
(Chef Boy-Ar-Dee)	8 oz. (⅕ of 40-oz. can)	156	31.8
(Franco-American)	1 cup	185	35.4
Italian style (Franco-American)	1 cup	174	30.9
SpaghettiOs (Franco-American)	1 cup	183	34.5
(Heinz)	8½-oz. can	178	31.1
SPAM (Hormel), canned:			
Regular	3 oz.	260	3.2
Spread	1 oz.	80	0.
& cheese	3 oz.	260	2.1
SPANISH MACKEREL, raw (USDA):			
Whole	1 lb. (weighed whole)	490	0.
Meat only	4 oz.	201	0.

Food and Description	Measure or Quantity	Calories	Carbo-hydrates (grams)
SPANISH-STYLE VEGETABLES, frozen (Birds Eye)	⅓ of 10-oz. pkg. (3.3 oz.)	85	7.1
SPEARMINT, extract (Ehlers)	1 tsp.	12	
SPECIAL K, cereal (Kellogg's)	1¼ cups (1 oz.)	107	20.3
SPICE CAKE MIX:			
*(Duncan Hines)	½₂ of cake (2.7 oz.)	199	35.0
*Apple with raisins, layer (Betty Crocker)	½₂ of cake	206	37.7
*Layer (Betty Crocker)	½₂ of cake	202	36.1
Honey: (USDA)	1 oz.	126	21.6
*Prepared with eggs, water, caramel icing (USDA)	2 oz.	200	34.5
*Streusel (Pillsbury)	½₂ of cake	350	52.0
SPINACH:			
Raw (USDA):			
Untrimmed	1 lb. (weighed with large stems & roots)	85	14.0
Trimmed or packaged	1 lb.	118	19.5
Trimmed, whole leaves	1 cup (1.2 oz.)	9	1.4
Trimmed, chopped	1 cup (1.8 oz.)	14	2.2
Boiled, whole leaves, drained (USDA)	1 cup (5.5 oz.)	36	5.6
Canned, regular pack:			
Solids & liq. (USDA)	½ cup (4.1 oz.)	22	3.5
Drained solids (USDA)	½ cup (4 oz.)	27	4.0
Drained liq. (USDA)	4 oz.	7	1.5
Drained solids (Del Monte)	½ cup (4 oz.)	24	3.0
Solids & liq. (Stokely-Van Camp)	½ cup (3.9 oz.)	21	3.3

(USDA): United States Department of Agriculture
(HEW/FAO): Health, Education and Welfare/Food and Agriculture Organization
* Prepared as Package Directs

Food and Description	Measure or Quantity	Calories	Carbo-hydrates (grams)
Canned, dietetic pack, low sodium:			
Solids & liq. (USDA)	4 oz.	24	3.7
Drained solids (USDA)	4 oz.	29	4.5
Drained liq. (USDA)	4 oz.	9	2.3
Solids & liq. (Blue Boy)	4 oz.	22	2.4
Frozen:			
Chopped:			
Not thawed (USDA)	4 oz.	27	4.3
Boiled, drained (USDA)	4 oz.	26	4.2
(Birds Eye)	⅓ of 10-oz. pkg.	23	2.7
Deviled, with cheddar cheese, casserole (Green Giant)	⅓ of 10-oz. pkg.	70	5.9
In cream sauce (Green Giant)	⅓ of 10-oz. pkg.	57	5.4
Leaf:			
Not thawed (USDA)	4 oz.	28	4.8
Boiled, drained (USDA)	4 oz.	27	4.4
(Birds Eye)	⅓ of 10-oz. pkg.	23	3.1
Creamed (Birds Eye)	⅓ of 9-oz. pkg.	61	5.4
In butter sauce (Green Giant)	⅓ of 10-oz. pkg.	48	4.0
SPINACH, NEW ZEALAND (See NEW ZEALAND SPINACH)			
SPINACH SOUFFLÉ, frozen (Stouffer's)	12-oz. pkg.	484	29.0
SPINY LOBSTER (See CRAYFISH)			
SPLEEN, raw (USDA):			
Beef & calf	4 oz.	118	0.
Hog	4 oz.	121	0.
Lamb	4 oz.	130	0.
SPONGE CAKE, home recipe (USDA)	1/12 of 10″ cake (2.3 oz.)	196	35.7
SPOT, fillets (USDA):			
Raw	1 lb.	993	0.
Baked	4 oz.	335	0.
SPRITE, soft drink	6 fl. oz.	70	18.1

Food and Description	Measure or Quantity	Calories	Carbo-hydrates (grams)
SQUAB, pigeon, raw (USDA):			
Dressed	1 lb. (weighed with feet, inedible viscera & bones)	569	0.
Meat & skin	4 oz.	333	0.
Meat only	4 oz.	161	0.
Light meat only, without skin	4 oz.	142	0.
Giblets	1 oz.	44	.3
SQUASH SEEDS, dry (USDA):			
In hull	4 oz.	464	12.6
Hulled	1 oz.	157	4.3
SQUASH, SUMMER:			
Fresh (USDA):			
Crookneck & Straightneck, yellow:			
Whole	1 lb. (weighed untrimmed)	89	19.1
Boiled, drained, diced	½ cup (3.6 oz.)	15	3.2
Boiled, drained, slices	½ cup (3.1 oz.)	13	2.7
Scallop, white & pale green:			
Whole	1 lb. (weighed untrimmed)	93	22.7
Boiled, drained, mashed	½ cup (4.2 oz.)	19	4.5
Zucchini & Cocozelle, green:			
Whole	1 lb. (weighed untrimmed)	73	15.5
Boiled, drained slices	½ cup (2.7 oz.)	9	1.9
Canned, zucchini in tomato sauce (Del Monte)	½ cup (4.1 oz.)	25	5.6
Frozen:			
Not thawed (USDA)	4 oz.	24	5.3
Boiled, drained (USDA)	4 oz.	24	5.3
Fried, breaded, zucchini (Mrs. Paul's)	9-oz. pkg.	567	62.5
Parmesan, zucchini (Mrs. Paul's)	12-oz. pkg.	259	16.0
Summer squash, slices (Birds Eye)	½ cup (3.3 oz.)	20	3.8
Zucchini (Birds Eye)	⅓ of 10-oz. pkg.	20	2.3

(USDA) : United States Department of Agriculture
(HEW/FAO) : Health, Education and Welfare/Food and Agriculture Organization
* Prepared as Package Directs

Food and Description	Measure or Quantity	Calories	Carbo-hydrates (grams)
SQUASH, WINTER:			
Fresh (USDA):			
Acorn:			
Whole	1 lb. (weighed with skin & seeds)	152	38.6
Baked, flesh only, mashed	½ cup (3.6 oz.)	56	14.3
Boiled, mashed	½ cup (4.1 oz.)	39	9.7
Butternut:			
Whole	1 lb. (weighed with skin & seeds)	171	44.4
Baked, flesh only	4 oz.	77	19.8
Boiled, flesh only	4 oz.	46	11.8
Hubbard:			
Whole	1 lb. (weighed with skin & seeds)	117	28.1
Baked, flesh only	4 oz.	57	13.3
Baked, flesh only, mashed	½ cup (3.6 oz.)	51	11.9
Boiled, flesh only, diced	½ cup (4.2 oz.)	35	8.1
Boiled, flesh only, mashed	½ cup (4.3 oz.)	37	8.4
Frozen:			
Not thawed (USDA)	4 oz.	43	10.4
Heated (USDA)	½ cup (4.2 oz.)	46	11.0
(Birds Eye)	⅓ of 12-oz. pkg.	43	9.1
SQUID, raw, meat only (USDA)	4 oz.	95	1.7
STARCH (See **CORNSTARCH**)			
START, instant breakfast drink	½ cup (4.7 oz.)	60	14.9
STEINWEIN REBENGOLD, Franconia wine (Deinhard) 11% alcohol	3 fl. oz.	60	1.0
STOCKPOT SOUP, canned (Campbell)	1 cup	90	8.5
STOMACH, PORK, scalded (USDA)	4 oz.	172	0.

Food and Description	Measure or Quantity	Calories	Carbohydrates (grams)
STRAINED FOOD (See BABY FOOD)			
STRAWBERRY:			
Fresh, whole (USDA)	1 lb. (weighed with caps & stems)	161	36.6
Fresh, whole, capped (USDA)	1 cup (5.1 oz.)	53	12.1
Canned, unsweetened or low calorie:			
Water pack, solids & liq. (USDA)	4 oz.	25	6.4
Solids & liq. (Blue Boy)	4 oz.	16	7.8
Low calorie, solids & liq. (S and W) *Nutradiet*	4 oz.	23	5.3
Frozen:			
Sweetened, whole, not thawed:			
(USDA)	16-oz. can	418	106.7
(USDA)	½ cup (4.5 oz.)	116	29.7
Sweetened, sliced, not thawed (USDA)	10-oz. pkg.	310	79.0
Sweetened, sliced, not thawed (USDA)	½ cup (4.5 oz.)	138	35.3
Whole (Birds Eye)	¼ of 16-oz. pkg.	101	26.6
Halves (Birds Eye)	½ cup (5.3 oz.)	162	39.9
Quick-thaw (Birds Eye)	½ cup (5 oz.)	122	30.7
*STRAWBERRY CAKE:			
Mix (Duncan Hines)	1/12 of cake (2.7 oz.)	207	35.6
Frozen (Mrs. Smith's)	1/8 of 9" cake (5.7 oz.)	379	51.7
STRAWBERRY DRINK MIX:			
Quik	2 heaping tsps. (.6 oz.)	62	15.9
*(Wyler's)	6 fl. oz.	64	15.8

(USDA): United States Department of Agriculture
(HEW/FAO): Health, Education and Welfare/Food and Agriculture Organization
Prepared as Package Directs

Food and Description	Measure or Quantity	Calories	Carbohydrates (grams)
STRAWBERRY EXTRACT & FLAVORING:			
Imitation (Ehlers)	1 tsp.	13	
Imitation (French's)	1 tsp.	16	
STRAWBERRY ICE CREAM:			
(Meadow Gold) 10% fat	¼ pt.	126	16.0
(Sealtest)	¼ pt. (2.3 oz.)	133	19.5
STRAWBERRY LIQUEUR,			
*(Leroux) 50 proof	1 fl. oz.	74	8.3
STRAWBERRY PIE:			
Home recipe (USDA)	⅛ of 9" pie (5.6 oz.)	313	48.8
Creme (Tastykake)	4-oz. pie	356	50.7
Frozen:			
Cream (Banquet)	2½-oz. serving	187	27.2
Cream (Morton)	¼ of 16-oz. pie	183	24.0
Cream (Mrs. Smith's)	⅙ of 8" pie (4.2 oz.)	221	30.0
STRAWBERRY PIE FILLING:			
(Comstock)	½ cup (5.4 oz.)	159	39.0
(Lucky Leaf)	8 oz.	248	60.0
STRAWBERRY PRESERVE or JAM:			
Sweetened (Bama)	1 T. (.7 oz.)	54	13.5
Dietetic or low calorie:			
(Diet Delight)	1 T. (.6 oz.)	23	5.7
(Kraft)	1 oz.	36	8.9
(S and W) *Nutradiet*	1 T. (.5 oz.)	12	3.0
(Slenderella)	1 T. (.6 oz.)	25	6.4
(Smucker's)	1 T. (.7 oz.)	2	.4
(Tillie Lewis)	1 T. (.8 oz.)	12	3.
STRAWBERRY RENNET MIX:			
Powder:			
Dry (Junket)	1 oz.	115	27.
*(Junket)	4 oz.	108	14.
Tablet:			
Dry (Junket)	1 tablet (<1 gram)	1	
*& sugar (Junket)	4 oz.	101	13.

Food and Description	Measure or Quantity	Calories	Carbo-hydrates (grams)
STRAWBERRY-RHUBARB PIE:			
(Tastykake)	4-oz. pie	399	63.5
Frozen:			
(Mrs. Smith's)	⅛ of 8″ pie (4.2 oz.)	319	46.7
(Mrs. Smith's) old-fashioned	⅛ of 9″ pie (5.8 oz.)	448	58.6
(Mrs. Smith's)	⅛ of 10″ pie (5.6 oz.)	411	60.6
STRAWBERRY-RHUBARB PIE FILLING, canned			
(Lucky Leaf)	8 oz.	258	62.8
STRAWBERRY SOFT DRINK:			
Sweetened:			
(Canada Dry)	6 fl. oz.	89	22.2
(Clicquot Club)	6 fl. oz.	98	20.0
(Cott)	6 fl. oz.	98	20.0
(Fanta)	6 fl. oz.	88	22.7
(Hoffman)	6 fl. oz.	89	22.3
(Mission)	6 fl. oz.	98	20.0
(Shasta)	6 fl. oz.	80	20.3
(Yoo-Hoo)	6 fl. oz.	90	18.0
(Yoo-Hoo) high-protein	6 fl. oz.	114	24.6
(Yukon Club)	6 fl. oz.	92	23.0
Low calorie:			
(Canada Dry)	6 fl. oz.	4	0.
(Clicquot Club)	6 fl. oz.	3	.5
(Cott)	6 fl. oz.	3	.5
(Hoffman)	6 fl. oz.	<1	.2
(Mission)	6 fl. oz.	3	.5
(Shasta)	6 fl. oz.	<1	<.1
STRAWBERRY SYRUP, low calorie (No-Cal)	1 tsp.	<1	0.
STRAWBERRY TURNOVER, frozen (Pepperidge Farm)	1 turnover (3.3 oz.)	326	34.5

(USDA): United States Department of Agriculture
(HEW/FAO): Health, Education and Welfare/Food and Agriculture Organization
* Prepared as Package Directs

Food and Description	Measure or Quantity	Calories	Carbo hydrate (grams
STRUDEL, frozen (Pepperidge Farm):			
Apple	⅛ of strudel (2.5 oz.)	202	26.0
Blueberry	⅛ of strudel (2.5 oz.)	240	28.4
Cherry	⅛ of strudel (2.5 oz.)	204	26.8
Pineapple-cheese	⅛ of strudel (2.3 oz.)	209	21.2
STURGEON (USDA):			
Raw, section	1 lb. (weighed with skin & bones)	362	0.
Raw, meat only	4 oz.	107	0.
Smoked	4 oz.	169	0.
Steamed	4 oz.	181	0.
SUCCOTASH, frozen:			
Not thawed (USDA)	4 oz.	110	24.4
Boiled, drained (USDA)	½ cup (3.4 oz.)	89	19.7
(Birds Eye)	½ cup (3.3 oz.)	87	19.4
SUCKER, CARP, raw (USDA):			
Whole	1 lb. (weighed whole)	196	0.
Meat only	4 oz.	126	0.
SUCKER, including WHITE and MULLET, raw (USDA):			
Whole	1 lb. (weighed whole)	203	0.
Meat only	4 oz.	118	0.
SUET, raw (USDA)	1 oz.	242	0.
SUGAR, beet or cane (there are no differences in calories and carbohydrates among brands):			
Brown:			
(USDA)	1 lb.	1692	437.3
Brownulated (USDA)	1 cup (5.4 oz.)	567	146.5
Firm-packed (USDA)	1 cup (7.5 oz.)	791	204.4
Firm-packed (USDA)	1 T. (.5 oz.)	48	12.5

SUGAR SPARKLED TWINKLES   [329]

Food and Description	Measure or Quantity	Calories	Carbo-hydrates (grams)
Confectioners':			
(USDA)	1 lb.	1746	451.3
Unsifted (USDA)	1 cup (4.3 oz.)	474	122.4
Unsifted (USDA)	1 T. (8 grams)	30	7.7
Sifted (USDA)	1 cup (3.4 oz.)	366	94.5
Sifted (USDA)	1 T. (6 grams)	23	5.9
Stirred (USDA)	1 cup (4.2 oz.)	462	119.4
Stirred (USDA)	1 T (8 grams)	29	7.5
Granulated:			
(USDA)	1 lb.	1746	451.3
(USDA)	1 cup (6.9 oz.)	751	194.0
(USDA)	1 T. (.4 oz.)	46	11.9
(USDA)	1 lump (1⅛" x ¾" x ⅜", 6 grams)	23	6.0
Maple (USDA)	1 lb.	1579	408.0
Maple (USDA)	1¾" x 1¼" x ½" piece (1.2 oz.)	104	27.0
SUGAR APPLE, raw (USDA):			
Whole	1 lb. (weighed with skin & seeds)	192	48.4
Flesh only	4 oz.	107	26.9
SUGAR CHEX, cereal	⅞ cup (1 oz.)	119	23.4
SUGAR FROSTED FLAKES, cereal (Kellogg's)	¾ cup (1 oz.)	108	25.5
SUGAR JETS, cereal (General Mills)	1 cup (1 oz.)	111	23.7
SUGAR POPS, cereal (Kellogg's)	1 cup (1 oz.)	109	25.7
SUGAR SMACKS, cereal (Kellogg's)	1 cup (1 oz.)	111	24.8
SUGAR SPARKLED TWINKLES, cereal (General Mills)	1 cup (1 oz.)	112	24.2

USDA): United States Department of Agriculture
HEW/FAO): Health, Education and Welfare/Food and Agriculture
     Organization
* Prepared as Package Directs

Food and Description	Measure or Quantity	Calories	Carbo hydrate. (grams
SUGAR SUBSTITUTE:			
(Adolph's)	1 tsp. (4 grams)	14	3.:
Superose (Whitlock)	1 packet (1 gram)	4	.:
Sweetness & Light	1 tsp. (1 gram)	4	.:
Sweetnin' (Tillie Lewis)	1 tsp. (5 grams)	0	0.
(Weight Watchers)	1 packet or ⅓ tsp. (1 gram)	4	.:
SUKI-YAKI MIX:			
(Durkee)	1¾-oz. pkg.	82	20.(
*With meat & vegetables (Durkee)	6 cups (1¾-oz. pkg.)	1757	75.:
SUNFLOWER SEED (USDA):			
In hulls	4 oz. (weighed in hull)	343	12.:
Hulled	1 oz.	159	5.(
SUNFLOWER SEED FLOUR (See **FLOUR**)			
SUNNY DOODLE:			
(Drake's)	1 cake (1.1 oz.)	141	21.
(Drake's)	1 cake (1 oz.)	121	18.:
SUPER ORANGE CRISP WHEAT PUFFS, (Post)	1 cup (1 oz.)	109	25.
SUPER SUGAR CRISP WHEAT PUFFS, (Post)	⅞ cup (1 oz.)	107	25.(
SURINAM CHERRY (See **PITANGA**)			
SUZY Q (Hostess)	1 cake (2¼ oz.)	268	38.
SWAMP CABBAGE (USDA):			
Raw, whole	1 lb. (weighed untrimmed)	107	19.
Boiled, trimmed, drained	4 oz.	24	4.
SWEETBREADS (USDA):			
Beef, raw	1 lb.	939	0.
Beef, braised	4 oz.	363	0.
Calf, raw	1 lb.	426	0.
Calf, braised	4 oz.	191	0.

Food and Description	Measure or Quantity	Calories	Carbo-hydrates (grams)
Hog (See **PANCREAS**)			
Lamb, raw	1 lb.	426	0.
Lamb, braised	4 oz.	198	0.
SWEET POTATO:			
Raw (USDA):			
All kinds, unpared	1 lb. (weighed whole)	419	96.6
All kinds, pared	4 oz.	129	29.8
Firm-fleshed, Jersey types, pared	4 oz.	116	25.5
Soft-fleshed, Puerto Rico variety, pared	4 oz.	133	31.0
Baked, peeled after baking (USDA)	3.9-oz. sweet potato (5" x 2")	155	35.8
Boiled, peeled after boiling (USDA)	5-oz. sweet potato (5" x 2")	168	38.7
Candied, home recipe (USDA)	6.2-oz. sweet potato (3½" x 2¼")	294	59.8
Canned, regular pack:			
In syrup, solids & liq. (USDA)	4 oz.	129	31.2
Vacuum or solid pack (USDA)	½ cup (3.8 oz.)	118	27.1
(King Pharr)	½ cup	118	22.5
Heavy syrup, solids & liq. (Del Monte)	½ cup (4.2 oz.)	138	33.7
Vacuum pack (Taylor's)	½ cup	135	32.0
Yam (King Pharr)	½ cup	114	27.0
Canned, dietetic pack, without added sugar & salt (USDA)	4 oz.	52	12.2
Dehydrated flakes, dry (USDA)	½ cup (2 oz.)	220	52.2
*Dehydrated flakes, prepared with water (USDA)	½ cup (4.4 oz.)	120	28.5

(USDA): United States Department of Agriculture
(HEW/FAO): Health, Education and Welfare/Food and Agriculture
             Organization
* Prepared as Package Directs

Food and Description	Measure or Quantity	Calories	Carbo-hydrates (grams)
Frozen:			
Candied (Mrs. Paul's)	⅓ of 12-oz. pkg.	186	45.0
Sweets & Apples, candied (Mrs. Paul's)	⅓ of 12-oz. pkg.	145	34.7
Candied yams (Birds Eye)	⅓ of 12-oz. pkg.	215	53.3
With brown sugar, pine-apple glaze (Birds Eye)	½ cup (3.3 oz.)	145	30.7
SWEET POTATO PIE:			
Home recipe (USDA)	⅛ of 9″ pie (5.4 oz.)	324	36.0
(Tastykake)	4-oz. pie	359	50.0
SWEETSOP (See SUGAR APPLE)			
SWISS ROLL (Drake's)	1 roll (3 oz.)	376	52.9
SWISS STEAK, frozen:			
(Stouffer's)	10-oz. pkg.	569	14.0
Dinner (Swanson)	10-oz. dinner	361	35.0
With beef gravy (Holloway House)	1 steak (7 oz.)	236	5.0
SWORDFISH (USDA):			
Raw, meat only	1 lb.	535	0.
Broiled with butter or margarine	3″ x 3″ x ½″ steak (4.4 oz.)	218	0.
Canned, solids & liq.	4 oz.	116	0.
SYLVANER WINE (Louis M. Martini) 12½% alcohol	3 fl. oz.	90	.2
SYRUP (See individual listings by kind, such as **PANCAKE & WAFFLE SYRUP** or by brand name, such as *LOG CABIN*)			

T

Food and Description	Measure or Quantity	Calories	Carbo-hydrates (grams)
TABASCO SAUCE (McIlhenny)	¼ tsp. (1 gram)	<1	<.

Food and Description	Measure or Quantity	Calories	Carbohydrates (grams)
TACO, beef, frozen:			
Regular size:			
(Patio)	2¼-oz. taco (from 13½-oz. pkg.)	179	15.1
(Rosarita)	2-oz. taco (from 12-oz. pkg.)	138	
Cocktail (Patio)	½-oz. taco (from 12-oz. pkg.)	39	4.8
Cocktail (Rosarita)	½-oz. taco (from 5½-oz. pkg.)	30	
TACO FILLING, canned:			
(Gebhardt)	1 oz.	63	3.0
Beef (Rosarita)	4 oz.	244	
TACO SAUCE (See SAUCE, Taco)			
TACO SEASONING MIX:			
(French's)	1¾-oz. pkg.	123	23.8
(Lawry's)	1¼-oz. pkg.	120	21.8
TAHITIAN TREAT, soft drink (Canada Dry)	6 fl. oz.	96	24.0
TAMALE:			
Canned:			
(Armour Star)	15½-oz. can	620	63.2
(Gebhardt)	2 oz.	110	20.0
(Hormel)	1 tamale (2.1 oz.)	80	4.9
(Rutherford)	6-oz. can	242	
(Wilson)	15½-oz. can	601	63.3
Frozen:			
(Banquet) cookin' bag	2 tamales with sauce (3 oz. each)	279	26.0
(Banquet) buffet	2-lb. pkg.	1488	138.8
(Rosarita)	10-oz. pkg. (3 pieces)	768	
With beef chili gravy (Patio)	1 piece	175	6.3

(USDA): United States Department of Agriculture
(HEW/FAO): Health, Education and Welfare/Food and Agriculture Organization

* Prepared as Package Directs

Food and Description	Measure or Quantity	Calories	Carbohydrates (grams)
TAMARIND, fresh (USDA):			
Whole	1 lb. (weighed with pods & seeds)	520	136.1
Flesh only	4 oz.	271	70.9
TANDY TAKE (Tastykake):			
Chocolate	.7-oz. cake	147	21.0
Choc-o-mint	.6-oz. cake	102	13.0
Dandy Kake	.6-oz. cake	102	13.0
Karamel	.7-oz. cake	100	12.2
Orange	.6-oz. cake	103	13.6
Peanut butter	.7-oz. cake	194	32.1
*TANG, instant breakfast drink:			
Grape	½ cup (4.7 oz.)	61	15.8
Grapefruit	½ cup (4.7 oz.)	61	15.0
Orange	½ cup (4.7 oz.)	61	14.7
TANGELO, fresh (USDA):			
Juice from whole fruit	1 lb. (weighed with peel, membrane & seeds)	104	24.6
Juice	½ cup (4.4 oz.)	51	12.0
TANGERINE or **MANDARIN ORANGE,** fresh:			
Whole (USDA)	1 lb. (weighed with peel, membrane & seeds)	154	38.9
Whole (USDA)	4.1-oz. tangerine (2⅜″ dia.)	39	10.0
Peeled (Sunkist)	1 large tangerine (4.1 oz.)	39	10.0
Sections, without membranes (USDA)	1 cup (6.8 oz.)	89	22.4
TANGERINE JUICE:			
Fresh (USDA)	½ cup (4.4 oz.)	53	12.5
Canned, unsweetened (USDA)	½ cup (4.4 oz.)	53	12.6
Canned, sweetened (USDA)	½ cup (4.4 oz.)	62	14.9
Frozen concentrate, unsweetened:			
Undiluted (USDA)	6-oz. can	340	80.4

Food and Description	Measure or Quantity	Calories	Carbohydrates (grams)
*Prepared with 3 parts water by volume (USDA)	½ cup (4.4 oz.)	57	13.4
Frozen concentrate, sweetened:			
*(Minute Maid)	½ cup (4.2 oz.)	57	13.1
*(Snow Crop)	½ cup (4.2 oz.)	57	13.1
TAPIOCA, dry, quick cooking, granulated:			
(USDA)	1 cup (5.4 oz.)	535	131.3
(USDA)	1 T. (10 grams)	35	8.6
(Minute Tapioca)	1 T.	40	10.0
TAPIOCA PUDDING:			
Apple, home recipe (USDA)	½ cup (4.4 oz.)	146	36.8
Cream, home recipe (USDA)	½ cup (2.9 oz.)	110	14.0
Chilled (Sealtest)	4 oz.	130	21.7
Canned (Hunt's)	5-oz. can	166	25.6
Mix:			
*All flavors (Jell-O)	½ cup (5.1 oz.)	166	27.6
*Chocolate (Royal)	½ cup (5.1 oz.)	186	29.9
*Fluffy recipe (Minute Tapioca)	½ cup (4.4 oz.)	150	20.1
*Vanilla (My-T-Fine)	½ cup (5 oz.)	144	25.2
*Vanilla (Royal)	½ cup (5.1 oz.)	169	27.9
TARO, raw (USDA):			
Tubers, whole	1 lb. (weighed with skin)	373	90.3
Tubers, skin removed	4 oz.	111	26.9
Leaves & stems	1 lb.	181	33.6
TAUTOG or **BLACKFISH**, raw:			
Whole (USDA)	1 lb. (weighed whole)	149	0.
Meat only (USDA)	4 oz.	101	0.
TEA:			
Bag (Lipton)	1 bag	0	0.
Bag (Tender Leaf)	1 bag	1	

(USDA): United States Department of Agriculture
(HEW/FAO): Health, Education and Welfare/Food and Agriculture Organization
* Prepared as Package Directs

Food and Description	Measure or Quantity	Calories	Carbo-hydrates (grams)
Canned (Lipton)	12 fl. oz. (12.8 oz.)	147	36.6
Instant:			
Dry powder, slightly sweetened (USDA)	1 tsp. (<1 gram)	1	.4
*Beverage, slightly sweetened (USDA)	1 cup (8.4 oz.)	5	.9
*(Lipton)	1 cup	0	0.
Nestea	1 tsp. (<1 gram)	<1	<.1
(Tender Leaf)	1 rounded tsp.	1	
*Lemon flavored (Lipton)	1 cup	3	.9
TEAM, cereal	1⅓ cups (1 oz.)	107	24.2
TEA MIX, iced:			
All flavors, Nestea	3 tsps. (.6 oz.)	58	15.1
*All flavors (Salada)	1 cup (.5 oz. dry)	57	13.6
*(Tender Leaf)	1 cup	57	14.2
*(Wyler's)	1 cup	56	14.0
Lemon flavored:			
*(Lipton)	1 cup	102	25.5
*Low calorie (Lipton)	1 cup	4	.7
*Low calorie (Tender Leaf)	1 cup (8.4 oz.)	12	3.1
TEE UP, soft drink	6 fl. oz.	64	16.1
TEMPTYS (Tastykake):			
Butter creme	⅔-oz. cake	94	12.9
Chocolate	⅔-oz. cake	95	17.1
Lemon	⅔-oz. cake	95	17.3
TENDERGREEN (See MUSTARD SPINACH)			
TEQUILA (See DISTILLED LIQUOR)			
TEXTURED VEGETABLE PROTEIN:			
Breakfast links, Morning-star Farms	.8-oz. link	54	2.3
Breakfast patties, Morning-star Farms	1.3-oz. pattie	98	4.9
Breakfast slices, Morning-star Farms	1-oz. slice	50	1.0
Burger Builder (Betty Crocker)	¼ cup	60	5.0

Food and Description	Measure or Quantity	Calories	Carbo-hydrates (grams)
Chili seasoning (Williams)	4-oz. pkg.	428	47.4
Hamburger seasoning (Williams)	4-oz. pkg.	385	53.6
Meat loaf seasoning (Williams)	4-oz. pkg.	393	54.2
Pathmark Plus:			
Dry	⅓ oz.	28	3.0
*Prepared	4 oz.	178	2.9
Sloppy Joe Seasoning (Williams)	4-oz. pkg.	382	55.8
Spaghetti sauce (Williams)	4-oz. pkg.	366	56.6
Taco seasoning (Williams)	4-oz. pkg.	378	48.7
TERRAPIN, DIAMOND BACK, raw (USDA):			
In shell	1 lb. (weighed in shell)	106	0.
Meat only	4 oz.	126	0.
THICK & FROSTY (General Foods)	1 cup (8.3 oz.)	314	37.7
THUNDERBIRD WINE (Gallo):			
14% alcohol	3 fl. oz.	86	8.1
20% alcohol	3 fl. oz.	106	7.5
THURINGER, sausage:			
(USDA)	1 oz.	87	.5
(Hormel) Old Smokehouse	1 oz.	100	<1.0
Summer sausage, all meat (Oscar Mayer)	.8-oz. slice	74	.3
Summer sausage, pure beef (Oscar Mayer)	.8-oz. slice	68	.5
TIA MARIA, liqueur (Hiram Walker) 63 proof	1 fl. oz.	92	10.0
TIKI, soft drink (Shasta):			
Sweetened	6 fl. oz.	84	21.3
Low calorie	6 fl. oz.	<1	<.1

(USDA): United States Department of Agriculture
(HEW/FAO): Health, Education and Welfare/Food and Agriculture Organization
* Prepared as Package Directs

Food and Description	Measure or Quantity	Calories	Carbo-hydrates (grams)
TILEFISH (USDA):			
Raw, whole	1 lb. (weighed whole)	183	0.
Baked, meat only	4 oz.	156	0.
TOASTER CAKE:			
Corn Treats (Arnold)	1.1-oz. piece	111	17.1
Toastee (Howard Johnson's):			
Blueberry	1 piece (1¼ oz.)	121	17.0
Cinnamon raisin	1 piece (1.1 oz.)	114	17.3
Corn	1 piece (1¼ oz.)	112	18.2
Orange	1 piece (1 oz.)	113	15.5
Pound	1 piece (1 oz.)	111	15.9
Toastette (Nabisco):			
Apple	1 piece (1⅔ oz.)	184	32.3
Blueberry	1 piece (1⅔ oz.)	184	33.0
Brown sugar, cinnamon	1 piece (1⅔ oz.)	189	31.9
Cherry	1 piece (1⅔ oz.)	182	32.7
Orange marmalade	1 piece (1⅔ oz.)	181	32.1
Peach	1 piece (1⅔ oz.)	183	32.7
Strawberry	1 piece (1⅔ oz.)	184	32.7
Toast-r-Cake (Thomas):			
Bran	1 piece (1.2 oz.)	116	19.6
Corn	1 piece (1.2 oz.)	118	18.1
Orange	1 piece (1.2 oz.)	117	17.9
TOASTERINO, frozen (Buitoni):			
Cheese, grilled	4 oz.	286	37.9
Pizzaburger	4 oz.	298	29.8
Sloppy Joe	4 oz.	295	33.8
TODDLER FOOD (See **BABY FOOD**)			
TOFFEE KRUNCH BAR (Sealtest)	3 fl. oz. (1.7 oz.)	149	11.9
TOFU (See **SOYBEAN CURD**)			
TOKAY WINE:			
(Gallo)	3 fl. oz.	107	7.4
(Gallo) 14% alcohol	3 fl. oz.	86	8.1
(Taylor) white, 18½% alcohol	3 fl. oz.	144	11.3

Food and Description	Measure or Quantity	Calories	Carbo-hydrates (grams)
TOMATO:			
Fresh, green whole, untrimmed (USDA)	1 lb. (weighed with core & stem end)	99	21.1
Fresh, green, trimmed, unpeeled (USDA)	4 oz.	27	5.8
Fresh, ripe (USDA):			
Whole, eaten with skin	1 lb.	100	21.3
Whole, peeled	1 lb. (weighed with skin, stem ends & hard core)	88	18.8
Whole, peeled	1 med. (2" x 2½", 5.3 oz.)	33	7.0
Whole, peeled	1 small (1¾" x 2½", 3.9 oz.)	24	5.2
Sliced, peeled	½ cup (3.2 oz.)	20	4.2
Boiled (USDA)	½ cup (4.3 oz.)	31	6.7
Canned, regular pack:			
Whole, solids & liq. (USDA)	½ cup (4.2 oz.)	25	5.1
(Contadina)	½ cup (4 oz.)	28	5.6
Solids & liq. (Del Monte)	½ cup (4.2 oz.)	30	5.0
Diced, in puree (Contadina)	½ cup (4 oz.)	44	9.2
Sliced (Contadina)	½ cup (4 oz.)	36	8.4
Stewed (Contadina)	½ cup (4 oz.)	36	8.0
Stewed (Del Monte)	½ cup (4.2 oz.)	30	6.8
Wedges, solids & liq. (Del Monte)	½ cup (4.1 oz.)	28	6.3
Whole, peeled (Hunt's)	½ cup (4.2 oz.)	24	5.6
Whole, solids & liq. (Stokely-Van Camp)	½ cup (4.1 oz.)	23	4.7
Canned, dietetic pack, low sodium:			
Solids & liq. (USDA)	4 oz.	23	4.8
Solids & liq. (Blue Boy)	4 oz.	25	4.8
Solids & liq. (Tillie Lewis)	½ cup (4.3 oz.)	25	4.6

(USDA): United States Department of Agriculture
(HEW/FAO): Health, Education and Welfare/Food and Agriculture Organization
* Prepared as Package Directs

Food and Description	Measure or Quantity	Calories	Carbohydrates (grams)
Whole, peeled (Diet Delight)	½ cup (4.3 oz.)	39	5.4
Whole, unseasoned (S and W) *Nutradiet*	4 oz.	24	5.2
TOMATO JUICE:			
Canned, regular pack:			
(USDA)	6 fl. oz. (6.4 oz.)	35	7.8
(USDA)	½ cup (4.3 oz.)	23	5.2
(Campbell)	6 fl. oz.	33	6.6
(Del Monte)	½ cup (4.3 oz.)	22	4.9
(Heinz)	5½-fl.-oz. can	34	6.6
(Hunt's)	5½-fl.-oz. can	30	7.2
(Libby's)	½ cup (4.3 oz.)	23	4.8
(Musselman's)	½ cup (4.2 oz.)	25	
(Stokely-Van Camp)	½ cup (4.3 oz.)	28	5.2
Canned, dietetic pack, low sodium:			
(USDA)	4 oz. (by wt.)	22	4.9
(Blue Boy)	4 oz. (by wt.)	24	4.5
(Diet Delight)	½ cup (3.9 oz.)	24	4.9
Unseasoned (S and W) *Nutradiet*	4 oz. (by wt.)	25	5.0
Concentrate, canned (USDA)	4 oz. (by wt.)	86	19.4
*Concentrate, canned, diluted with 3 parts water by volume (USDA)	4 oz. (by wt.)	23	5.1
Dehydrated (USDA)	1 oz.	86	19.3
*Dehydrated (USDA)	½ cup (4.3 oz.)	24	5.4
TOMATO JUICE COCKTAIL:			
(USDA)	4 oz. (by wt.)	24	5.7
Snap-E-Tom	6 fl. oz. (6.5 oz.)	36	7.5
TOMATO PASTE, canned:			
(USDA)	6-oz. can	139	31.6
(USDA)	½ cup (4.6 oz.)	106	24.0
(USDA)	1 T. (.6 oz.)	13	3.0
(Contadina)	1 T. (.5 oz.)	12	2.4
(Del Monte)	1 T. (.6 oz.)	14	3.3
(Hunt's)	½ cup (4.6 oz.)	108	25.7
(Hunt's)	1 T. (.6 oz.)	14	3.2
(Stokely-Van Camp)	½ cup (4.6 oz.)	106	24.1
TOMATO PUREE:			
Canned, regular pack:			
(USDA)	1 cup (8.8 oz.)	98	22.2

Food and Description	Measure or Quantity	Calories	Carbo-hydrates (grams)
(Contadina)	1 cup	96	20.0
(Hunt's)	1 cup (8.8 oz.)	92	21.9
Canned, dietetic pack (USDA)	8 oz.	88	20.0
TOMATO SALAD, jellied			
(Contadina)	½ cup	60	13.6
TOMATO SAUCE, canned:			
(Contadina)	1 cup	80	16.8
(Del Monte) plain	1 cup (8.8 oz.)	60	12.7
(Del Monte) with mushrooms	1 cup (8.8 oz.)	75	17.0
(Del Monte) with onions	1 cup (8.8 oz.)	90	18.5
(Del Monte) with tomato tidbits	1 cup (8.8 oz.)	90	21.8
(Hunt's) plain	1 cup (8.7 oz.)	78	18.7
(Hunt's) herb	1 cup (8.8 oz.)	186	27.0
(Hunt's) special	1 cup (8.7 oz.)	94	27.2
(Hunt's) with bits	1 cup (8.7 oz.)	82	19.4
(Hunt's) with cheese	1 cup (8.8 oz.)	107	20.6
(Hunt's) with mushrooms	1 cup (8.8 oz.)	83	19.8
(Hunt's) with onions	1 cup (8.8 oz.)	102	24.5
(Rosarita) hot	8 oz.	56	
TOMATO SOUP:			
Canned, regular pack:			
Condensed (USDA)	8 oz. (by wt.)	163	28.8
*Prepared with equal volume water (USDA)	1 cup (8.6 oz.)	88	15.7
*Prepared with equal volume milk (USDA)	1 cup (8.8 oz.)	172	22.5
*(Campbell)	1 cup	79	14.0
*(Heinz) California	1 cup (8.5 oz.)	81	17.3
(Heinz) *Great American*	1 cup (8¾ oz.)	168	26.3
*(Manischewitz)	1 cup	60	9.1
*Beef (Campbell) *Noodle-O's*	1 cup	109	15.5
*Bisque (Campbell)	1 cup	115	20.9
*Rice, old-fashioned (Campbell)	1 cup	99	16.7
*Rice (Manischewitz)	1 cup	78	12.8

(USDA): United States Department of Agriculture
(HEW/FAO): Health, Education and Welfare/Food and Agriculture
* Prepared as Package Directs

Food and Description	Measure or Quantity	Calories	Carbo-hydrates (grams)
With vegetables (Heinz)			
Great American	1 cup (8¾ oz.)	126	17.6
Canned, dietetic pack:			
Low sodium (Campbell)	7¼-oz. can	97	16.9
*With rice (Claybourne)	8 oz.	73	14.6
*With rice (Slim-ette)	8 oz. (by wt.)	34	7.2
(Tillie Lewis)	1 cup (8 oz.)	70	11.8
TOMATO SOUP MIX:			
(Lipton) *Cup-a-Soup*	1 pkg. (.8 oz.)	79	17.3
Vegetable:			
With noodles (USDA)	1 oz.	98	17.8
*With noodles (USDA)	1 cup (8 oz.)	62	11.6
*(Golden Grain)	1 cup	80	13.3
*With noodles (Lipton)	1 cup (8 oz.)	68	12.9
TOMCOD, ATLANTIC, raw (USDA):			
Whole	1 lb. (weighed whole)	136	0.
Meat only	4 oz.	87	0.
TOM COLLINS:			
Canned (Party Tyme)			
10% alcohol	2 fl. oz.	58	5.9
Mix (Party Tyme)	½-oz. pkg.	50	13.3
TOM COLLINS or COLLINS MIXER SOFT DRINK:			
(Canada Dry)	6 fl. oz.	60	15.0
(Dr. Brown's)	6 fl. oz.	64	16.1
(Hoffman)	6 fl. oz.	64	16.1
(Kirsch)	6 fl. oz.	60	15.1
(Shasta)	6 fl. oz.	56	16.5
(Yukon Club)	6 fl. oz.	60	15.0
TONGUE (USDA):			
Beef, medium fat, raw, untrimmed	1 lb.	714	1.4
Beef, medium fat, braised	4 oz.	277	.5
Calf, raw, untrimmed	1 lb.	454	3.1
Calf, braised	4 oz.	181	1.1
Hog, raw, untrimmed	1 lb.	741	1.7
Hog, braised	4 oz.	287	.6
Lamb, raw, untrimmed	1 lb.	659	1.7
Lamb, braised	4 oz.	288	.6
Sheep, raw, untrimmed	1 lb.	877	7.9
Sheep, braised	4 oz.	366	2.7

Food and Description	Measure or Quantity	Calories	Carbohydrates (grams)
TONGUE, CANNED:			
Pickled (USDA)	1 oz.	76	<.1
Potted or deviled (USDA)	1 oz.	82	.2
(Hormel)	1 oz. (12-oz. can)	67	<.1
TOPPING (See also **CHOCOLATE SYRUP**):			
Sweetened:			
Butterscotch (Kraft)	1 oz.	84	18.9
Butterscotch (Smucker's)	1 T. (.7 oz.)	66	16.6
Caramel:			
(Smucker's)	1 T. (.7 oz.)	65	16.4
Chocolate (Kraft)	1 oz.	84	18.7
Vanilla (Kraft)	1 oz.	84	19.2
Cherry (Smucker's)	1 T. (.6 oz.)	53	13.5
Chocolate or chocolate flavored:			
(Kraft)	1 oz.	73	18.0
Fudge (Hershey's)	1 T. (.5 oz.)	54	.6
Fudge (Kraft)	1 oz.	74	15.9
Fudge (Smucker's)	1 T. (.7 oz.)	54	13.0
Fudge, mint (Smucker's)	1 T. (.6 oz.)	55	13.0
Milk (Smucker's)	1 T. (.7 oz.)	68	15.1
Marshmallow creme (Kraft)	1 oz.	90	22.9
Mint (Marzetti)	1 T.	38	9.4
Pecan (Kraft)	1 oz.	122	13.6
Pecan in syrup (Smucker's)	1 T. (.7 oz.)	61	14.0
Pineapple (Kraft)	1 oz.	80	19.7
Pineapple (Smucker's)	1 T. (.6 oz.)	53	13.3
Spoonmallow (Kraft)	1 oz.	83	21.9
Strawberry (Kraft)	1 oz.	80	19.7
Strawberry (Smucker's)	1 T. (.6 oz.)	49	12.4
Walnut (Kraft)	1 oz.	113	14.3
Walnut in syrup (Smucker's)	1 T. (.6 oz.)	61	13.5
Dietetic, chocolate (Diet Delight)	1 T. (.6 oz.)	20	4.7
Dietetic, chocolate (Tillie Lewis)	1 T. (.6 oz.)	8	1.5

(USDA): United States Department of Agriculture
(HEW/FAO): Health, Education and Welfare/Food and Agriculture Organization
* Prepared as Package Directs

Food and Description	Measure or Quantity	Calories	Carbo-hydrates (grams)
TOPPING, WHIPPED:			
(USDA) pressurized	1 cup (2.5 oz.)	190	9.0
(USDA) pressurized	1 T. (4 grams)	10	Tr.
(Birds Eye) *Cool Whip*	1 T. (4 grams)	16	1.1
(Kraft)	1 oz.	79	4.3
(Lucky Whip)	1 T. (4 grams)	12	.5
(Sealtest) *Big Top*	1.5 fl. oz. (.5 oz.)	15	.7
(Sealtest) *Zip Whipt*, real cream	1.5 fl. oz. (.4 oz.)	26	1.7
TOPPING, WHIPPED, MIX:			
*(D-Zerta)	1 T.	7	.3
*(Dream Whip)	1 T. (.2 oz.)	14	1.2
*(Lucky Whip)	1 T. (4 grams)	10	1.0
TORTILLA (USDA)	.7-oz. tortilla (5″)	42	9.7
TOTAL, cereal (General Mills)	1¼ cups (1 oz.)	100	23.0
TOWEL GOURD, raw (USDA):			
Unpared	1 lb. (weighed with skin)	69	15.8
Pared	4 oz.	20	4.6
TREET (Armour)	1 oz.	84	.3
TRIPE, beef (USDA):			
Commercial	4 oz.	113	0.
Pickled	4 oz.	70	0.
TRIPLE JACK WINE (Gallo) 20% alcohol	3 fl. oz.	102	6.5
TRIPLE SEC LIQUEUR:			
(Bols) 78 proof	1 fl. oz.	101	8.8
(Garnier) 60 proof	1 fl. oz.	83	8.5
(Hiram Walker) 80 proof	1 fl. oz.	105	9.8
(Leroux) 80 proof	1 fl. oz.	102	8.9
(Old Mr. Boston) 42 proof	1 fl. oz.	97	10.1
(Old Mr. Boston) 60 proof	1 fl. oz.	105	10.1
TRIX, cereal (General Mills)	1 cup (1 oz.)	110	25.2
TROPICAL PUNCH SOFT DRINK (Yukon Club)	6 fl. oz.	90	22.5
TROUT:			
Brook, fresh, whole (USDA)	1 lb. (weighed whole)	224	0.

Food and Description	Measure or Quantity	Calories	Carbo-hydrates (grams)
Brook, fresh, meat only (USDA)	4 oz.	115	0.
Lake (See **LAKE TROUT**)			
Rainbow (USDA):			
Fresh, meat with skin	4 oz.	221	0.
Canned	4 oz.	237	0.
Frozen (1000 Springs):			
Boned	5-oz. trout	135	2.7
Dressed	5-oz. trout	164	3.2
Boned & breaded	5-oz. trout	245	
TUNA:			
Raw, bluefin, meat only (USDA)	4 oz.	164	0.
Raw, yellowfin, meat only (USDA)	4 oz.	151	0.
Canned in oil:			
Solids & liq.:			
(USDA)	6½-oz. can	530	0.
(Breast O' Chicken)	6½-oz. can	540	0.
Chunk (Star-Kist)	6½-oz. can	535	0.
Chunk (Star-Kist)	3¼-oz. can	268	0.
Chunk, light (Chicken of the Sea)	6½-oz. can	405	<1.8
Chunk, light (Del Monte)	6½-oz. can	478	0.
Chunk, light (Del Monte)	1 cup (4.7 oz.)	346	0.
Solid (Star-Kist)	7-oz. can	577	0.
White albacore (Del Monte)	6½-oz. can	543	0.
White albacore (Del Monte)	1 cup (4.7 oz.)	392	0.
Drained solids:			
(USDA)	6½-oz. can	309	0.
Albacore (Del Monte)	1 cup (5.6 oz.)	306	0.
Chunk, light (Chicken of the Sea)	6½-oz. can	294	0.
Chunk, light (Del Monte)	1 cup (5.6 oz.)	374	0.

(USDA): United States Department of Agriculture
(HEW/FAO): Health, Education and Welfare/Food and Agriculture Organization
* Prepared as Package Directs

Food and Description	Measure or Quantity	Calories	Carbohydrates (grams)
Chunk, light (Icy Point)	6½-oz. can	280	0.
Chunk, light (Pillar Rock)	6½-oz. can	280	0.
Chunk, light (Snow Mist)	6½-oz. can	280	0.
Solid, white (Icy Point)	7-oz. can	286	0.
Solid, white (Pillar Rock)	7-oz. can	286	0.
Canned in water:			
Solids & liq. (USDA)	6½-oz. can	234	0.
(Breast O' Chicken)	6½-oz. can	230	0.
Solids & liq. (Star-Kist)	7-oz. can	210	0.
Drained, solid, light (Chicken of the Sea)	6½-oz. can	224	0.
Drained, solid, white (Chicken of the Sea)	6½-oz. can	216	0.
Canned, dietetic:			
Drained, chunk, white (Chicken of the Sea)	6½-oz. can	200	0.
Solids & liq. (Star-Kist)	6½-oz. can	207	0.
Solids & liq. (Star-Kist)	3¼-oz. can	112	0.
TUNA CAKE, frozen, thins (Mrs. Paul's)	10-oz. pkg.	689	47.1
TUNA & NOODLE DINNER (Star-Kist)	15-oz. can	364	
TUNA PIE, frozen:			
(Banquet)	8-oz. pie	479	42.7
(Morton)	8-oz. pie	384	34.0
(Star-Kist)	8-oz. pie	450	
TUNA SALAD, home recipe, made with tuna, celery, mayonnaise, pickle, onion & egg (USDA)	4 oz.	193	4.0
TUNA SOUP, Creole, canned (Crosse & Blackwell)	6½ oz. (½ can)	57	6.6
TURBOT, GREENLAND, raw (USDA):			
Whole	1 lb. (weighed whole)	344	0.

Food and Description	Measure or Quantity	Calories	Carbo-hydrates (grams)
Meat only	4 oz.	166	0.
Frozen (Weight Watchers)	18-oz. dinner	426	17.4
Frozen, with apple (Weight Watchers)	9½-oz. luncheon	277	11.0
TURKEY:			
Raw, ready-to-cook (USDA)	1 lb. (weighed with bones)	722	0.
Raw, light meat (USDA)	4 oz.	132	0.
Raw, dark meat (USDA)	4 oz.	145	0.
Raw, skin only (USDA)	4 oz.	459	0.
Roasted (USDA):			
Flesh, skin & giblets	From 13½-lb. raw ready-to-cook turkey	9678	0.
Flesh & skin	From 13½-lb. raw ready-to-cook turkey	7872	0.
Flesh & skin	4 oz.	253	0.
Meat only:			
Chopped	1 cup (5 oz.)	268	0.
Diced	1 cup (4.8 oz.)	256	0.
Light	4 oz.	200	0.
Light	1 slice (4″ x 2″ x ¼″, 3 oz.)	75	0.
Dark	4 oz.	230	0.
Dark	1 slice (2½″ x 1⅝″ x ¼″, .7 oz.)	43	0.
Skin only	1 oz.	128	0.
Giblets, simmered (USDA)	2 oz.	132	.9
Smoked, cooked, pressed (Oscar Mayer)	.8-oz. slice	23	0.
Canned, boned:			
(USDA)	4 oz.	229	0.
Solids & liq. (Lynden Farms)	5-oz. jar	239	0.
(Swanson) with broth	5-oz. jar	217	0.
Canned, roast (Wilson)			
Tender Made	4 oz.	117	0.

(USDA): United States Department of Agriculture
(HEW/FAO): Health, Education and Welfare/Food and Agriculture
    Organization
* Prepared as Package Directs

Food and Description	Measure or Quantity	Calories	Carbo-hydrates (grams)
TURKEY DINNER:			
Canned, noodle (Lynden Farms)	15-oz. can	463	34.0
Frozen:			
Sliced turkey, mashed potato, peas (USDA)	12 oz.	381	43.2
(Banquet)	11-oz. dinner	293	27.8
(Morton)	11-oz. dinner	346	28.1
(Morton) 3-course	16¾-oz. dinner	613	76.0
(Swanson)	11½-oz. dinner	401	43.7
(Swanson) 3-course	16-oz. dinner	501	54.5
With gravy, dressing & potato (Swanson)	8¾-oz. pkg.	292	27.5
(Weight Watchers)	18-oz. dinner	302	12.4
TURKEY FRICASSEE, canned (Lynden Farms)	14.5-oz. can	366	28.8
TURKEY GIZZARD (USDA):			
Raw	4 oz.	178	1.2
Simmered	4 oz.	222	1.2
TURKEY PIE:			
Home recipe, baked (USDA)	⅓ of 9″ pie (8.2 oz.)	550	42.2
Frozen:			
Commercial, unheated (USDA)	8 oz.	447	45.6
(Banquet)	8-oz. pie	415	40.6
(Banquet)	2-lb. 4-oz. pie	1327	135.2
(Morton)	8-oz. pie	411	34.0
(Swanson)	8-oz. pie	422	37.5
(Swanson) deep-dish	1-lb. pie	746	63.8
TURKEY, POTTED (USDA)	1 oz.	70	0.
TURKEY SOUP, canned:			
(Campbell) *Chunky*	1 cup	112	10.8
Broth (Lynden Farms)	1 cup (8 oz.)	14	0.
Noodle:			
Condensed (USDA)	8 oz. (by wt.)	147	15.9
*Prepared with equal volume water (USDA)	1 cup (8.8 oz.)	82	8.8
*(Campbell)	1 cup	72	7.5
*(Heinz)	1 cup (8½ oz.)	83	10.0
(Heinz) *Great American*	1 cup (8¾ oz.)	97	12.1
Low sodium (Campbell)	7½-oz. can	78	9.2

Food and Description	Measure or Quantity	Calories	Carbohydrates (grams)
Rice, with mushrooms (Heinz) *Great American*	1 cup (8½ oz.)	101	13.2
*Vegetable (Campbell)	1 cup	73	8.0
Vegetable (Heinz) *Great American*	1 cup (8½ oz.)	98	13.2
*TURKEY SOUP MIX, noodle (Lipton)	1 cup (8 oz.)	61	7.4
TURKEY TETRAZZINI, frozen (Stouffer's)	12-oz. pkg.	694	68.7
TURNIP (USDA):			
Fresh, without tops	1 lb. (weighed with skins)	117	25.7
Fresh, pared, diced	½ cup (2.4 oz.)	20	4.4
Fresh, pared, slices	½ cup (2.3 oz.)	19	4.2
Boiled, drained, diced	½ cup (2.8 oz.)	18	3.8
Boiled, drained, mashed	½ cup (4 oz.)	26	5.6
TURNIP GREENS, leaves & stems:			
Fresh (USDA)	1 lb. (weighed untrimmed)	107	19.0
Boiled, in small amount water, short time, drained (USDA)	½ cup (2.5 oz.)	14	2.6
Boiled, in large amount water, long time, drained (USDA)	½ cup (2.5 oz.)	14	2.4
Canned, solids & liq.:			
(USDA)	½ cup (4.1 oz.)	21	3.7
(Stokely-Van Camp)	½ cup (3.9 oz.)	20	3.5
Frozen:			
Not thawed (USDA)	4 oz.	26	4.5
Boiled, drained (USDA)	½ cup (2.9 oz.)	19	3.2
Chopped (Birds Eye)	½ cup (3.3 oz.)	22	2.7

TURNOVER (See individual kinds)

(USDA): United States Department of Agriculture
(HEW/FAO): Health, Education and Welfare/Food and Agriculture Organization
* Prepared as Package Directs

Food and Description	Measure or Quantity	Calories	Carbo-hydrates (grams)
TURTLE, GREEN (USDA):			
Raw, in shell	1 lb. (weighed in shell)	97	0.
Raw, meat only	4 oz.	101	0.
Canned	4 oz.	120	0,
TV DINNER (See individual listing such as **BEEF DINNER, CHICKEN DINNER, CHINESE DINNER, ENCHILADA DINNER,** etc.)			
20/20 WINE (Mogen David)			
20% alcohol	3 fl. oz.	105	9.8
TWINKIE (Hostess)	1 cake (1½ oz.)	162	25.5
TWISTER, wine (Gallo)			
20% alcohol	3 fl. oz.	109	8.2

U

UPPER-10, soft drink	6 fl. oz. (6.5 oz.)	78	18.5

V

VALPOLICELLA WINE, Italian red (Antinori)	3 fl. oz.	84	6.3
VANDERMINT, Dutch liqueur, (Park Avenue Imports)			
60 proof	1 fl. oz.	90	10.2
VANILLA:			
Extract (Ehlers)	1 tsp.	8	
Pure extract (French's)	1 tsp.	13	
Imitation (French's)	1 tsp.	12	
VANILLA CAKE, frozen (Pepperidge Farm)	⅛ of cake (3.1 oz.)	332	47.3

Food and Description	Measure or Quantity	Calories	Carbohydrates (grams)
VANILLA ICE CREAM (See also individual brand names):			
(Borden) 10.5% fat	¼ pt. (2.3 oz.)	132	15.8
Lady Borden, 14% fat	¼ pt. (2.5 oz.)	162	17.0
(Meadow Gold) 10% fat	¼ pt.	126	15.0
(Sealtest) *Party Slice*	¼ pt. (2.3 oz.)	133	15.8
(Sealtest) 10.2% fat	¼ pt. (2.3 oz.)	133	15.8
(Sealtest) 12.1% fat	¼ pt. (2.3 oz.)	144	16.1
French (Prestige)	¼ pt. (2.6 oz.)	183	15.8
Fudge royale (Sealtest)	¼ pt. (2.3 oz.)	132	18.2
VANILLA ICE MILK			
(Borden) *Lite-line*	¼ pt.	108	17.2
VANILLA PIE FILLING MIX (See **VANILLA PUDDING MIX**)			
VANILLA PUDDING:			
Blancmange, home recipe, with starch base (USDA)	½ cup (4.5 oz.)	142	20.4
Canned (Betty Crocker)	½ cup	170	29.5
Canned (Del Monte)	5-oz. can	190	32.8
Canned (Hunt's)	5-oz. can	238	30.2
Canned (My-T-Fine) *Rich 'N Ready*	5-oz. can	192	34.4
Canned (Thank You)	½ cup (4.5 oz.)	169	29.2
Chilled (Breakstone)	5-oz. container	252	32.5
Chilled (Sealtest)	4 oz.	125	20.9
(Sanna) *Swiss Miss*	4¼-oz. container	172	25.7
VANILLA PUDDING or PIE FILLING MIX:			
Sweetened:			
*Regular, plain or French (Jell-O)	½ cup (5.2 oz.)	173	29.3
*Instant, plain or French (Jell-O)	½ cup (5.3 oz.)	178	30.5
*Regular (My-T-Fine)	½ cup (5 oz.)	176	32.7
*Regular (Royal)	½ cup (5.1 oz.)	163	26.4
*Instant (Royal)	½ cup (5.1 oz.)	176	28.8
*Low calorie (D-Zerta)	½ cup (4.6 oz.)	107	12.2

(USDA): United States Department of Agriculture
(HEW/FAO): Health, Education and Welfare/Food and Agriculture Organization
* Prepared as Package Directs

Food and Description	Measure or Quantity	Calories	Carbo-hydrates (grams)
VANILLA RENNET MIX:			
Powder:			
Dry (Junket)	1 oz.	116	28.0
*(Junket)	4 oz.	108	14.7
Tablet:			
Dry (Junket)	1 tablet (<1 gram)	1	.2
*& sugar (Junket)	4 oz.	101	13.5
VANILLA SOFT DRINK,			
(Yoo-Hoo) high-protein	6 fl. oz. (6.4 oz.)	100	18.9
VEAL, medium fat (USDA):			
Chuck, raw	1 lb. (weighed with bone)	628	0.
Chuck, braised, lean & fat	4 oz.	266	0.
Flank, raw	1 lb. (weighed with bone)	1410	0.
Flank, stewed, lean & fat	4 oz.	442	0.
Foreshank, raw	1 lb. (weighed with bone)	368	0.
Foreshank, stewed, lean & fat	4 oz.	245	0.
Loin, raw	1 lb. (weighed with bone)	681	0.
Loin, broiled, medium done, chop, lean & fat	4 oz.	265	0.
Plate, raw	1 lb. (weighed with bone)	828	0.
Plate, stewed, lean & fat	4 oz.	344	0.
Rib, raw, lean & fat	1 lb. (weighed with bone)	723	0.
Rib, roasted, medium done, lean & fat	4 oz.	305	0.
Round & rump, raw	1 lb. (weighed with bone)	573	0.
Round & rump, broiled, steak or cutlet, lean & fat	4 oz. (weighed without bone)	245	0.
VEAL DINNER, frozen:			
Breaded veal with spaghetti in tomato sauce (Swanson)	8¼-oz. pkg.	272	24.9
Parmigiana (Kraft)	11-oz. dinner	474	25.9
Parmigiana (Swanson)	12¼-oz. dinner	492	47.7
Parmigiana (Weight Watchers)	9½-oz. luncheon	260	8.1

Food and Description	Measure or Quantity	Calories	Carbo-hydrates (grams)
VEGETABLE BOUILLON			
CUBE:			
(Herb-Ox)	1 cube (4 grams)	6	.5
(Steero)	1 cube (4 grams)	4	<.1
(Wyler's)	1 cube (4 grams)	7	.3
VEGETABLE FAT (See FAT)			
VEGETABLE JUICE			
COCKTAIL, canned:			
(USDA)	4 oz. (by wt.)	19	4.1
Unseasoned (S and W)			
Nutradiet	4 oz. (by wt.)	24	5.1
V-8 (Campbell)	¾ cup	31	6.0
VEGETABLES, MIXED:			
Canned, regular pack:			
(Veg-All)	½ cup (4 oz.)	39	7.8
Solids & liq. (Del Monte)	½ cup (4 oz.)	46	7.4
Drained solids (Del Monte)	½ cup (2.8 oz.)	41	7.4
Drained liq. (Del Monte)	4 oz.	22	3.7
Solids & liq. (Stokely-Van Camp)	½ cup (3.8 oz.)	71	15.0
Canned, Chinese:			
(La Choy)	1 cup	22	4.0
Chow Mein, drained (Chun King)	1 cup	23	3.5
Drained (Chun King)	1 cup	20	3.1
Chop Suey (Hung's)	4 oz.	20	3.0
Chop Suey (La Choy)	1 cup	30	5.0
Frozen:			
Not thawed (USDA)	4 oz.	74	15.5
Boiled, drained (USDA)	½ cup (3.2 oz.)	58	12.2
(Birds Eye)	½ cup (3.3 oz.)	50	12.4
In butter sauce (Green Giant)	⅓ of 10-oz. pkg.	67	10.3
Chinese (Birds Eye)	⅓ of 10-oz. pkg.	65	6.0
Jubilee (Birds Eye)	⅓ of 10-oz. pkg.	138	18.9
With onion sauce (Birds Eye)	½ cup (2.7 oz.)	117	13.6

(USDA): United States Department of Agriculture
(HEW/FAO): Health, Education and Welfare/Food and Agriculture Organization
* Prepared as Package Directs

Food and Description	Measure or Quantity	Calories	Carbo- hydrates (grams)
VEGETABLE OYSTER (See **SALSIFY**)			
VEGETABLE SOUP:			
Canned, regular pack:			
*(Campbell)	1 cup	77	12.6
(Campbell) *Chunky*	1 cup	105	16.5
*(Campbell) old-fashioned	1 cup	70	8.9
Beef, condensed (USDA)	8 oz. (by wt.)	147	17.9
*Beef, prepared with equal volume water (USDA)	1 cup (8.6 oz.)	78	9.6
*Beef (Campbell)	1 cup	75	7.3
*Beef (Heinz)	1 cup (8½ oz.)	66	9.6
Beef (Heinz) *Great American*	1 cup (8¾ oz.)	126	12.2
With beef broth, condensed (USDA)	8 oz. (by wt.)	145	24.9
*With beef broth, prepared with equal volume water (USDA)	1 cup (8.8 oz.)	80	13.8
With beef broth (Heinz) *Great American*	1 cup (8¾ oz.)	144	18.4
*With beef stock (Heinz)	1 cup (8½ oz.)	83	13.4
With ground beef (Heinz) *Great American*	1 cup (8¾ oz.)	139	12.1
*& *Noodle-O's* (Campbell)	1 cup	71	9.7
Vegetarian:			
Condensed (USDA)	8 oz. (by wt.)	145	24.0
*Prepared with equal volume water (USDA)	1 cup (8.6 oz.)	78	13.2
*(Campbell)	1 cup	71	11.8
*(Heinz)	1 cup (8¾ oz.)	83	14.2
(Heinz) *Great American*	1 cup (8½ oz.)	125	18.1
*(Manischewitz)	1 cup	63	10.2
Canned, dietetic pack:			
Low sodium (Campbell)	7½-oz. can	83	14.4
Beef, low sodium (Campbell)	7½-oz. can	78	8.8
*(Claybourne)	8 oz.	104	21.0
*(Slim-ette)	8 oz. (by wt.)	46	9.9
(Tillie Lewis)	1 cup (8 oz.)	62	11.1
Frozen:			
With beef, condensed (USDA)	8 oz. (by wt.)	159	15.9

Food and Description	Measure or Quantity	Calories	Carbohydrates (grams)
*With beef, prepared with equal volume water (USDA)	8 oz. (by wt.)	79	7.7
VEGETABLE SOUP MIX:			
*(Wyler's)	1 cup	56	9.6
*Beef (Lipton)	1 cup	58	8.2
*Chicken (Wyler's)	1 cup	37	5.7
Country (Lipton)	1 pkg. (2.4 oz.)	231	42.5
*& noodle (Goodman's)	1 cup	37	
*& noodle (Lipton) Country	1 cup	75	14.0
Spring (Lipton) *Cup-a-Soup*	½-oz. pkg.	42	7.5
VEGETABLE STEW, canned (Hormel) *Dinty Moore*	8 oz.	170	19.5
"VEGETARIAN FOODS":			
Canned or dry:			
Beans, rich brown (Loma Linda)	½ cup (3.7 oz.)	122	21.8
Bean, soy:			
Boston-style (Loma Linda)	½ cup (3.7 oz.)	141	14.9
Green, drained (Loma Linda)	½ cup (3.7 oz.)	109	7.9
Tomato sauce (Loma Linda)	½ cup (3.7 oz.)	118	8.7
Big franks, drained (Loma Linda)	1 frank (1.6 oz.)	86	2.4
Breading meal (Loma Linda)	1 cup (3.7 oz.)	364	61.3
Breading meal (Worthington)	¼ cup (1.1 oz.)	116	21.0
Burger Aid (Worthington)	1 oz.	102	9.0
Cheze-O-Soy (Worthington)	½" slice (2.5 oz.)	125	6.4
Chili (Worthington)	¼ can (5 oz.)	166	14.0
Chili with beans (Loma Linda)	½ cup (4.7 oz.)	158	22.0
Choplet (Worthington)	1 choplet (2.2 oz.)	72	3.1

(USDA): United States Department of Agriculture
(HEW/FAO): Health, Education and Welfare/Food and Agriculture Organization
* Prepared as Package Directs

Food and Description	Measure or Quantity	Calories	Carbo-hydrates (grams)
Choplet burger (Worthington)	⅓ cup (3.2 oz.)	118	11.5
Cutlet (Worthington)	1 cutlet (2.2 oz.)	71	3.1
Dinner bits, drained (Loma Linda)	1 bit (.5 oz.)	23	.6
Dinner cuts, drained (Loma Linda)	1 cut (1.6 oz.)	45	1.9
Dinner cuts, no salt added, drained (Loma Linda)	1 cup (1.6 oz.)	46	2.5
Fry stick (Worthington)	1 piece (2.3 oz.)	103	5.2
Garbanzo (Loma Linda)	½ cup (4.1 oz.)	145	25.5
GranBurger (Worthington)	1 oz.	96	6.3
Granola (Loma Linda)	½ cup (2 oz.)	246	36.0
Gravy Quik, brown (Loma Linda)	⅛ of pkg. (6 grams)	15	2.3
J-7901 or J-7901A (Worthington)	1 oz.	95	5.2
Jell Quik, dry (Loma Linda)	1 oz.	106	26.4
Kaffir Tea (Worthington)	1 bag (1 gram)	3	.6
Lentils, drained (Loma Linda)	¾ cup (3.5 oz.)	91	15.0
Linketts, drained (Loma Linda)	1 link (1.3 oz.)	76	.9
Little links, drained (Loma Linda)	1 link (.8 oz.)	45	1.3
Madison burger (Worthington)	⅓ cup (2 oz.)	86	2.3
Meat-like loaf (Loma Linda):			
Beef, drained	¼" slice (2 oz.)	120	2.8
Chicken	¼" slice (2 oz.)	114	1.7
Luncheon	¼" slice (2 oz.)	122	2.8
Turkey	¼" slice (2 oz.)	125	2.3
Meat loaf mix (Worthington)	2 oz.	236	22.0
Multigen powder (Loma Linda)	½ cup (2.1 oz.)	227	39.1
Non-meatballs (Worthington)	1 piece (.6 oz.)	35	1.1
Not meat with tomato (Worthington)	2⅓ oz.	214	18.1
Numete (Worthington)	½" slice (2.3 oz.)	163	7.0

Food and Description	Measure or Quantity	Calories	Carbo-hydrates (grams)
Nuteena (Loma Linda)	½" slice (2.5 oz.)	152	5.5
Oven-cooked wheat (Loma Linda)	½ cup (2.6 oz.)	263	53.1
Peanuts & soya (USDA)	4 oz.	269	15.2
Prime vegetable burger (Worthington)	½" slice (2.1 oz.)	74	3.5
Proteena (Loma Linda)	½" slice (2.6 oz.)	141	4.1
Protose, canned (Worthington)	½" slice (2.7 oz.)	175	5.9
Rediburger (Loma Linda)	½" slice (2.5 oz.)	153	3.9
Redi-loaf mix, beef (Loma Linda)	⅓ cup (1.2 oz.)	160	8.2
Redi-loaf mix, chicken (Loma Linda)	⅓ cup (1.2 oz.)	159	8.1
Ruskets, biscuits (Loma Linda)	1 biscuit (.6 oz.)	65	13.8
Ruskets, flakes (Loma Linda)	1 cup (1 oz.)	101	21.4
Sandwich spread (Loma Linda)	1 T. (.6 oz.)	23	1.8
Sandwich spread (Worthington)	3 T. (1.2 oz.)	79	3.5
Saucette (Worthington)	1 link (.6 oz.)	39	.5
Savita (Worthington)	1 tsp. (.4 oz.)	20	1.3
Savorex (Loma Linda)	1 oz.	52	5.6
Seasoning, chicken (Loma Linda)	1 T. (3 grams)	8	1.0
Soyagen:			
A.P. & malt powder (Loma Linda)	¼ cup (1.4 oz.)	184	18.7
Carob, powder (Loma Linda)	¼ cup (1.4 oz.)	184	19.4
Liquid (Loma Linda)	1 cup (8.6 oz.)	146	11.0
Soyalac, concentrate, liquid (Loma Linda)	1 fl. oz. (1.1 oz.)	41	3.6
Soyalac, infant powder (Loma Linda)	1 oz.	136	12.4
Soyalac, ready-to-use (Loma Linda)	1 oz.	19	1.7

(USDA): United States Department of Agriculture
(HEW/FAO): Health, Education and Welfare/Food and Agriculture Organization
* Prepared as Package Directs

Food and Description	Measure or Quantity	Calories	Carbohydrates (grams)
Soyamel, any kind (Worthington)	1 oz.	129	12.3
Soyameat (Worthington):			
Slice beef	1 slice (1 oz.)	69	3.3
Diced beef	1 oz.	30	1.4
Dice chicken	1 oz.	30	.6
Fried chicken	1 piece (1.2 oz.)	64	.5
Sliced chicken	1 slice (1.1 oz.)	34	.1
Salisbury steak	1 slice (2.5 oz.)	157	7.0
Soy flour (Loma Linda)	¼ cup (.9 oz.)	115	7.0
Stew pac, drained (Loma Linda)	½ cup (3 oz.)	138	5.4
Stripple Zips (Worthington)	1 oz.	131	2.9
Tamales (Worthington)	1 oz.	23	4.0
Tastee cuts (Loma Linda)	1 cut (1.5 oz.)	42	1.5
Tenderbit (Loma Linda)	1 piece (.9 oz.)	28	1.6
Vegeburger (Loma Linda)	½ cup (3.9 oz.)	126	4.6
Vegeburger, no salt added (Loma Linda)	½ cup (3.9 oz.)	132	5.9
Vegechee (Loma Linda)	½" slice (2.5 oz.)	106	3.2
Vegelona (Loma Linda)	½" slice (3.3 oz.)	154	5.2
Vegetable skallop (Worthington)	1 piece (.7 oz.)	26	.9
Vegetable steaks (Worthington)	1 piece (.7 oz.)	21	1.8
Vegetarian burger (Worthington)	⅓ cup (2.5 oz.)	104	3.2
Veja-links (Worthington)	1 link (1.2 oz.)	72	1.2
Wham, sliced or loaf (Worthington)	1 slice (1 oz.)	46	1.3
Wheat germ, natural or toasted (Loma Linda)	1 T. (.4 oz.)	40	4.6
Wheat protein (USDA)	4 oz.	124	10.0
Wheat protein, nuts or peanuts (USDA)	4 oz.	240	20.1
Wheat protein, vegetable oil (USDA)	4 oz.	214	5.9
Wheat & soy protein (USDA)	4 oz.	118	8.6
Wheat & soy protein, soy or other vegetable oil (USDA)	4 oz.	170	10.8
Worthington 209	1 slice (.5 oz.)	18	.5
Yum (Worthington)	1 serving (1.5 oz.)	89	3.2

Food and Description	Measure or Quantity	Calories	Carbo-hydrates (grams)
Frozen (Worthington):			
Beef pie	1 pie (7.9 oz.)	506	51.5
Beef style, loaf or sliced	1 slice (1 oz.)	52	1.4
Chicken pie	1 pie (7.9 oz.)	450	41.4
Chicken style, diced, roll or sliced	1 oz. or 1 slice	72	.8
Chic-Ketts	1 oz.	55	1.1
Chili	¼ can (5 oz.)	176	16.8
Corned beef, loaf or sliced	1 slice (.5 oz.)	36	1.2
Croquettes	1 croquette (1 oz.)	69	5.0
FriPats	1 pat (2.6 oz.)	198	11.5
Holiday roast	1 slice (2 oz.)	142	3.7
Non-meatballs	1 piece (.6 oz.)	55	1.7
Prosage	⅜" slice (1.2 oz.)	81	3.5
Salisbury steak	1 slice (2 oz.)	111	6.5
Smoked beef, roll or sliced	1 slice (7 grams)	15	.4
Stripples	1 slice (7 grams)	17	.3
Turkey, smoked, loaf or sliced	1 slice (.7 oz.)	46	1.2
Wham, diced, sliced or loaf	1 slice (1 oz.)	53	1.2
VENISON, raw, lean meat only (USDA)	4 oz.	143	0.
VERMOUTH:			
Dry & extra dry:			
(C & P) 19% alcohol	3 fl. oz.	90	3.0
(Gallo) 18% alcohol	3 fl. oz.	75	1.7
(Gancia) 21% alcohol	3 fl. oz.	126	
(Lejon) 18.5% alcohol	3 fl. oz.	99	2.2
(Noilly Pratt) 19% alcohol	3 fl. oz.	101	1.6
(Taylor) 17% alcohol	3 fl. oz.	102	.9
Rosso (Gancia) 21% alcohol	3 fl. oz.	153	6.9
Sweet:			
(C & P) 16% alcohol	3 fl. oz.	120	14.4
(Gallo) 18% alcohol	3 fl. oz.	118	12.3
(Lejon) 18.5% alcohol	3 fl. oz.	134	11.4
(Noilly Pratt) 16% alcohol	3 fl. oz.	128	12.1
(Taylor) 17% alcohol	3 fl. oz.	132	10.4
White (Gancia) 16.8% alcohol	3 fl. oz.	132	7.8

(USDA): United States Department of Agriculture
(HEW/FAO): Health, Education and Welfare/Food and Agriculture Organization
* Prepared as Package Directs

Food and Description	Measure or Quantity	Calories	Carbo- hydrates (grams)
White (Lejon) 18.5% alcohol	3 fl. oz.	101	2.6
VERNORS, soft drink:			
Regular	6 fl. oz. (6.2 oz.)	70	16.8
Low calorie	6 fl. oz. (6.2 oz.)	1	<.1
VICHYSSOISE SOUP (Crosse & Blackwell)	½ can (6½ oz.)	94	9.4
VIENNA SAUSAGE, canned:			
(USDA)	1 oz.	68	<.1
(USDA)	1 sausage (from 5-oz. can, .6 oz.)	38	<.1
(Armour Star)	5-oz. can	393	0.
(Armour Star)	1 sausage (.6 oz.)	45	0.
(Hormel)	1 sausage (.6 oz.)	42	.5
(Libby's)	4 oz.	318	1.6
(Van Camp)	1 oz.	68	<.1
(Wilson)	1 oz.	85	<.1
VILLA ANTINORI, Italian white wine, 12½% alcohol	3 fl. oz.	87	6.3
VINEGAR:			
Cider:			
(USDA)	½ cup (4.2 oz.)	17	7.1
(USDA)	1 T. (.5 oz.)	2	.9
Distilled:			
(USDA)	½ cup (4.2 oz.)	14	6.0
(USDA)	1 T. (.5 oz.)	2	.8
Red or white wine (Regina)	1 T. (.5 oz.)	3	5.1
VINESPINACH or **BASELLA**, raw (USDA)	4 oz.	22	3.9
VINO PRIMO WINE (United Vintners) 12% alcohol	3 fl. oz.	66	1.6
VIN ROSÉ (See **ROSÉ WINE**)			
VIRGIN SOUR MIX (Party Tyme)	½-oz. pkg.	50	13.2
VODKA, unflavored (See **DISTILLED LIQUOR**)			

Food and Description	Measure or Quantity	Calories	Carbo-hydrates (grams)
VODKA, FLAVORED (Old Mr. Boston):			
Wild cherry, grape, lemon, lime or orange, 70 proof	1 fl. oz.	100	8.0
Peppermint, 70 proof	1 fl. oz.	90	5.0
VODKA SCREWDRIVER (Old Mr. Boston) 25 proof	3 fl. oz.	117	10.5
VODKA SOFT DRINK, sweetened (Shasta)	6 fl. oz.	66	16.7
VODKA & TONIC, canned (Party Tyme) 10% alcohol	2 fl. oz.	55	5.1
VOIGNY WINE (Chanson) 13% alcohol	3 fl. oz.	96	7.5

W

Food and Description	Measure or Quantity	Calories	Carbo-hydrates (grams)
WAFER (See **COOKIE** or **CRACKER**)			
WAFFLE:			
Home recipe (USDA)	2.6-oz. waffle (7" dia.)	209	28.1
Frozen:			
(USDA)	1.6-oz. waffle (8 in 13-oz. pkg.)	116	19.3
(USDA)	.8-oz. waffle (6 in 5-oz. pkg.)	61	10.1
Original (Aunt Jemima)	2 sections (1.5 oz.)	117	16.2
WAFFLE MIX (USDA) (See also **PANCAKE & WAFFLE MIX**):			
Dry, complete mix	1 oz.	130	18.5

(USDA): United States Department of Agriculture
(HEW/FAO): Health, Education and Welfare/Food and Agriculture Organization
* Prepared as Package Directs

d ...ption	Measure or Quantity	Calories	Carbo- hydrates (grams)
*Prepared with water	2.6-oz. waffle (½" x 4½" x 5½", 7" dia.)	229	30.2
Dry, incomplete mix	1 oz.	101	21.5
*Prepared with egg & milk	2.6-oz. waffle (7" dia.)	206	27.2
*Prepared with egg & milk	7.1-oz. waffle (9" x 9" x ⅝", 1⅛ cup batter)	550	72.4

WAFFLE SYRUP (See **SYRUP**)

WALNUT:
Black:

In shell, whole (USDA)	1 lb. (weighed in shell)	627	14.8
Shelled, whole (USDA)	4 oz.	712	16.8
Chopped (USDA)	½ cup (2.1 oz.)	377	8.9
Kernels (Hammons)	4 oz.	746	11.6

English or Persian:

In shell, whole (USDA)	1 lb. (weighed in shell)	1329	32.2
Shelled, whole (USDA)	4 oz.	738	17.9
Chopped (USDA)	½ cup (2.1 oz.)	391	9.5
Chopped (USDA)	1 T. (8 grams)	49	1.2
Halves (USDA)	½ cup (1.8 oz.)	326	7.9
(Diamond)	3-oz. bag (¾ cup)	564	15.0
(Diamond)	15 halves (.5 oz.)	99	2.7

WALNUT, BLACK, EXTRACT:

(Ehlers)	1 tsp.	4	
Imitation (French's)	1 tsp.	12	

*WALNUT CAKE MIX, BLACK (Betty Crocker) | ¹⁄₁₂ of cake | 202 | 36.3 |

WATER CHESTNUT, CHINESE, raw (USDA):

Whole	1 lb. (weighed unpeeled)	272	66.4
Peeled	4 oz.	90	21.5

WATERCRESS, raw (USDA):

Untrimmed	½ lb. (weighed untrimmed)	40	6.2
Trimmed	½ cup (.6 oz.)	3	.5

Food and Description	Measure or Quantity	Calories	Carbo-hydrates (grams)
WATERMELON, fresh (USDA):			
Whole	1 lb. (weighed with rind)	54	13.4
Wedge	2-lb. wedge (4" x 8" measured with rind)	111	27.3
Slice	½ slice (12.2 oz., ¾" x 10")	41	10.2
Diced	1 cup (5.6 oz.)	42	10.2
WATERMELON RIND (Crosse & Blackwell)	1 T. (.6 oz.)	38	9.3
WATERMELON SOFT DRINK, sweetened:			
(Hoffman)	6 fl. oz.	91	22.6
(Nedick's)	6 fl. oz.	91	22.6
WAX GOURD, raw (USDA):			
Whole	1 lb. (weighed with skin & cavity contents)	41	9.4
Flesh only	4 oz.	15	3.4
WEAKFISH (USDA):			
Raw, whole	1 lb. (weighed whole)	263	0.
Broiled, meat only	4 oz.	236	0.
WELSH RAREBIT:			
Home recipe (USDA)	1 cup (8.2 oz.)	415	14.6
Canned (Snow)	4 oz.	171	8.4
WEST INDIAN CHERRY (See **ACEROLA**)			
WHALE MEAT, raw (USDA)	4 oz.	177	0.
WHEAT CHEX, cereal	⅔ cup (1 oz.)	108	23.0
WHEATENA, cereal	½ cup (.9 oz. dry)	88	18.1
WHEAT FLAKES, cereal, crushed (USDA)	1 cup (2.5 oz.)	248	56.4

(USDA): United States Department of Agriculture
(HEW/FAO): Health, Education and Welfare/Food and Agriculture Organization
* Prepared as Package Directs

Food and Description	Measure or Quantity	Calories	Carbo-hydrates (grams)
WHEAT GERM, crude, commercial, milled (USDA)	1 oz.	103	13.2
WHEAT GERM, CEREAL:			
(USDA)	¼ cup (1 oz.)	110	14.0
(Kretschmer)	¼ cup (1 oz.)	106	12.6
With sugar & honey (Kretschmer)	¼ cup (1 oz.)	107	26.9
WHEATIES, cereal	1¼ cups (1 oz.)	101	23.1
WHEAT OATA, cereal	¼ cup (1 oz.)	104	19.6
WHEAT, PUFFED, cereal:			
Added nutrients (USDA)	1 cup (.4 oz.)	44	9.4
Frosted with sugar and honey (USDA)	1 cup (.4 oz.)	45	10.6
(Checker)	½ oz.	51	11.0
(Quaker)	1⅓ cups (½ oz.)	51	11.2
(Sunland)	½ oz.	51	11.0
(Whiffs)	½ oz.	51	11.0
WHEAT, ROLLED (USDA):			
Uncooked	1 cup (3.1 oz.)	296	66.3
Cooked	1 cup (7.7 oz.)	163	36.7
WHEAT, SHREDDED, cereal (See **SHREDDED WHEAT**)			
WHEY, fluid (USDA)	1 cup (8.6 oz.)	63	12.4
***WHIP 'N CHILL** (Jell-O):*			
All flavors except chocolate	½ cup (3 oz.)	135	19.3
Chocolate	½ cup (3 oz.)	144	22.0
WHISKEY or **WHISKY** (See **DISTILLED LIQUOR**)			
WHISKEY SOUR:			
Canned (Hiram Walker)	3 fl. oz.	177	12.0
(National Distillers) *Duet,* canned 12½ % alcohol	8-fl.-oz. can	256	17.6
Mix (Bar-Tender's)	1 serving (⅝ oz.)	70	17.2
Mix (Party Tyme)	½-oz. pkg.	50	13.5
WHISKEY SOUR SOFT DRINK, sweetened (Shasta)	6 fl. oz.	65	16.5

Food and Description	Measure or Quantity	Calories	Carbohydrates (grams)
WHITEFISH, LAKE (USDA):			
Raw, whole	1 lb. (weighed whole)	330	0.
Raw, meat only	4 oz.	176	0.
Baked, stuffed, made with bacon, butter, onion, celery & bread crumbs, home recipe	4 oz.	244	6.6
Smoked	4 oz.	176	0.
WHITEFISH & PIKE (See **GEFILTE FISH**)			
WIENER (See **FRANKFURTER**)			
WILD BERRY, fruit drink (Hi-C)	6 fl. oz. (6.3 oz.)	90	21.8
WILD RICE, raw (USDA)	½ cup (2.9 oz.)	289	61.7
WINE (most wines are listed by kind, brand, vineyard, region or grape name):			
Cooking, Sauterne or Burgundy (Regina)	½ cup (3.9 oz.)	93	4.6
Cooking, Sherry (Regina)	½ cup (3.9 oz.)	158	11.5
Dessert (USDA) 18.8% alcohol	3 fl. oz. (3.1 oz.)	122	6.9
Dessert (Petri)	3 fl. oz.	124	
Flavored (Petri)	3 fl. oz.	124	
Table:			
(USDA) 12.2% alcohol	3 fl. oz. (3.1 oz.)	75	3.7
(Petri)	3 fl. oz.	59	
(Great Western) red or white, *Pleasant Valley*, 12% alcohol	3 fl. oz.	88	4.7
WINK, soft drink (Canada Dry)	6 fl. oz. (6.4 oz.)	85	22.8

(USDA): United States Department of Agriculture
(HEW/FAO): Health, Education and Welfare/Food and Agriculture Organization
* Prepared as Package Directs

Food and Description	Measure or Quantity	Calories	Carbo-hydrates (grams)
WINTERGREEN EXTRACT:			
(Ehlers)	1 tsp.	11	
(French's)	1 tsp.	24	
WON TON SOUP, canned			
(Mow Sang)	10-oz. can	134	21.0
WORCESTERSHIRE SAUCE (See **SAUCE,** Worcestershire)			
WRECKFISH, raw, meat only			
(USDA)	4 oz.	129	0.

Y

YAM (USDA):			
Raw, whole	1 lb. (weighed with skin)	394	90.5
Raw, flesh only	4 oz.	115	26.3
Canned & frozen (See **SWEET POTATO**)			
YAM BEAN, raw (USDA):			
Unpared tuber	1 lb. (weighed unpared)	225	52.2
Pared tuber	4 oz.	62	14.5
YANKEE DOODLES:			
(Drake's)	1 cake (1 oz.)	120	18.0
(Drake's)	1 cake (1.1 oz.)	140	21.0
YEAST:			
Baker's:			
Compressed (USDA)	1 oz.	24	3.1
Compressed (Fleischmann's)	⅗-oz. cake	19	1.9
Dry (USDA)	1 oz.	80	11.0
Dry (USDA)	1 pkg. (7 grams)	20	2.7
Dry (Fleischmann's)	¼ oz. (pkg. or jar)	24	2.9
Brewer's dry, debittered (USDA)	1 oz.	80	10.9
Brewer's dry, debittered (USDA)	1 T. (8 grams)	23	3.1

Food and Description	Measure or Quantity	Calories	Carbo- hydrates (grams)
YELLOWTAIL, raw, meat only (USDA)	4 oz.	156	0.
YODEL (Drake's) chocolate	1 roll (.9 oz.)	116	14.6
YOGURT:			
Made from whole milk (USDA)	½ cup (4.3 oz.)	76	6.0
Made from partially skimmed milk, plain or vanilla:			
(USDA)	½ cup (4.3 oz.)	61	6.3
(USDA)	8-oz. container	113	11.8
Plain:			
(Borden) Swiss style	5-oz. container	82	9.9
(Borden) Swiss style	8-oz. container	131	15.9
(Breakstone)	8-oz. container	141	12.7
(Breakstone)	1 T. (.5 oz.)	9	.8
(Dannon)	8-oz. container	136	14.1
(Dean)	8-oz. container	143	18.4
Apple, Dutch (Dannon)	8-oz. container	258	51.1
Apple, Dutch (Dean)	8-oz. container	228	41.3
Apricot:			
(Breakstone)	8-oz. container	220	37.4
(Breakstone) *Swiss Parfait*	8-oz. container	249	42.9
(Dannon)	8-oz. container	258	51.1
Black cherry (Breakstone) *Swiss Parfait*	8-oz. container	256	44.9
Blueberry:			
(Axelrod's)	8-oz. container	226	41.0
(Breakstone)	8-oz. container	252	46.3
(Breakstone) *Swiss Parfait*	8-oz. container	286	5
(Dannon)	8-oz. container	258	
(Dean)	8-oz. container	259	
(Meadow Gold)	8-oz. container	24	
(Meadow Gold) Swiss style	8-oz. container	2	
(Sanna) *Swiss Miss*	4-oz. container		
(Sealtest) *Light n' Lively*	8-oz. container		
(SugarLo)	8-oz. contain		
Boysenberry:			
(Dannon)	8-oz. con		

(USDA): United States Department of Ag
(HEW/FAO): Health, Education and
               Organization
* Prepared as Package Directs

Food and Description	Measure or Quantity	Calories	Carbo- hydrates (grams)
(Meadow Gold)	8-oz. container	249	54.0
Cherry:			
(Dannon)	8-oz. container	258	51.1
(Dean)	8-oz. container	245	47.9
(Meadow Gold)	8-oz. container	249	54.0
Black (SugarLo)	8-oz. container	117	14.6
Cinnamon apple			
(Breakstone)	8-oz. container	229	39.9
Coffee (Dannon)	8-oz. container	198	33.3
Danny (Dannon):			
Cuplet, any flavor	4-oz. container	129	25.5
Frozen pop	2½-oz. pop	127	18.0
Honey (Breakstone)			
Swiss Parfait	8-oz. container	277	51.5
Lemon:			
(Breakstone) *Swiss Parfait*	8-oz. container	254	44.9
(Dannon)	8-oz. container	198	33.3
(Sealtest) *Light n' Lively*	8-oz. container	229	43.4
Lime (Breakstone) *Swiss Parfait*	8 oz. container	243	40.1
Mandarin orange:			
(Borden) Swiss style	5-oz. container	142	28.7
(Borden) Swiss style	8-oz. container	227	45.9
(Breakstone) *Swiss Parfait*	8-oz. container	263	48.3
Orange (Dean)	8-oz. container	311	62.9
Peach:			
(Axelrod's)	8-oz. container	220	39.6
(Borden) Swiss style	5-oz. container	138	27.8
(Borden) Swiss style	8-oz. container	221	44.5
(Breakstone) *Swiss Parfait*	8-oz. container	254	47.4
(Dean)	8-oz. container	259	49.1
lba (Breakstone)			
ss Parfait	8-oz. container	268	49.4
w Gold)	8-oz. container	249	54.0
Light n' Lively	8-oz. container	252	49.3
	8-oz. container	118	14.6
	8-oz. container	220	37.9
	8-oz. container	265	48.7
	8-oz. container	249	54.0
ly	8-oz. container	241	47.2
	8-oz. container	118	14.8
od's)	8-oz. container	229	42.2
annon)	8-oz. container	258	51.1

Food and Description	Measure or Quantity	Calories	Carbo-hydrates (grams)
Prune whip (Breakstone)	8-oz. container	231	41.1
Prune whip (Dannon)	8-oz. container	258	51.1
Raspberry:			
(Axelrod's)	8-oz. container	227	40.6
(Borden) Swiss style	5-oz. container	147	29.5
(Borden) Swiss style	8-oz. container	236	47.2
(Breakstone)	8-oz. container	249	45.8
(Dannon)	8-oz. container	258	51.1
Red (Breakstone) *Swiss Parfait*	8-oz. container	263	46.5
Red (Dean)	8-oz. container	272	53.6
(Meadow Gold) Swiss style	8-oz. container	245	49.0
(Sanna) *Swiss Miss*	4-oz. container	125	19.0
Red (Sealtest) *Light n' Lively*	8-oz. container	225	41.8
(SugarLo)	8-oz. container	118	14.8
Strawberry:			
(Axelrod's)	8-oz. container	224	40.6
(Borden) Swiss style	5-oz. container	142	27.8
(Borden) Swiss style	8-oz. container	227	44.5
(Breakstone)	8-oz. container	225	43.5
(Breakstone) *Swiss Parfait*	8-oz. container	259	50.6
(Dannon)	8-oz. container	258	51.1
(Dean)	8-oz. container	256	46.8
(Meadow Gold)	8-oz. container	249	54.0
(Meadow Gold) Swiss style	8-oz. container	245	49.0
(Sanna) *Swiss Miss*	4-oz. container	125	19.0
(Sealtest) *Light n' Lively*	8-oz. container	234	44.3
(SugarLo)	8-oz. container	111	13.2
Vanilla:			
(Borden) Swiss style	5-oz. container	148	
(Borden) Swiss style	8-oz. container	235	
(Breakstone)	8-oz. container	195	
(Dannon)	8-oz. container	198	

YOUNGBERRY, fresh (See
BLACKBERRY, fresh)

(USDA): United States Department of A
(HEW/FAO): Health, Education and
Organization
* Prepared as Package Directs

Food and Description	Measure or Quantity	Calories	Carbo-hydrates (grams)
ZELTINGER ANGLERWEIN, German Moselle wine (Deinhard) 11% alcohol	3 fl. oz.	60	1.0
ZELLER SCHWARZE KATZ, wine (Julius Kayser) 9% alcohol	3 fl. oz.	57	3.0
ZINFANDEL WINE: (Inglenook) Estate, 12% alcohol	3 fl. oz. (2.9 oz.)	58	.3
(Inglenook) Vintage, 12% alcohol	3 fl. oz. (2.9 oz.)	59	.3
(Italian Swiss Colony) 13% alcohol	3 fl. oz. (2.9 oz.)	61	.9
(Louis M. Martini) 12½% alcohol	3 fl. oz.	90	.2
ZING, cereal beverage, 0.4% alcohol	12 fl. oz. (12 oz.)	62	15.0
ZITI, baked, with sauce, frozen (Buitoni)	4 oz.	128	21.4
ZUCCHINI (See **SQUASH, SUMMER**)			
...BACK: ...A):	1 oz.	120	21.1
	1 piece (7 grams)	31	5.4

BIBLIOGRAPHY

Dawson, Elsie H., Gilpin, Gladys L., and Fulton, Lois H. *Average weight of a measured cup of various foods.* U.S.D.A. ARS 61–6, February 1969. 19 pp.

Leung, W. T. W., Busson, F., and Jardin, C. *Food composition table for use in Africa.* U.S. Department of Health, Education and Welfare and Food and Agriculture Organization of the United Nations. 1968. 306 pp.

Leung, W. T. W., Butrum, R. V., and Chang, F. H. *Food composition table for use in East Asia.* U.S. Department of Health, Education and Welfare and Food and Agriculture Organization of the United Nations. December 1972. 334 pp.

Merrill, A. L. and Watt, B. K., *Energy value of foods—basis and derivation.* U.S.D.A. Handb. 74, 105 pp. 1955.

Pecot, Rebecca K., Jaeger, Carol M., and Watt, Bernice K., *Proximate composition of beef from carcass to cooked meat: Method of derivation and tables of values.* U.S.D.A. Home Economics Research Report 31, 32 pp. 1965.

Pecot, Rebecca K. and Watt, Bernice K., *Food yields: Summarized by different stages of preparaton.* U.S.D.A. Handb. 102, 93 pp. 1956.

U.S.D.A. Nutritive value of foods. Home and Garden Bul. 72, 36 pp. 1964 and revised edition, 1970. 41 pp.

U.S.D.A. Unpubl. Data 1969.

Watt, Bernice K., Merrill, Annabel L., et. al., *Composition of foods: Raw, processed, prepared.* U.S.D.A. Agriculture Handb. 8, 190 pp. 1963.

BARBARA KRAUS is the author of a number of guides to food and nutrition, including *The Barbara Kraus Dictionary of Protein*, as well as several cookbooks. Ms. Kraus is a New York University graduate with a master's in anthropology specializing in the study of food habits. She resides in New York and is working on her fourteenth book.